# PHYSIOLOGY AND PHARMACOLOGY OF THE AIRWAYS

## LUNG BIOLOGY IN HEALTH AND DISEASE

*Executive Editor:* **Claude Lenfant**
*Director, Division of Lung Diseases*
*National Institutes of Health*
*Bethesda, Maryland*

**Volume 1** IMMUNOLOGIC AND INFECTIOUS REACTIONS IN THE LUNG, *edited by Charles H. Kirkpatrick and Herbert Y. Reynolds*

**Volume 2** THE BIOCHEMICAL BASIS OF PULMONARY FUNCTION, *edited by Ronald G. Crystal*

**Volume 3** BIOENGINEERING ASPECTS OF THE LUNG, *edited by John B. West*

**Volume 4** METABOLIC FUNCTIONS OF THE LUNG, *edited by Y. S. Bakhle and John R. Vane*

**Volume 5** RESPIRATORY DEFENSE MECHANISMS (in two parts), *edited by Joseph D. Brain, Donald F. Proctor, and Lynne M. Reid*

**Volume 6** DEVELOPMENT OF THE LUNG, *edited by W. Alan Hodson*

**Volume 7** LUNG WATER AND SOLUTE EXCHANGE, *edited by Norman C. Staub*

**Volume 8** EXTRAPULMONARY MANIFESTATIONS OF RESPIRATORY DISEASE, *edited by Eugene Debs Robin*

**Volume 9** CHRONIC OBSTRUCTIVE PULMONARY DISEASE, *edited by Thomas L. Petty*

**Volume 10** PATHOGENESIS AND THERAPY OF LUNG CANCER, *edited by Curtis C. Harris*

**Volume 11** GENETIC DETERMINANTS OF PULMONARY DISEASE, *edited by Stephen D. Litwin*

**Volume 12** THE LUNG IN THE TRANSITION BETWEEN HEALTH AND DISEASE, *edited by Peter T. Macklem and Solbert Permutt*

**Volume 13** EVOLUTION OF RESPIRATORY PROCESSES: A COMPARATIVE APPROACH, *edited by Stephen C. Wood and Claude Lenfant*

**Volume 14** PULMONARY VASCULAR DISEASES, *edited by Kenneth M. Moser*

**Volume 15** PHYSIOLOGY AND PHARMACOLOGY OF THE AIRWAYS, *edited by Jay A. Nadel*

*Other volumes in preparation*

REGULATION OF BREATHING, *edited by Thomas F. Hornbein*

DIAGNOSTIC TECHNIQUES IN PULMONARY DISEASE, *edited by Marvin A. Sackner*

OCCUPATIONAL LUNG DISEASES: RESEARCH APPROACHES AND METHODS, *edited by Margaret Turner-Warwick and Hans Weill*

# PHYSIOLOGY AND PHARMACOLOGY OF THE AIRWAYS

***Edited by***

**Jay A. Nadel**

*University of California, San Francisco*
*School of Medicine*
*San Francisco, California*

MARCEL DEKKER, INC. New York • Basel

**Library of Congress Cataloging in Publication Data**

Main entry under title:

Physiology and pharmacology of the airways.

(Lung biology in health and disease ; v. 15)
Includes bibliographical references and indexes.
1. Airway (Medicine) 2. Airway (Medicine)--
Drug effects. I. Nadel, Jay A., [date]
II. Series.
RC756.L83 vol. 15 [QP121] 616.2'4s [612'.2]
ISBN 0-8247-6382-3 80-16046



MARCEL DEKKER, INC.
270 Madison Avenue, New York, New York 10016

Current printing (last digit):
10 9 8 7 6 5 4 3 2 1

PRINTED IN THE UNITED STATES OF AMERICA

# CONTRIBUTORS

**David S. Covert, Ph.D.** Assistant Professor, Department of Environmental Health, School of Public Health and Community Medicine, University of Washington School of Medicine, Seattle, Washington

**C. Claudia Ferguson** Lecturer, Department of Pathology, McGill University, Montreal, Quebec, Canada

**Jerome H. Fleisch, Ph.D.** Research Scientist, Department of Immunology and Connective Tissue Research, Lilly Research Laboratories, Eli Lilly and Company, Indianapolis, Indiana

**N. Robert Frank, M.D.** Professor, Department of Environmental Health, School of Public Health and Community Medicine, University of Washington School of Medicine, Seattle, Washington

**Warren M. Gold, M.D.** Professor, Department of Medicine; Senior Staff Member, Cardiovascular Research Institute, University of California, San Francisco, School of Medicine, San Francisco, California

**Roland H. Ingram, Jr., M.D.** Director, Respiratory Division, Peter Bent Brigham Hospital; Associate Professor, Department of Medicine, Harvard Medical School, Boston, Massachusetts

**Edwin A. Kroeger, Ph.D.** Associate Professor, Department of Physiology, Faculty of Medicine, University of Manitoba, Winnipeg, Manitoba, Canada

**E. R. McFadden, Jr., M.D.** Associate Professor, Department of Medicine, Peter Bent Brigham Hospital, Harvard Medical School, Boston, Massachusetts

**Jay A. Nadel, M.D.** Chief, Section of Pulmonary Diseases; Professor, Departments of Medicine and Physiology, Cardiovascular Research Institute, University of California, San Francisco, School of Medicine, San Francisco, California

**John B. Richardson, B.Sc., M.D., Ph.D.** Professor and Chairman, Department of Pathology, McGill University, Montreal, Quebec, Canada

**Newman L. Stephens, M.D.** Professor, Department of Physiology, Faculty of Medicine, University of Manitoba, Winnipeg, Manitoba, Canada

# FOREWORD

Most of us who are asked to name how the great advances in modern medicine and surgery have come about, would probably respond by listing some Nobel laureates and the discoveries closely linked with their names: for example, Roentgen and X-rays; Koch and the tubercle bacillus; Fleming and penicillin; Enders and culture of polio virus; Banting and insulin. Yet, once in awhile, an event that is ineligible for a Nobel Prize has had just as important an impact on medical advance as one that was eligible and won an award. One such event was Abraham Flexner's 1910 report "Medical Education in the United States and Canada" that resulted in a considerable decrease in the number of American medical schools and a considerable increase in their quality and in the scientific content of their curricula. Another was the opening of the Johns Hopkins Medical School in 1893, staffed by four professors, each outstanding as a scientist in his specialty and each believing in joining scientific research, medical education, and patient care.

Sometimes a book or a series of books has had a strong influence on the advance of medical science. One such book was the first edition of Osler's *Medicine* (1892) because Osler's emphasis on how little physicians knew for sure led John Rockefeller's adviser on philanthropy to recommend the building of the great Institute for Medical Research, which opened in 1904 and for decades was the foremost institution for research in basic medical sciences in the United States. Another was the first (1941) edition of Goodman and Gilman's *Pharmacological Basis for Medical Practice* that revolutionized teaching and research on the action and use of drugs; as one professor of pharmacology stated in 1941, no professional pharmacologist could from then on teach at a lower level than that of the superb text used by his students!

In the field of respiration and the lungs, there are some classic monographs and a comprehensive *Handbook of Physiology* that have heightened the interest of scientists, students, and physicians in this subject and stimulated them to enter pulmonary research. One can safely predict that this new series of monographs, "Lung Biology in Health and Disease," will have an even greater impact on young (and older) researchers because it is the first truly comprehensive, monumental work in this field. It does not deal just with cellular processes or just with clinical problems but with the entire spectrum of basic sciences and of lung function, metabolic functions, and respiratory defense mechanisms. The series will also include volumes that apply to modern biological knowledge to elucidate mechanisms of pulmonary and respiratory disorders (immunologic, infectious, and genetic disorders, physiology and pharmacology of airways, genesis and resolution of pulmonary edema, and abnormalities of respiratory regulation). Other volumes will deal with the biology of specific pulmonary diseases (e.g., cancer, chronic obstructive pulmonary disease, disorders of the pulmonary circulation, and abnormalities associated with occupational and environmental factors) and with early detection and specific diagnosis.

This series shows the lung as a challenging organ, with many problems calling for innovative research. If it attracts some imaginative, creative, and perceptive young scientists to attack these difficult problems, the tremendous effort in writing, editing, and publishing these volumes will be well worthwhile. The volumes cannot win the Nobel Prize, but someone may who was challenged by them.

**Julius H. Comroe, Jr.**
San Francisco, California

# INTRODUCTION

During the last decade, our conception of airway disease has evolved along with remarkable advances in our knowledge of the physiology and pharmacology of the airways. Indeed, it is probable that this new knowledge led to the development of these new concepts. Looking back, it is clear that our current understanding of airway function has emerged because of the mutual interests of a great number of scientists from many disciplines. Morphologists, physiologists, biologists, molecular biologists, clinicians, and pharmacologists, as well as mathematicians and physicists, have all studied the airways. It is, therefore, no surprise that Dr. Nadel, the editor of the monograph *Physiology and Pharmacology of the Airways* of the series "Lung Biology in Health and Disease," called upon scientists with such a variety of interests to contribute to his volume. It is a personal privilege to introduce this new volume and to outline its content.

The monograph reviews the relationships between the lungs and airway structure and function and the mechanisms which regluate the airways. This remarkable and complex distributing system includes the nasal passages, the mouth, the trachea, and its two major subdivisions, the right and left bronchi, and each of their twenty to twenty-three subdivisions, which produce approximately one million terminal tubes. Some of these airways are close, some are far from the hila, but they must simultaneously distribute fresh air to the alveoli and remove wasted air from them and this must be accomplished with minimal dead space, minimal resistance, and maximal uniformity of distribution that must match an equally complex distributing system involving the pulmonary circulation. The airways must also be capable of filtering and conditioning the air to defend the lung (and body) against a vast array of potentially dangerous inhaled particles, liquids, and gases.

The first chapter of the volume reviews the ultrastructural morphology of the airways. Epithelium, glands, smooth muscle, nerve endings, cartilage, and connective tissue are discussed. When possible, a correlation is made between physiological functions and ultrastructural characteristics, and species differences are identified when they influence the function of the airways. Although it is recognized that we "still lack sufficient morphological data," this chapter emphasizes the great contribution that these data have made, especially when coupled with physiological studies.

The second chapter relates this underlying structure to function, beginning with the biophysics and biochemistry of the airways and continuing with length-tension relationships and their modification by hydrogen ion, carbon dioxide, and oxygen, and stress relaxation of airway smooth muscle and connective tissues.

The next chapter, which examines current concepts of the biochemistry of contraction of airway smooth muscle, discusses the role of ion fluxes, calcium metabolism, and actomyosin, and the relationship of changes in the levels of cyclic nucleotides to the electromechanical physiologic contractile process. It also reviews mechanisms involving cyclic AMP and cyclic GMP, and the possible relationship of changes in cyclic nucleotide levels to airway function.

Chapter 4 reviews the airway pharmacology, including the significance of $\alpha$-adrenergic, $\beta$-adrenergic ($\beta_1$ and $\beta_2$), and cholinergic receptors. In addition, other drug effects on bronchial smooth muscle are discussed, including the roles of histamine, prostaglandins, bradykinin, serotonin, and antigen-induced mediator release mechanisms on airway function.

Chapter 5 discusses the regulation of airway function by nervous mechanisms, including the anatomy and physiology of sympathetic and parasympathetic nerves, evidence for nonadrenergic inhibitory nerves, the possible modulation of parasympathetic ganglion output by sympathetic innervation, the possible relationship between sympathetic innervation and vascular as distinct from airway smooth muscle, and the pulmonary reflexes initiated in the airways and their relationship to the phenomenon of hyperirritability.

The next chapter reviews the properties and effects on respiratory function of airborne particles. As these particles are part of our ambient environment, the airway responses they elicit are most important. The chapter first describes the particles and their deposition, then examines the changes that occur after the particles enter the airways. Finally, there is a comprehensive review of factors that modulate the response of the airways to the inhalation of particles.

The final chapter reviews current concepts of airway physiology and includes two sections. One describes methods of assessment, which include use of flow-volume curves, resistance-volume curves, and so forth. The other section discusses physiologic implications of airway dynamics in both the uncompressed and compressed state, dynamic frequency effects on resistance, compliance and distribution of ventilation, the relationship of airway function to the distribution of ventilation and perfusion, the relative contributions of large and small airways to airflow resistance and static elastic properties of the lung, and then considers a teleologic rationale for the presence of airway tone, Finally, this chapter discusses the relationship between changes in airway structure and function and certain specific disease states.

**Claude Lenfant**
Bethesda, Maryland

# CONTENTS

*Contributors* iii
*Foreword* **Julius H. Comroe, Jr.** v
*Introduction* vii

1/ MORPHOLOGY OF THE AIRWAYS 1

*John B. Richardson and C. Claudia Ferguson*

I Epithelium 2
II Glands 6
III Smooth Muscle 7
IV Innervation 13
V Cartilage 22
VI Connective Tissue 23
References 24

2/ ULTRASTRUCTURE, BIOPHYSICS, AND BIOCHEMISTRY OF AIRWAY SMOOTH MUSCLE 31

*Newman L. Stephens and Edwin A. Kroeger*

I Structure and Ultrastructure 32
II Biophysics of Airway Smooth Muscle 65
III Biochemistry of Airway Smooth Muscle 90
References 111

3/ ROLE OF CYCLIC NUCLEOTIDES IN AIRWAY SMOOTH MUSCLE 123

*Warren M. Gold*

I General Considerations 124
II Problems in Evaluating Data 125
III Enzymes Related to Cyclic Nucleotide Metabolism 128
IV Cyclic Nucleotide Content of the Lung 138
V Cyclic Nucleotide Metabolism in Mast Cells 151
VI Cyclic Nucleotide Metabolism in Smooth Muscle 158
VII Summary 176
References 177

4/ PHARMACOLOGIC ASPECTS OF AIRWAY SMOOTH MUSCLE **191**

*Jerome H. Fleisch*

I Drug Receptors in Airway Smooth Muscle 192
II Antigen-Induced Mediator Release 202
III Alteration of Drug-Receptor Systems in Disease 204
References 206

5/ AUTONOMIC REGULATION OF AIRWAY SMOOTH MUSCLE **217**

*Jay A. Nadel*

I Parasympathetic Nervous System 217
II Sympathetic Nervous System: General Considerations 235
References 239

6/ ATMOSPHERIC PARTICLES: BEHAVIOR AND FUNCTIONAL EFFECTS **259**

*David S. Covert and N. Robert Frank*

I Atmospheric Aerosols 261
II Aerosol Changes Following Inhalation 268
III Interactions with Other Pollutants: $SO_2$ Model 275
IV Factors That May Modulate Response 281
V Air Quality Standards 289
References 290

7/ CLINICAL APPLICATION AND INTERPRETATION OF AIRWAY PHYSIOLOGY **297**

*E. R. McFadden, Jr., and Roland H. Ingram, Jr.*

I Measurements of Pulmonary Mechanics 298
II Determinants of Maximum Expiratory Flow 300
III Airway-Parenchyma Interaction 304
IV Regional Nonuniformities of Resistance and Compliance 307
V Airway Responsivity 312
VI Clinical Physiology 315
VII Summary 319
References 319

Author Index 325
Subject Index 353

# PHYSIOLOGY AND PHARMACOLOGY OF THE AIRWAYS

# 1

# Morphology of the Airways

*JOHN B. RICHARDSON and C. CLAUDIA FERGUSON*

McGill University
Montreal, Quebec, Canada

This review deals chiefly with recent work on the ultrastructural morphology of the airways. The morphology of the human lung will be emphasized, and differences between the human morphology and that of other species will be pointed out when it is felt that these differences influence the function of the airways. An attempt will be made to correlate physiological studies on the nerves and smooth muscle in the airways with the ultrastructure of these two components. This approach is not possible with the epithelium since less is known about the physiology of the airway epithelium.

The trachea and the distal airways arise from the foregut and might be expected to share some of the morphological and physiologic characteristics of the gastrointestinal tract. When neuroblasts migrate with the vagus nerve the septum between the esophagus and the trachea is still intact [1] and thus the neural control of the smooth muscle in the airways may be similar to that in the gastrointestinal tract. Evidence to support the similarity between the two will be given in the sections on smooth muscle and innervation (Secs. III and IV).

The growth of the airways has been reviewed recently and the differences between the airways of children and adults with respect to the quantity of muscle, which increases with age, and the proportion of mucous glands, which decreases with age, has been pointed out [2]. The difference in the rate of growth of the central and peripheral airways was proposed as a reason why croup or bronchiolitis is not a serious or life-threatening condition in children after the age of 5 to 6 years [3]. The airways resistance in children below the age of 5 years is mainly in the peripheral airways and there is a change to the adult pattern at, or after, the age of 5 years [3].

The local production and secretion of immunoglobulins in the lung and in the gastrointestinal tract has also been an area of recent work [4-6]. There are similarities between these two systems in the production of immunoglobulins [5] and in the uptake of antigen from the epithelial surface under normal and disease conditions [7-9].

## I. Epithelium

The epithelium of the trachea and the main bronchi is a pseudostratified epithelium with at least four distinct cell types: ciliated, basal, goblet, and Kultschitzky's cells. In the more distal airways this pattern simplifies to a simple cuboidal epithelium. A fifth cell type, the Clara cell, is found in the bronchi and bronchioles. Other cell types have been described in the epithelium and their presence varies with different species. A recent review discusses the lining cells of the pulmonary airways in more detail [10]. The neuroendocrine cell, the Kulschitzky's-type cell, which has been described in human tissue, has counterparts in the gastrointestinal tract. A recent review discusses their structure and possible function [11]. One study on human fetal, newborn and childhood tissue demonstrated these cells in the tracheal epithelium and showed that they took up L-dopa and subsequently fluoresced when treated with the Falck technique [12]. The uptake of L-dopa places these cells in the APUD (amine, precursor, uptake, decarboxylation) series of cells found throughout the body [13]. Three types of neuroendocrine cells were found in the human fetal tissue, but a definite difference between these cells has not been shown [12]. Collections of these cells are also found in the lung and these have been termed neuroepithelial bodies [11,14]. Since secretion by the cells was not demonstrated it was concluded that they probably had a receptor function [12]. Kultschitzky's cells may also be the source of the vasoactive peptide (VIP) [15] which was isolated from intestinal cells [12].

While neuroepithelial bodies have been described in the human respiratory epithelium [10,12,16], they have been described in more detail in the rabbit [14]. In the rabbit they are found throughout the entire bronchial and bronchiolar epithelium and in particular in regions of bifurcation. The cells have a cylindrical shape and extend from the luminal surface to the basement membrane. When there are several cells, they form a distinct body with the cells slightly inclined toward each other so that they form a trapezoidal structure [14]. The cells have a dense, somewhat eosinophilic cytoplasm and no cilia. Beneath the basement membrane, at the base of this trapezoid-shaped collection of cells, there is a capillary. Unmyelinated nerve endings with agranular vesicles are seen between the cells of these neuroepithelial bodies. Vesicles with dense-cores of variable morphology are present in the cells; some dense-core vesicles have a halo around the core, others are oval with no halo. These two types of vesicles have been called type 1 and type 2 vesicles. Type 1, the vesicle with the halo, has a dense core when fixed with glutaraldehyde and does not when fixed with osmic acid alone. The preservation of the dense core within the vesicle by glutaraldehyde and not be osmic acid has been taken as evidence of primary amino groups in the dense core [17,18]. With the Falck technique, the neuro-epithelial cells emitted an intense yellow fluorescence. It was concluded that the type 1 vesicle contained a primary amine which was probably serotonin since the dense core was preserved by glutaraldehyde and yellow fluorescence is characteristic of serotonin [14]. A receptor function has been proposed for these neuro-epithelial bodies on the basis of their innervation and the possible presence of serotonin [14].

A brush cell, described in the trachea of the rat [19], has rarely been seen in the human tracheal epithelium [20], but brush cells are found in the human bronchiolar epithelium. On the basis of the numerous basal bodies located directly below the microvilli of these cells, it was proposed that brush cells may be transitional cells in the formation of ciliated cells [21].

A nonciliated cell, which contained vesicles filled with electron-dense material near its luminal surface, was described in the mouse tracheal epithelium [22]. This cell was frequently seen in the epithelium, whereas few goblet cells were found. Since this nonciliated cell contained secretory-like granules which demonstrated a positive reaction for polysaccharides, it was felt that this cell was the secretory cell responsible for mucous production in the mouse trachea rather than the goblet cell [22]. In the guinea pig tracheal epithelium a nonciliated elongated cell was found to take up tracer proteins and transport them to the basal portion of the cell [8]. This cell, in the guinea pig, unlike the nonciliated cell in the mouse, did not protrude into the lumen, but rather had a narrow and flat-surfaced neck with very small microvilli (Fig. 1). It had the ultrastructural characteristics of both the intermediate cell described by Rhodin [20] and the brush cell [19]. The function of this cell in the guinea pig is unknown [8].

There are species differences in the respiratory epithelium, but the ciliated, basal, goblet, and Kultschitzky's cells are rather constant in all species examined. The structure of the ciliated, basal, intermediate, and goblet cells in the human respiratory epithelium has been described in detail by Rhodin [20]. The human

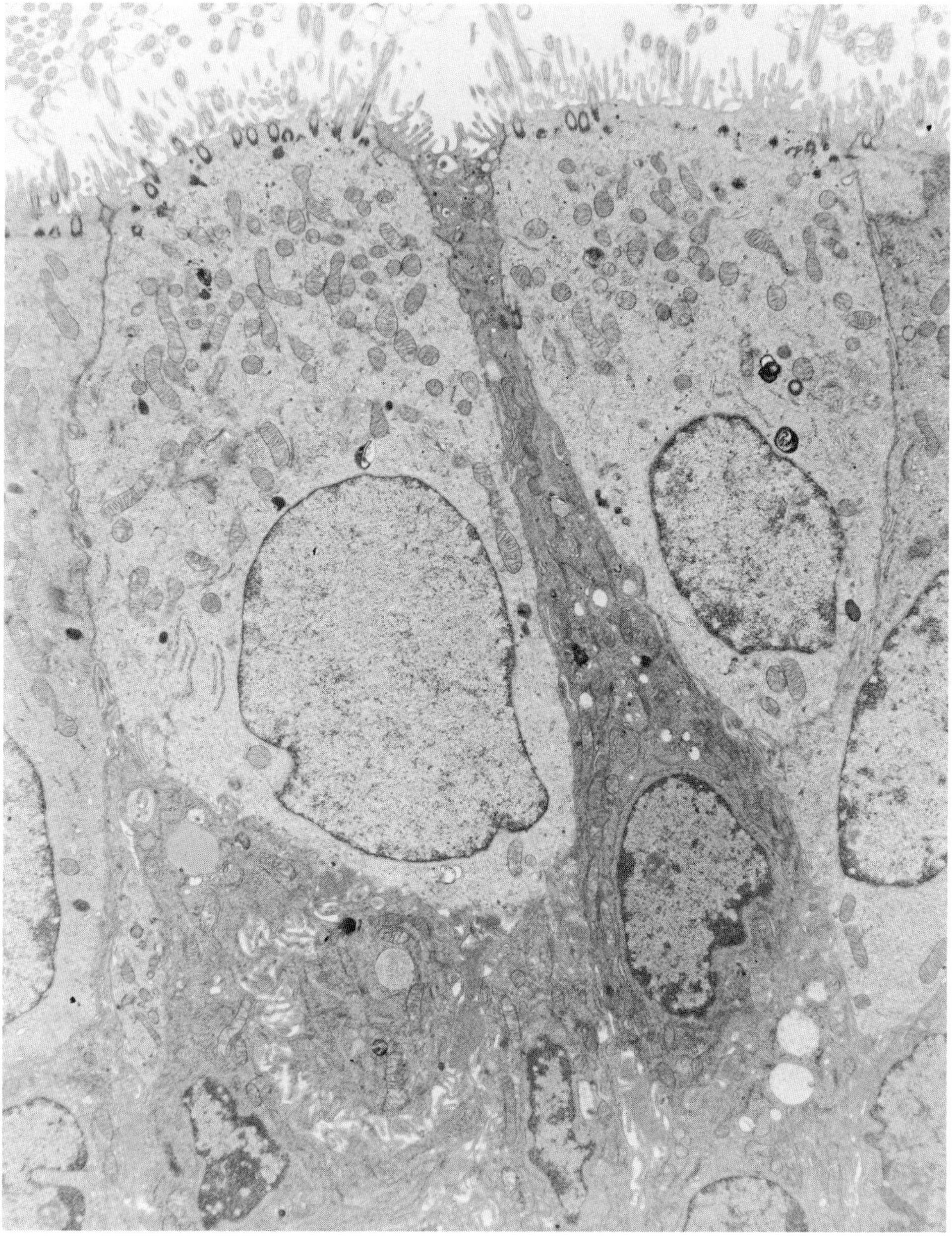

**FIGURE 1** Guinea pig tracheal epithelium. A darker-staining cell with small microvilli is seen between two ciliated cells. This dark cell has been associated with the uptake of tracer protein (×6000) [8].

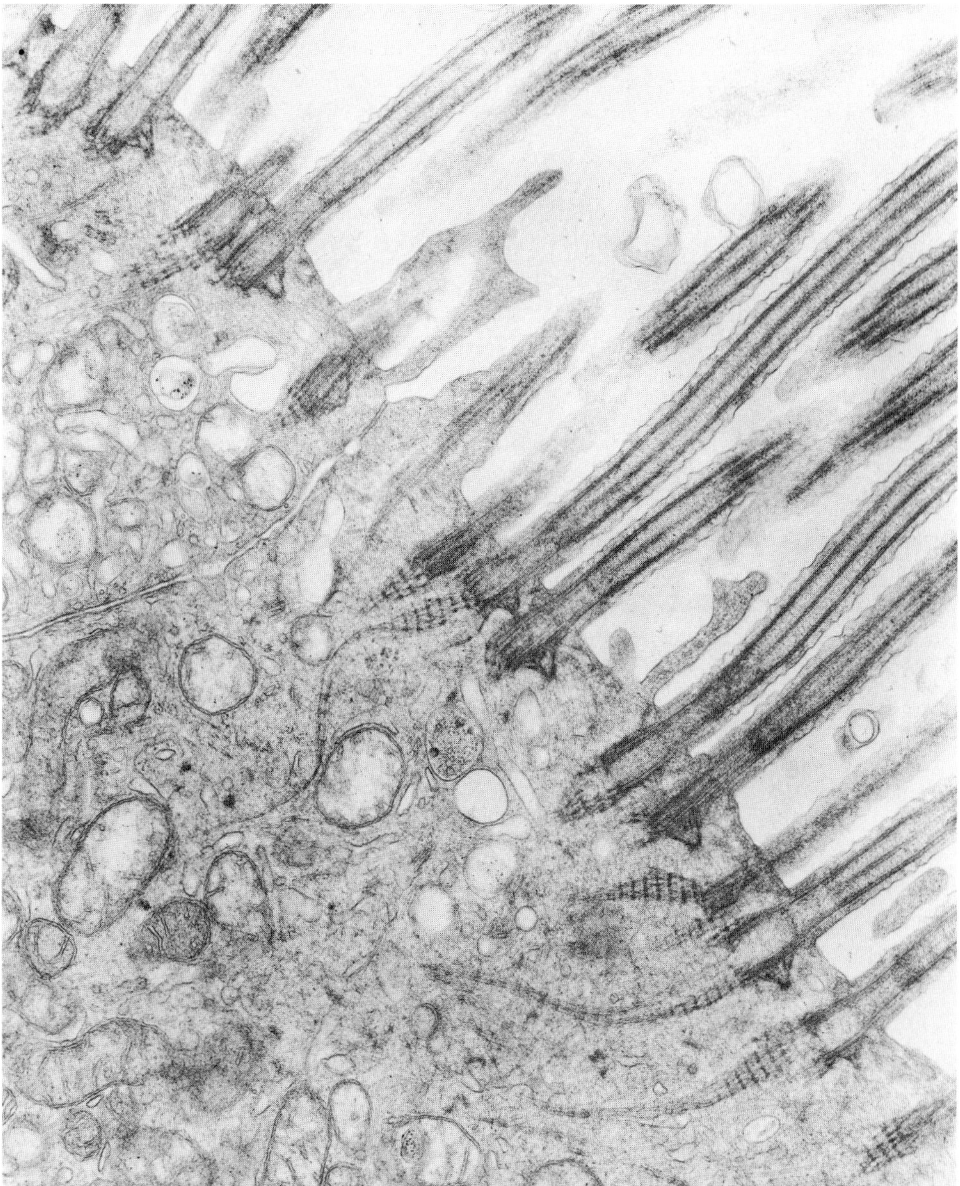

**FIGURE 2** Ciliated human tracheal epithelium showing wispy, striated basal bodies extending into the cytoplasm. The function of these striated bodies is not known (×29,000).

ciliated epithelium has an elaborate basal body, the triplets of which extend down into the cytoplasm and have a banded structure [20]. Banded extensions of the triplet bodies of the cilia are also seen in the chicken [23], the cat, and the horse [24]. The purpose of these structures, which resemble striated muscle (Fig. 2), is not clear, and whether they aid or even alter mucus transport has not been investigated.

Recent studies with freeze-fracture techniques have shown a variety of junctions between epithelial cells. Tight junctions, with multiple strands, have been demonstrated in the guinea pig [25]. These tight junctions can be rendered permeable to tracer proteins by ether [8], cigarette smoke [26], cholinergic agonists, and histamine [27]. Freeze-fracture techniques have shown that these agents degrade and fragment the structure of the tight junctions. How this fragmentation occurs or what effect the degradation of the junctions has on the protective function of the epithelium is not clear.

Another cell junction in the epithelial junctional complex is the desmosome, and the structure of this junction is well known. Several new junctions are the nexus or gap junction, and the orthogonal arrays or rectolinear entities. The nexus is thought to be important in cell-to-cell communication and developmental coordination [28,29]. The structure of the nexus has been determined with the transmission electron microscope and freeze-fracture techniques [30]. The nexus has been found in the tracheal epithelium of the guinea pig [25,26], where it is relatively common. What function it plays in the respiratory epithelium is not known but it may be to coordinate the movement of the cilia. The orthogonal array or rectolinear entity has been seen in the tracheal epithelium of the guinea pig [25]. This structure has been described in striated muscle, where it is thought to be of importance in the electrogenic mechanism [31], and in the epithelium of the intestine, where its function is unknown [32]. What purpose the orthogonal array plays in the epithelium is not clear, but since nerve endings with granular and agranular vesicles have been described in the epithelium of the chicken [33] and the rat [34], the orthogonal arrays may represent the terminals of cholinergic nerves on the epithelium or play a role in the electrical and contractile properties of the epithelial cells [25]. The purpose of such nerve terminals remains obscure.

## II. Glands

There are well-developed glands beneath the epithelium which open into the lumen of the large airways. These glands consist of three distinct parts: (1) an acinus composed of mucus cells, serous cells, and, in some areas, lymphocytes [35,36]; (2) a tubule; and (3) an excretory duct [36]. The openings of these excretory ducts are lined by stratified, ciliated columnar epithelium which merges into nonciliated cuboidal epithelium. Each duct admits several glandular tubules, the cells of which are rich in mitochondria [36,37]. It has been suggested that the cells of the tubules play a role in the regulation of fluid [36], as has also been suggested for the collecting ducts of the pancreas [37]. Myoepithelial cells surround the tubules or collecting ducts. Unmyelinated axons are seen adjacent to the mucus cells and the myoepithelial cells [36]. When examined with the electron microscope, human serous cells show granules of variable densities. These granules range in size from 100 to 1740 nm. The mucus cells are usually filled with secretory granules of a moderate electron density. These granules vary in size from 300 to 1800 nm [36]. Meyrick and Reid proposed that the lymphocytes found in the human bronchial submucosal glands may have a role in the secretion of immunoglobulins [36].

The glands beneath the epithelium appear at week 25 of gestation. Their number is fixed at birth. Both adult and infant trachea have about 4000 glands and the density of these glands changes from between 7.7 to 10 glands/mm$^2$ at birth and 0.7 to 0.9 glands/mm$^2$ in the adult [38]. The glands are larger in the posterior or membranous portion of the trachea where they are in the muscle as well as in the submucosa [35].

There are few ultrastructural studies on the glands of the human airways and little is known about the changes that take place in disease other than the increase in the size of the glands, which is presumably due to hyperplasia of the cells since no new glands appear to be formed [39]. Little is known about the innervation of these glands in humans or of the local or systemic factors which control their secretion [40].

## III. Smooth Muscle

The gross and light microscopic features of the airway smooth muscle have been well described and are reviewed by Nagaishi [41].

One of the similarities between the lung and the gastrointestinal tract is the distribution of the smooth muscle. In a study of four full-term human fetuses, where the trachea was sectioned both transversally and longitudinally, the circumferential muscles were found in an inner and an outer layer [42]. The inner fibers were circular and the outer were longitudinal and arranged in bundles (Fig. 3a). A muscularis mucosa was present beneath the tracheal mucosa and was similar to the muscularis mucosa of the intestine [42]. The longitudinal bundles are quite evident in newborn and young children but they are not noticeable in the adult, where the transverse fibers predominate (Fig. 3b). Thus, at birth, the smooth muscle of the human trachea and main bronchi has a gross morphological pattern similar to the smooth muscle of the gastrointestinal tract.

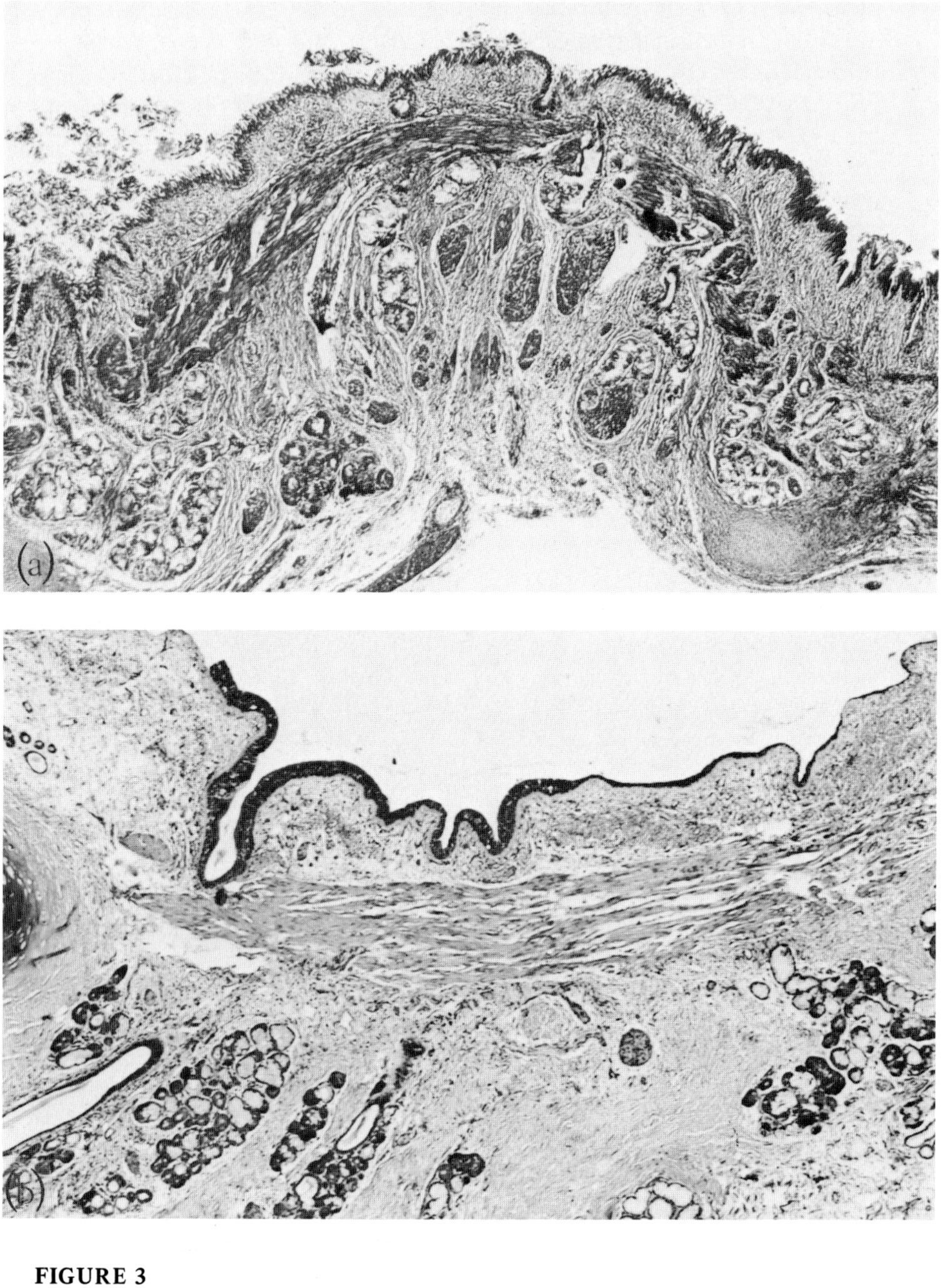


**FIGURE 3**

There are few electron microscope studies of human airway smooth muscle. We have studied the human tracheal smooth muscle and others have studied canine [43] and bovine [44] tracheal smooth muscle. The human smooth muscle has a scanty innervation, with two basic axon profiles which will be described in the next section. The smooth muscle cells of the human airways resemble those of the mammalian intestine [45,46] in that they have numerous cell-to-cell connections (Fig. 4), many of which are of the gap junction type (Figs. 5 and 6). The presence of gap junctions implies that the smooth muscle cells are electrically coupled. Gap junctions are common in human airway smooth muscle whereas in the canine, bovine, and guinea pig tracheal muscle they are rare (Fig. 7) [43,44,47]. A complete ultrastructural study of the smooth muscle and the cell junctions in the distal human airways has not been performed.

Electrically active smooth muscle cells may act in unison as a single unit if the cells are coupled, or as multiple units if they are not coupled. In a multiple unit type of muscle each cell responds differently than the next cell and the degree of response depends on the stimulation that the cell has received. Smooth muscle which acts as a single unit, such as that in the intestine, has a relatively scanty innervation in comparison to smooth muscle which acts as a multiple unit since stimulation of one cell in the single unit is passed on to the other cells to which it is connected. Electrophysiological studies on the canine and bovine trachealis muscle have not shown action potentials nor have they shown coupled cells under normal circumstances [43,44,48]. Action potentials were recorded from human bronchial smooth muscle during an asthmatic attack [49], but in vitro studies on airway smooth muscle from asthmatic patients have not been done to confirm this finding. While the basic structure of human airway smooth muscle is similar to that of the gastrointestinal tract, the physiological characteristics of the muscle have not been determined and it is not known if there are pacemaker cells and action potentials in the normal human airway smooth muscle or if the smooth muscle responds as a single or a multiple unit.

---

**FIGURE 3** (a) A photomacrograph of a cross section from the trachea of a human neonate. A transverse layer of smooth muscle is seen directly beneath the epithelium. Below the transverse layer of smooth muscle there are longitudinal bundles of smooth muscle (×55). (b) A photomacrograph from a similar section of an adult human trachea. No longitudinal bundles of smooth muscle are seen beneath the transverse layer of smooth muscle (×52).

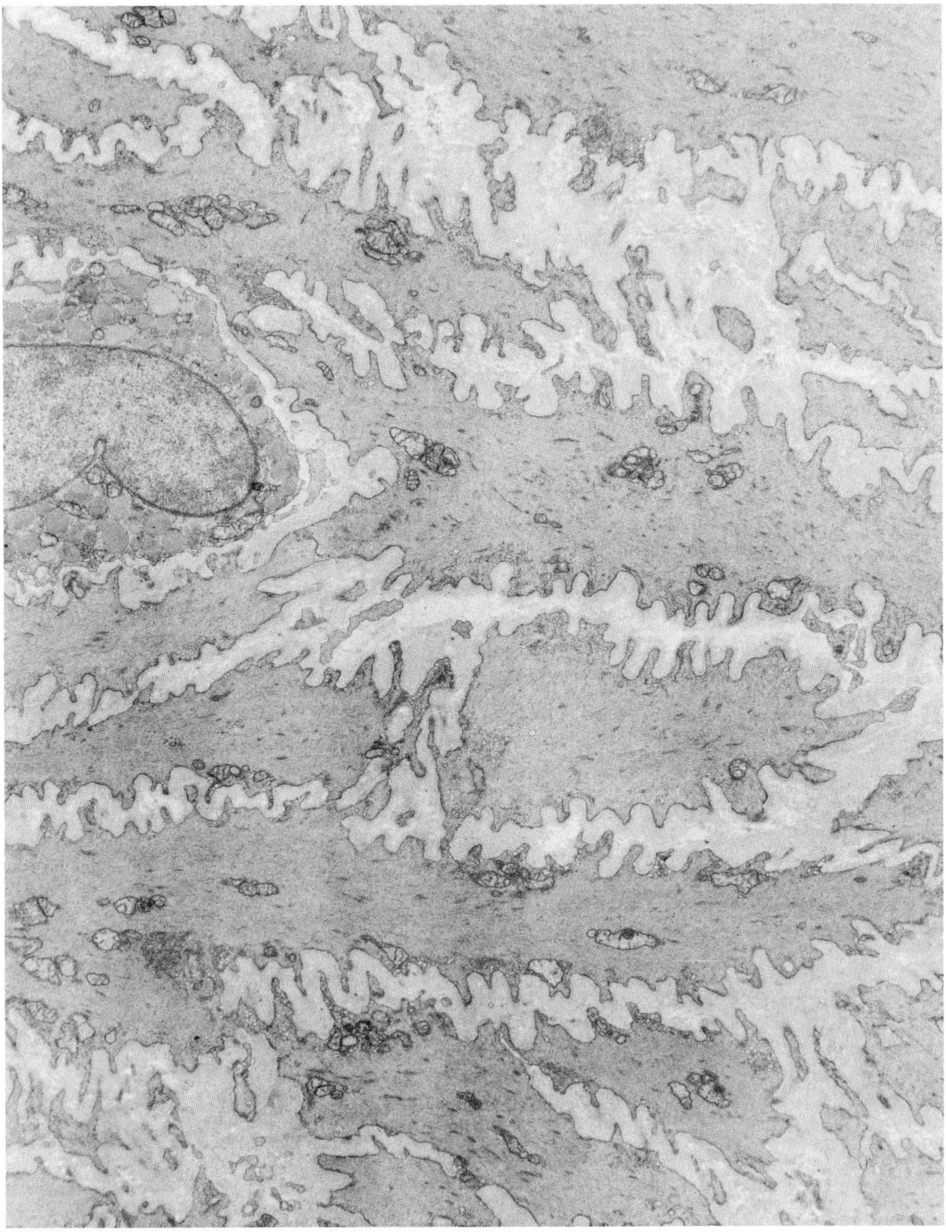

**FIGURE 4** An electron micrograph of human tracheal smooth muscle which shows numerous cell-to-cell connections. Most of the connections are of the nexus type (×6500).

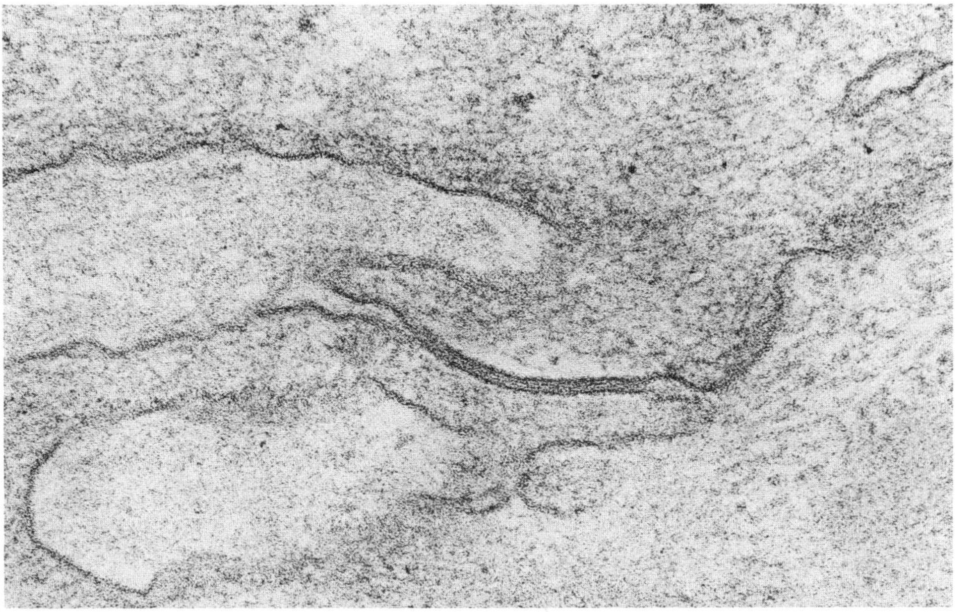

**FIGURE 5** A gap junction or nexus between two human tracheal smooth muscle cells (×107,000).

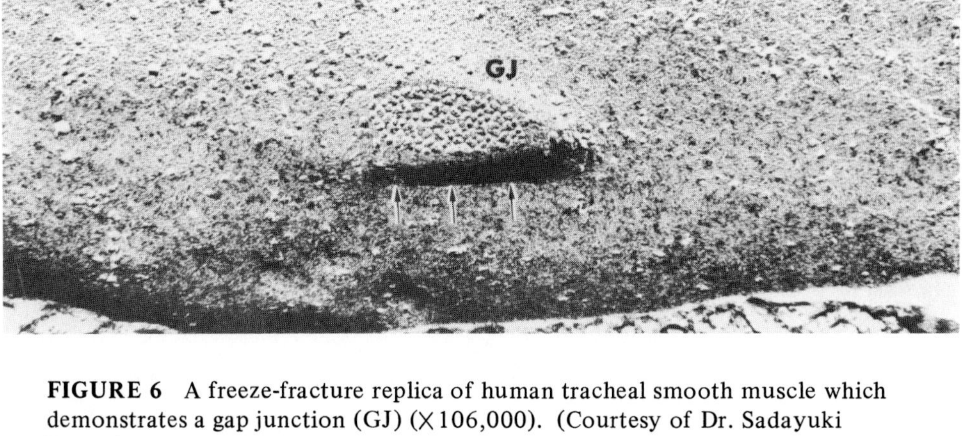


**FIGURE 6** A freeze-fracture replica of human tracheal smooth muscle which demonstrates a gap junction (GJ) (×106,000). (Courtesy of Dr. Sadayuki Inoue.)

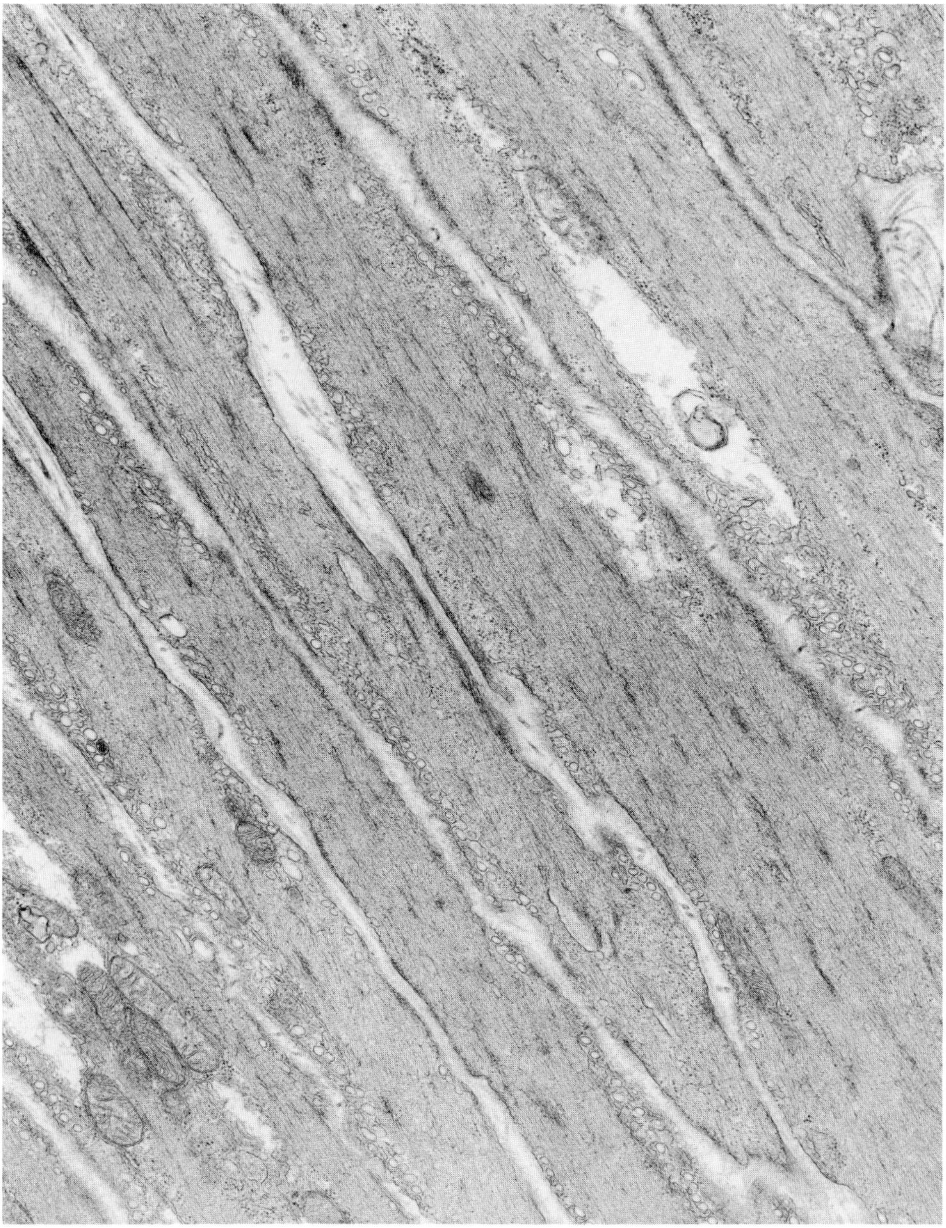

**FIGURE 7** A representative area from guinea pig trachealis muscle. The smooth muscle cells are often found in close apposition, but no cell-to-cell connections are seen. This type of pattern has also been described in canine and bovine trachealis muscle (×19,000) [43,44].

## IV. Innervation

Extensive work has been done on the innervation of the human lung at the level of the light microscope, and the basic outline of the innervation as derived from studies in the nineteenth and twentieth centuries was reviewed by Larsell and Dow [50], Blümcke [51], and Gaylor [52]. Since these reviews there has been little additional information at this level of microscopy and what there has been was reviewed by Nagaishi [41].

The general pattern consists of afferent and efferent pathways. The extensive afferent or sensory innervation originates in the epithelium of the airways, the interalveolar spaces, the muscle, and the submucosal layer [41]. The afferent fibers are myelinated and unmyelinated or nonmyelinated and terminate in the vagal nuclei. The efferent fibers, which run to the smooth muscle and the glands, arise from ganglia. These ganglia receive preganglionic fibers from the vagal nuclei and are part of the parasympathetic system. The ganglia are mainly located external to the smooth muscle and the cartilage (Fig. 8). There are a few ganglia in the submucosa but these are generally smaller and have fewer neurons than the larger ganglia in the extrachondrial region. The existence of sympathetic innervation has been less clearly established, particularly in the human, but the accepted pattern in the human is that preganglionic fibers leave the spinal cord

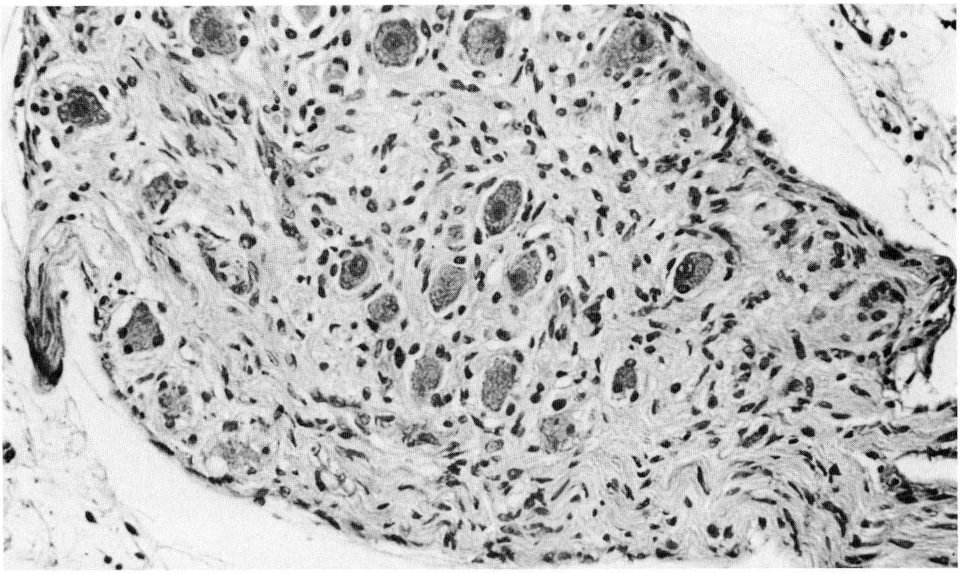

**FIGURE 8** A photomicrograph of a large ganglion in the extrachondrial region of the main-stem bronchus. The ganglion arises from one side of a nerve which is seen in the lower right-hand corner (X750).

and synapse with the prevertebral ganglia. Postganglionic fibers leave the ganglia and proceed to the airways where they innervate the smooth muscle and presumably the glands of the airways as well as the pulmonary vasculature.

The accepted interpretation of this morphology is that the excitation of the glands and smooth muscle of the airways is under the control of the vagus nerve and is cholinergic. The inhibition of the glands and the smooth muscle is presumed to be under the control of the adrenergic system. However, autonomic innervation of the glands is not well studied. The normal tone of the smooth muscle is a result of the opposite actions of these systems. This was the general interpretation of gastrointestinal tract innervation until recent years, when the concept of myogenic activity was introduced [45]. No detailed studies, however, have been completed on human airway smooth muscle to determine if myogenic activity plays a role in the production of smooth muscle tone.

There are few ultrastructural studies on nerves in the lung. Rhodin [20], in his paper on the tracheal epithelium of humans, found unmyelinated nerves entering the basement membrane of the epithelium, but not actually penetrating it. Rhodin did, however, find unmyelinated nerve endings between the basal portion of ciliated and mucus-producing cells [20]. Studies on the innervation of the tracheal epithelium in animals are not extensive. Ultrastructural studies on rat tracheal epithelium demonstrated unmyelinated nerves in the epithelium [34]. Most of the axons lay between the basal cells, but some axons were also seen directly beneath the tight junctions [34]. Axon profiles which contained granular and agranular vesicles were found in rat epithelium, and the presence of these vesicles suggested that some of the axons were efferent [34]. The remainder of the axons had no vesicles, contained only mitochondria, and were thought to be sensory or afferent [34].

There have been several studies on the innervation of the chicken lung [33, 53-56]. These studies have shown unmyelinated axons between epithelial cells which were thought to have a sensory function [55]. The interepithelial axons in the chicken tracheal epithelium were related to the ciliated cells. No association was found between the axons and the mucous cells in the chicken, in contrast to the rat tracheal epithelium where similar axons were associated with mucous cells. Many axons in the chicken tracheal epithelium contain granular and agranular vesicles which may indicate that these nerves have an efferent action on the epithelium (Fig. 9). However, it is not as yet known whether these axon profiles belong to the afferent or the efferent system, but from a morphological basis their structure is more in keeping with an efferent action than a sensory or afferent action.

The smooth muscle of the chicken has a mixed innervation [53,56]. Four basic types of vesicles were described. Type 1 were large, irregular or oval vesicles up to 120 nm in diameter. Type 2 were small, round, granular vesicles 50 to 85

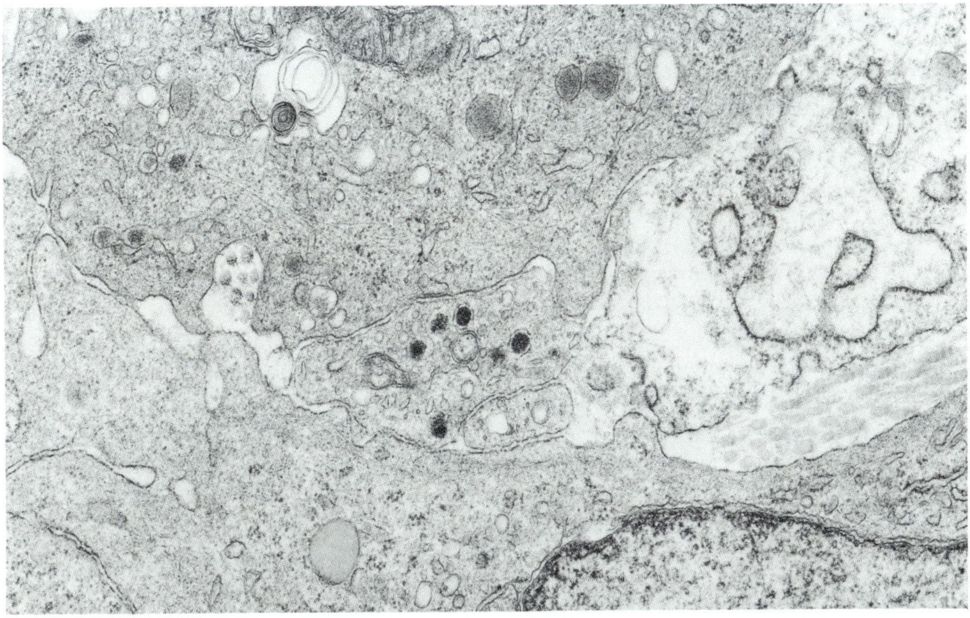

**FIGURE 9** A small axon is seen beneath the basal cells of the epithelium in the chicken trachea. Small agranular and large granular vesicles are present in the axon profile (X22,000).

nm in diameter with a dense central core 45 to 70 nm in diameter. Type 3 were small granular vesicles 50 to 110 nm in diameter with an eccentric core 25 to 50 nm in diameter. Type 4 were round, agranular vesicles 40 to 55 nm in diameter. These vesicles were seen in three basic types of axon profiles. The first contained agranular vesicles, the second contained granular vesicles of one or more of the types described, and the third contained numerous agranular and granular vesicles [53]. Neurons were found in the connective tissue and there was synaptic contact between unmyelinated axons and the neurons [53]. A study on the intrapulmonary airways of the monkey described axon profiles with dense-core vesicles, but no definite function was assigned to these axons [57].

A detailed study on innervation in the cat lung demonstrated both cholinergic and adrenergic nerves in the smooth muscle [58]. These nerves were demonstrated by electron microscopy and by histochemical techniques [58]. The histochemical technique for the demonstration of adrenergic nerves has been applied to the airways of many different animals [59-64]. These studies have demonstrated a great species variation in adrenergic innervation. In the cat, there is abundant adrenergic innervation of the smooth muscle [58,61], but in the guinea pig, the adrenergic innervation of the smooth muscle is mainly in the proximal portion of the trachea [59,60]. Cholinergic innervation, however, is a constant feature in all airways examined [65].

Coburn and Tomita first demonstrated the presence of nonadrenergic or purinergic inhibitory nerves in mammalian airway smooth muscle [59]. This initial demonstration was in the guinea pig trachealis muscle, and the findings were confirmed and enlarged upon by others [66-68]. These inhibitory nerves are part of a third autonomic nervous system present throughout the body [45]. In the gastrointestinal tract these nerves are the principal inhibitory nerves, whereas in the bladder they are excitatory [45]. The nonadrenergic inhibitory system of the gastrointestinal tract develops in conjunction with the cholinergic excitatory system, and both the cholinergic and nonadrenergic systems are functional well before the arrival of adrenergic nerves to the intestine [69]. In the upper portion of the gastrointestinal tract, there are preganglionic fibers which run in the vagus nerve and terminate on inhibitory neurons within the ganglia. Postganglionic fibers from inhibitory neurons go to the smooth muscle, and stimulation of these nerves produces a characteristic depolarization of the smooth muscle membrane potential [45]. The chemical mediator of this inhibitory nervous system is not known, but there is extensive evidence to support adenosine triphosphate or another purine nucleotide as the mediator [45]. There is also some evidence against the proposal that adenosine triphosphate is the mediator [70,71]. The axon profiles of the postganglionic fibers of this system are thought to be morphologically distinct from other profiles in that they contain large (180-220 nm) opaque vesicles which are not destroyed by 6-hydroxydopamine or depleted by reserpine [45]. The exact composition of these vesicles is, however, not known.

Our work on the innervation of human airway smooth muscle is incomplete, but there are certain morphological features which may be of importance. We have demonstrated the presence of nonadrenergic inhibitory nerves in the smooth muscle of the human trachea and bronchi [72]. In this study, no adrenergic inhibitory fibers were demonstrated by either physiologic or histochemical techniques [72]. Ultrastructural morphological studies of the nerves in the human airways have to date confirmed these initial findings, and the only evi-

---

**FIGURE 10** An electron micrograph of a part of a large ganglion from a human trachea. The tissue was not placed in a warm physiologic solution before fixation, and the preservation of the ultrastructural morphology is poor. An axon profile filled with small granular vesicles of the type associated with adrenergic neurotransmission is seen in the large circle. This location within the ganglia is the only area in the human trachea and main-stem bronchi where adrenergic nerves have been seen. A synapse is seen in the smaller circle (×9000).

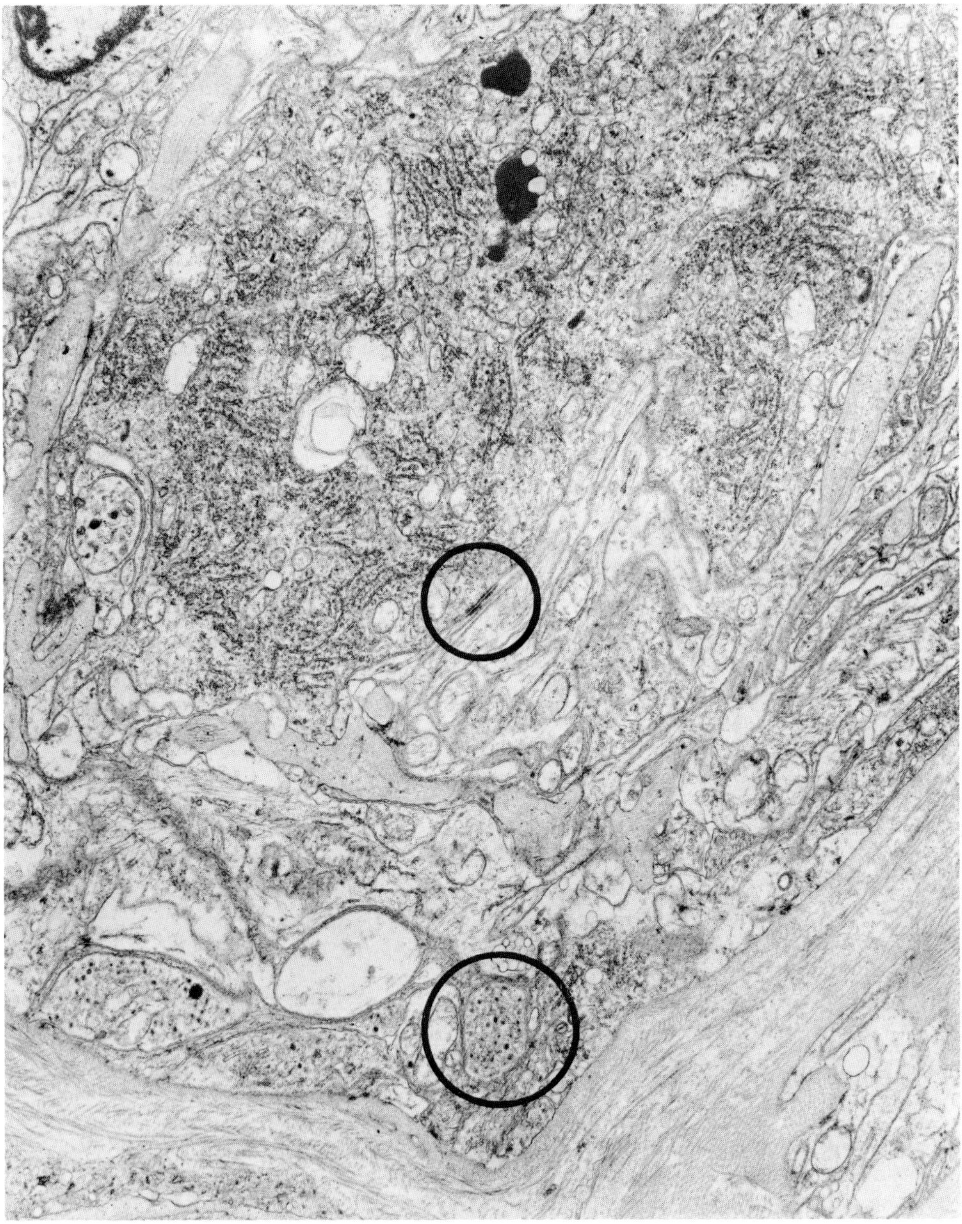

**FIGURE 10**

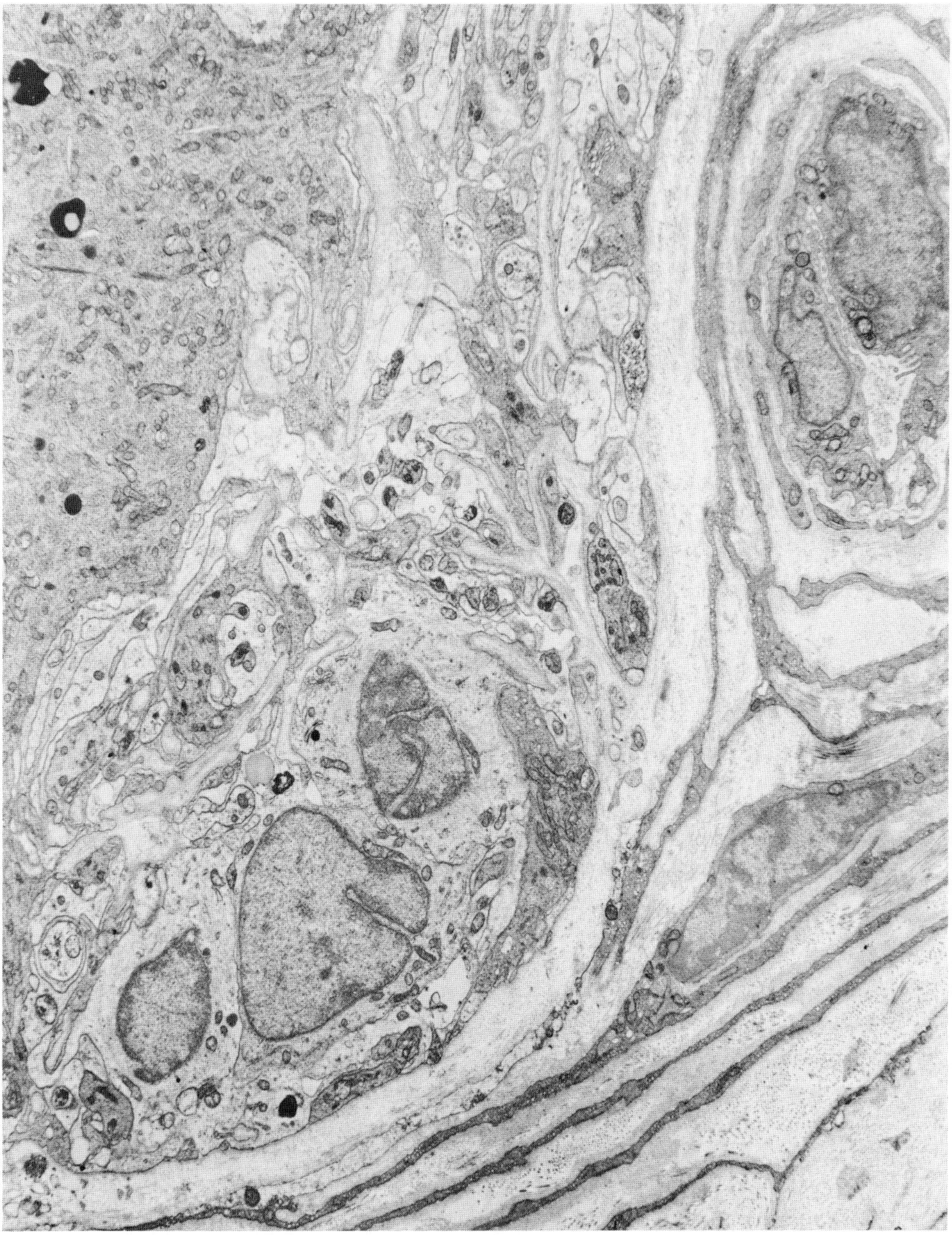

**FIGURE 13** This electron micrograph shows the edge of a large ganglion. Part of a neuron is seen in the upper left-hand corner. The nuclei of glial cells are seen in the lower portion of the micrograph. The ganglion is surrounded by a basal lamina. No blood vessels or collagen fibers are seen within the ganglion. The neuron is surrounded by a complex neuropil. This type of ganglion morphologically resembles those in the myenteric plexus of the gastrointestinal tract (×6,000).

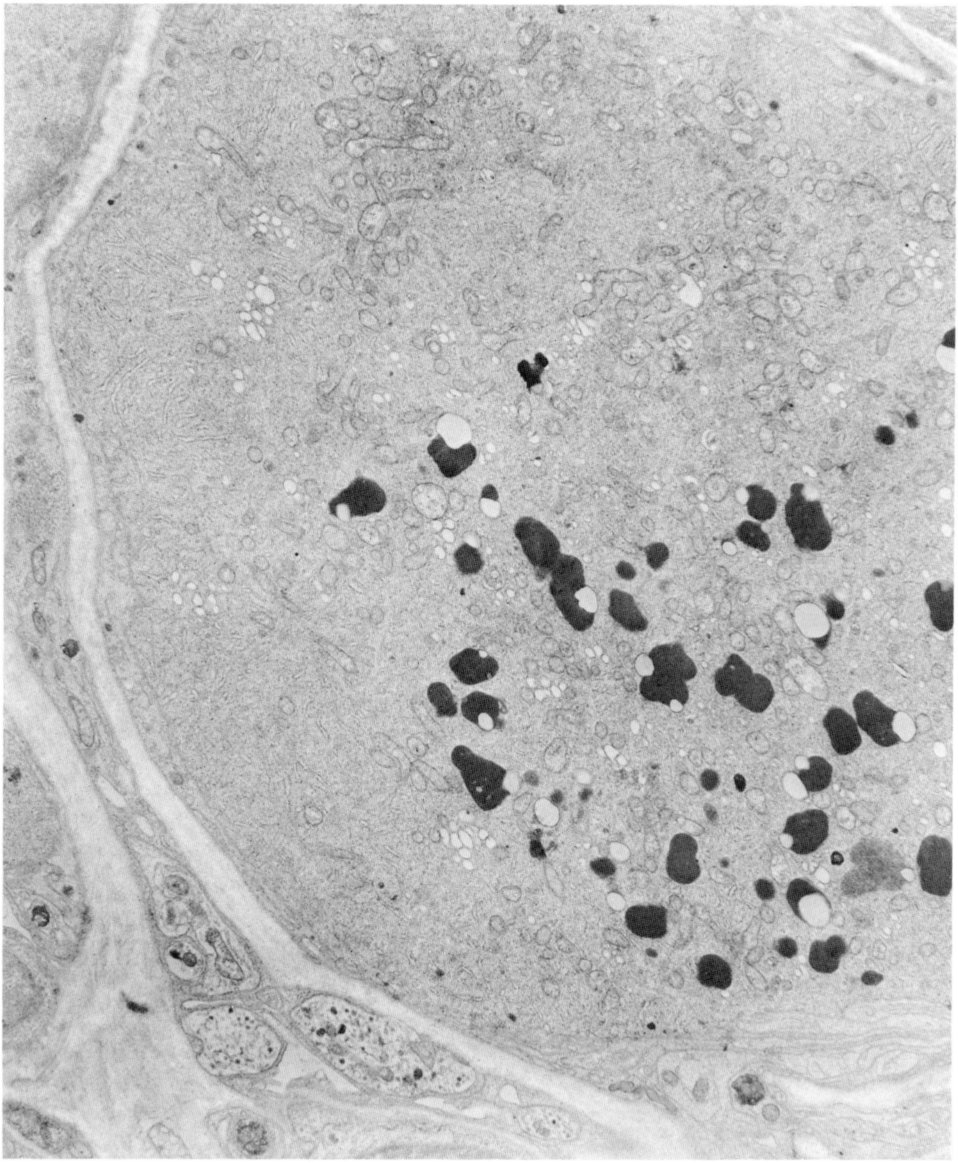

**FIGURE 14** This ganglion is of the simplified type. A satellite cell surrounds the neuron. A nerve is present in the lower left-hand corner of the micrograph, and this nerve is connected to the neuron. Other nerves are seen adjacent to, but not connected to, the neuron. This simplified ganglion is quite unlike the complex ganglion, in which there is a dense neuropil surrounding the neurons (×8000).

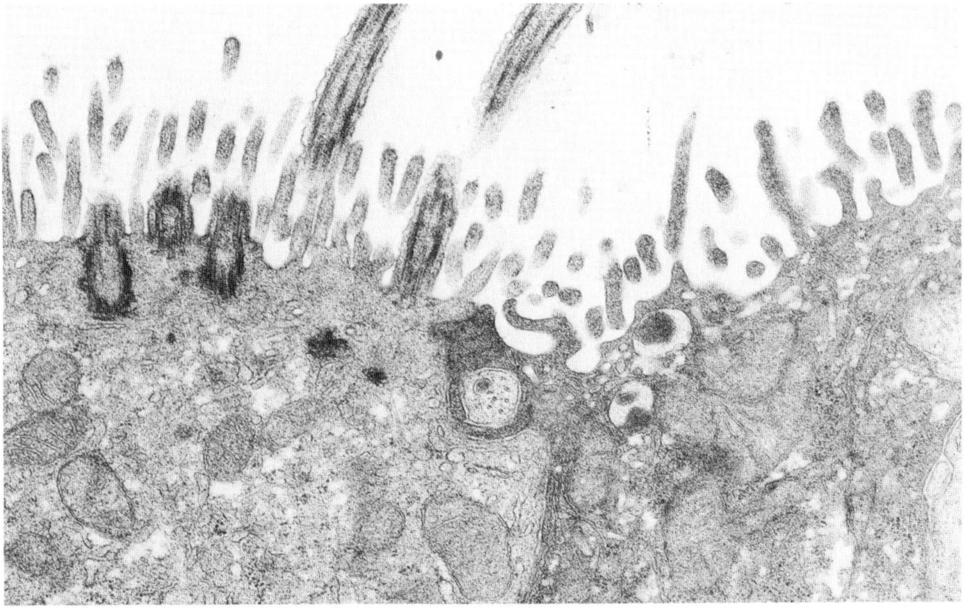

**FIGURE 15** Guinea pig tracheal epithelium. An axon is present beneath the tight junction between a ciliated and a nonciliated cell. This type of axon profile has been associated with irritant reflexes (X24,000).

Unmyelinated axons are found in human tracheal epithelium [20] and are sometimes seen between the epithelial cells near the lumen of the airway. These axons are similar to those found in the guinea pig epithelium (Fig. 15). No axon profiles with vesicles have been seen in human epithelium, but a systematic search for them has not been done. It is not clear if the axons without vesicles, which are seen in the epithelium, originate in the ganglia of the airways or whether they are only related to the vagal nuclei. Most evidence to date would suggest that they originate in the vagal nuclei [77].

## V. Cartilage

The cartilaginous structure of the human lung has been extensively described [78-80]. The cartilage rings in the trachea and main bronchi are C shaped, and this structure becomes modified where the cartilage plates begin. The main bronchi are symmetrical [78]. Characteristic secondary carinal cartilage plates are found at the terminal bifurcation of the main-stem bronchi, and these plates are felt to be essential to the support of the airways at the bifurcation [78]. Cartilaginous rings cease and plates begin precisely along the line where the airways enter the lung [78]. In fetal life, precartilage is seen at week 10 of gestation [80], and the plates of cartilage are usually complete by week 28 of gestation [79].

There is species variation in the cartilaginous airway skeleton. In birds, the cartilage completely surrounds the trachea and the main bronchi and there is no membranous portion [78]. In the dog, the cartilage rings almost touch each other at the dorsal surface and leave only a small membranous part [78]. Within the lung parenchyma the cartilage may be absent as in birds, amphibia, rodents, and reptiles, or it may have a distinctive form easily differentiated from that present in the trachea and main-stem bronchi [78]. The embryological events which account for these differences and the physiological meaning of the species variation are not clear [78].

## VI. Connective Tissue

Little work has been done on the morphology of the connective tissue of the airways. It is frequently referred to as a loose network of collagen and elastic fibers with fibroblasts, mast cells, lymphocytes, macrophages, and eosinophils [20].

Collections of lymphoid tissue, either as nodules or aggregates, are found in the submucosal tissue. Some species have a modification of the epithelium over these areas of lymphoid tissue which is similar to the modified surface of the epithelium in the gastrointestinal tract over Peyer's patches [81,82]. This modified airway epithelium may play a role as a portal for antigenic material to the lymphoid tissue below [81,82]. In the distal airways the lymphoid aggregates are not seen in the normal human at birth unless there has been an intrauterine infection [83]. It is generally believed that the airways produce immunoglobulins locally, and this topic has been recently reviewed [5]. The route by which the antigens penetrate the epithelium to gain access to the lymphoid tissue is not clear. The route may be by way of the modified epithelium [81] or it may be by uptake from the lumen by certain cells [8]. Studies of the lymphoid tissue under a variety of conditions are needed.

Little morphological information is available on lymphatics in the human lung. One study of human and rabbit pulmonary tissue showed that the lymphatics of the two species were similar [84]. The lymphatics are lined by flat endothelial cells which often contain small (7 to 10 nm) round, coated vesicles. The lymphatic endothelium rests on a thin, interrupted basement membrane. The junctions between these cells are simple end-to-end junctions or junctions formed by the overlapping of the endothelial cells [84]. The endothelial cells have a close association with the collagen fibers. Fine filaments pass through the basement membrane of the endothelial cells to the collagen and presumably act as anchors [84]. A recent review has dealt with the structure in more detail [85].

On gross examination of the trachea, longitudinal corrugations are seen on the posterior surface and these corrugations continue into the bronchi [86]. The corrugations are developed in utero before week 23 of gestation and are formed by submucosal bundles of elastic tissue embedded in collagen [86]. The function of these bundles, which are seen in a variety of animals, is obscure [86]. They may provide an increased surface area for the mucosa or act as conduits for secretions. They may also have a role in the equalization of tension during inspiration and provide elastic recoil during expiration [86].

In summary, we still lack sufficient morphological data for a complete understanding of the functions of the airways. It is evident from the marked species variation that extrapolation from one animal to another may not be valid. The morphology of the human airways has been the least studied. The lack of human material is likely due to the difficulty in obtaining suitable human tissue for ultrastructural studies. We have found that we can use material from recent autopsies which, after a suitable period in a warm physiological solution, shows remarkably good ultrastructural detail [87]. Morphological studies are best coupled to physiologic studies of the airways. It is now evident that we know little about the function of many of the cells or even of parts of these, such as cilia. The nervous system in the airways now seems more complicated than before, and physiologic studies of this system will have to be performed before we can correlate the normal structure with the function. Until such studies are done, it will be difficult to understand the abnormalities which occur in disease states.

## Acknowledgments

The authors wish to thank Mr. Charles P. Hodge, consultant photographer to the department of pathology, for his expert advice and help in the preparation of the photographic material; Miss A. De Notariis for her assistance in the preparation of the human tissue for electron microscopy; and Miss L. Surette and Miss K. Morham for their patient help in the preparation of the manuscript.

## References

1. Okamoto, E., and T. Ueda, Embryogenesis of intramural ganglia of the gut and its relation to Hirschsprung's disease, *J. Pediatr. Surg.,* **2**:437-443 (1967).
2. Thurlbeck, W. M., Structure of the lung, *Int. Rev. Physiol.,* **14**:1-36 (1977).

3. Hogg, J. C., J. Williams, J. B. Richardson, P. T. Macklem, and W. M. Thurlbeck, Age as a factor in the distribution of lower airway conductance in the pathologic anatomy of obstructive lung disease, *N. Engl. J. Med.,* **282**: 1283-1287 (1970).
4. Tada, T., and K. Ishizaka, Distribution of γE-forming cells in lymphoid tissues of the human and monkey, *J. Immunol.,* **104**:377-387 (1970).
5. Kaltreider, H. B., Expression of immune mechanisms in the lung, *Am. Rev. Resp. Dis.,* **113**:347-380 (1976).
6. Callerame, M. L., J. J. Condemi, K. Ishizaka, S. G. O. Johansson, and J. H. Vaughan, Immunoglobulins in bronchial tissues from patients with asthma, with special reference to immunoglobulin E, *J. Allergy,* **47**:187-197 (1971).
7. Richardson, J. B., R. C. Boucher, A. De Notariis, and C. C. Ferguson, The effects of laryngotracheitis on the permeability of the chicken airways and the subsequent antibody production. Submitted for publication (Unpublished).
8. Richardson, J. B., T. Bouchard, and C. C. Ferguson, Uptake and transport of exogenous proteins by respiratory epithelium, *Lab. Invest.,* **35**:307-314 (1976).
9. Perrotto, J. L., L. M. Hang, K. J. Isselbacher, and K. S. Warren, Systemic cellular hypersensitivity induced by an intestinally absorbed antigen, *J. Exp. Med.,* **140**:296-299 (1974).
10. Breeze, R. G., and E. B. Wheeldon, The cells of the pulmonary airways, *Am. Rev. Resp. Dis.,* **116**:705-777 (1977).
11. Cutz, E., and R. P. Orange, Mast cells and endocrine (APUD) cells of the lung. In *Asthma: Physiology, Immunopharmacology and Treatment.* Edited by L. M. Lichtenstein and K. F. Austen. New York, Academic, 1977.
12. Cutz, E., W. Chan, V. Wong, and P. E. Conen, Ultrastructure and fluorescence histochemistry of endocrine (APUD-type) cells in tracheal mucosa of human and various animal species, *Cell Tissue Res.,* **158**(4):425-437 (1975).
13. Pearse, A. G. E., The cytochemistry and ultrastructure of polypeptide hormone producing cells of the APUD series and the embryologic, physiologic and pathologic implications of the concept, *J. Histochem. Cytochem.,* **17**:303-313 (1969).
14. Lauweryns, J. M., M. Cokelaere, and P. Theunynck, Neuro-epithelial bodies in the respiratory mucosa of various mammals. A light optical, histochemical and ultrastructural investigation, *Z. Zellforsch. Mikrosk. Anat.,* **135**(4): 569-592 (1972).
15. Said, S. I., and V. Mutt, Polypeptide with broad biological activity: Isolation from small intestine, *Science,* **169**:1217-1218 (1970).
16. Lauweryns, J. M., and P. Goddeeris, Neuroepithelial bodies in the human child and adult lung, *Am. Rev. Resp. Dis.,* **111**:469-476 (1975).
17. Coupland, R., and D. Hopwood, The mechanism of the differential staining reaction for adrenaline and noradrenaline storing granules in tissue fixed in glutaraldehyde, *J. Anat.,* **100**:227-243 (1966).

18. Richardson, J. B., T. Bouchard, and G. Boyd, Polymers of biogenic amines, *Can. J. Physiol. Pharm.,* **55**:895-903 (1977).
19. Rhodin, J. A. G., and T. Dalhamn, Electron microscopy of the tracheal ciliated mucosa in rat, *Z. Zellforsch.,* **44**:345-412 (1956).
20. Rhodin, J. A. G., The ciliated cell. Ultrastructure and function of the human tracheal mucosa, *Am. Rev. Resp. Dis.,* **93**:1-15 (1966).
21. Basset, F., J. Poirier, M. Le Crom, and J. Turiaf, Etude ultrastructurale de l'épithelium bronchiolaire humain, *Z. Zellforsch. Mikrosk. Anat.,* **116**(3): 425-442 (1971).
22. Hansell, M. M., and R. L. Moretti, Ultrastructure of the mouse tracheal epithelium, *J. Morphol.,* **128**:159-170 (1969).
23. Purcell, D. A., The ultrastructure of tracheal epithelium in the fowl, *Res. Vet. Sci.,* **12**:455-458 (1971).
24. Pavelka, M., H. R. Ronge, and G. Stockinger, Vergleichende untersuchungen am trachealepithel verschiedener saüger, *Acta Anat. (Basel),* **94**(2): 262-282 (1976).
25. Inoue, S., and J. C. Hogg, Freeze-etch study of the tracheal epithelium of normal guinea pigs with particular reference to intercellular junctions, *J. Ultrastruct. Res.,* **61**:89-99 (1977).
26. Simani, A. S., S. Inoue, and J. C. Hogg, Penetration of the respiratory epithelium of guinea pigs following exposure to cigarette smoke, *Lab. Invest.,* **31**(1):75-81 (1974).
27. Boucher, R. C., V. Ranga, P. D. Pare, S. Inoue, L. A. Moroz, and J. C. Hogg, The effect of histamine and metacholine on respiratory mucosal permeability, *Am. Rev. Resp. Dis.,* **115**(2):307 (1977).
28. Gilula, N. B., Gap junctions and cell communication. In *International Cell Biology.* Edited by B. R. Brinckley and K. R. Porter. New York, The Rockefeller University Press, 1976-77.
29. Lowenstein, W. R., Cellular communication through membrane junctions: Special consideration of wound healing and carcinoma, *Arch. Intern. Med.,* **129**:209-305 (1972).
30. McNutt, S. N., and R. S. Weinstein, The ultrastructure of the nexus, *J. Cell Biol.,* **47**:666-688 (1970).
31. Rash, J. E., and M. H. Ellisman, Studies of excitable membranes. I. Macromolecular specialization of the neuromuscular junction and the non-junctional sarcolemma, *J. Cell Biol.,* **63**:567-586 (1974).
32. Staehelin, L. A., Three types of gap junctions interconnecting intestinal epithelial cells visualized by freeze-etching, *Proc. Natl. Acad. Sci. USA,* **69**: 1318-1321 (1972).
33. Walsh, C., and J. McLelland, Intraepithelial axons in the avian lung, *Z. Zellforsch. Mikrosk. Anat.,* **147**:209-217 (1974).
34. Jeffrey, P., and L. Reid, Intraepithelial nerves in normal rat airways: A quantitative electron microscopic study, *J. Anat.,* **114**:35-45 (1973).
35. Tos, M. K., Mucous glands of the trachea in man. Quantitative studies, *Anat. Anz.,* **128**(2):136-149 (1971).

36. Meyrick, B., and L. Reid, Ultrastructure of cells in the human bronchial submucosal glands, *J. Anat.*, **107**(2):281-299 (1970).
37. Case, R. M., A. A. Harper, and T. Scratcherd, Water and electrolyte secretion by pancreas. In *The Exocrine Glands.* Edited by S. Y. Botelho, F. P. Brooks, and W. B. Shelley. Philadelphia, University of Pennsylvania, 1969.
38. Tos, M., Mucous elements in the airways, *Acta Otolaryngol. (Stockh.)*, **82** (3-4):249-251 (1976).
39. Dunnill, M. S., G. R. Massarella, and J. A. Anderson, A comparison of the quantitative anatomy of the bronchi in normal subjects, in status asthmaticus, in chronic bronchitis and in emphysema, *Thorax*, **24**(2):176-179 (1969).
40. Widdicombe, J. G., Control of secretion of tracheobronchial mucus, *Br. Med. Bull.*, **34**:57-61 (1978).
41. Nagaishi, C., *Functional Anatomy and Histology of the Lung.* Baltimore, University Park Press, 1972.
42. Hakansson, C. H., U. Mercke, B. Sonesson, and N. G. Toremalm, Functional anatomy of the musculature of the trachea, *Acta Morphol. Neerl. Scand.*, **14**(4):291-297 (1976).
43. Stephens, N. L., Airway smooth muscle: Biophysics, biochemistry and pharmacology. In *Asthma: Physiology, Immunopharmacology and Treatment.* Edited by L. M. Lichtenstein and K. F. Austen. New York, Academic, 1977.
44. Cameron, A. R., and C. T. Kirkpatrick, A study of excitatory neuromuscular transmission in the bovine trachea, *J. Physiol. (Lond.)*, **270**:733-745 (1977).
45. Burnstock, G., Purinergic nerves, *Pharmacol. Rev.*, **24**:509-581 (1972).
46. Gabella, G., Quantitative morphological study of smooth muscle cells of the guinea-pig taenia coli, *Cell Tissue Res.*, **170**:161-186 (1976).
47. Richardson, J. B., and C. C. Ferguson, Neuromuscular structure and function in the airways, *Fed. Proc.*, **38**(2):202-208 (1979).
48. Suzuki, H., K. Morita, and H. Kuriyama, Innervation and properties of the smooth muscle of the dog trachea, *Jpn. J. Physiol.*, **26**(3):303-320 (1976).
49. Akasaka, K., K. Konno, Y. Ono, S. Mue, and C. Abe, Electromyographic study of bronchial smooth muscle in bronchial asthma, *Tohoku J. Exp. Med.*, **117**(1):55-59 (1975).
50. Larsell, G., and R. S. Dow, The innervation of the human lung, *Am. J. Anat.*, **52**(1):125-146 (1933).
51. Blümcke, S., Morphological aspects of the innervation of lungs, *Beitr. Klin. Tuberk.*, **138**:229-242 (1968).
52. Gaylor, J. B., The intrinsic nervous mechanism of the human lung, *Brain*, **57**:143-160 (1934).
53. Cook, R. D., and A. S. King, Observations of the ultrastructure of the smooth muscle and its innervation in the avian lung, *J. Anat.*, **106**:273-283 (1970).
54. McLelland, M., Observations with the light microscope on the ganglia and nerve plexuses of the intrapulmonary bronchi of the bird, *J. Anat.*, **105**:202 (1969).

55. Cook, R. D., and A. S. King, Nerves of the avian lung: Electron microscopy, *J. Anat.,* **105**:202 (1969).
56. Akester, A. R., and S. P. Mann, Ultrastructure and innervation of the tertiary bronchial unit in the lung of *Gallus domesticus, J. Anat.,* **105**:202-204 (1969).
57. Castelman, W. L., D. L. Dungworth, and W. S. Tyler, Intrapulmonary airway morphology in three species of monkeys: A correlated scanning and transmission electron microscopic study, *Am. J. Anat.,* **142**(1):107-121 (1975).
58. Silva, D. G., and G. Ross, Ultrastructural and fluorescence histochemical studies on the innervation of the tracheobronchial muscle of normal cats and cats treated with 6-hydroxydopamine, *J. Ultrastruct. Res.,* **47**:310-328 (1974).
59. Coburn, R. F., and Tomita, T., Evidence for non-adrenergic inhibitory nerves in the guinea pig trachealis muscle, *Am. J. Physiol.,* **224**:1072-1080 (1973).
60. O'Donnell, S. R., and N. Sarr, Histochemical localization of adrenergic nerves in the guinea pig trachea, *Br. J. Pharmacol.,* **47**:707-710 (1973).
61. Dahlstrom, A., K. Fuxe, T. Hokfelt, and K. Norbet, Adrenergic innervation of the bronchial muscle of the cat, *Acta Physiol. Scand.,* **66**:507-508 (1966).
62. El-Bermani, A., W. F. McNary, and D. E. Bradley, The distribution of acetylcholinesterase and catecholamine containing nerves in the rat lung, *Anat. Rec.,* **167**:207-212 (1970).
63. Mann, S. P., The formation of mammalian bronchial smooth muscle: The localization of catecholamines and cholinesterases, *Histochem. J.,* **3**:319-331 (1971).
64. Weiner, N., Adrenergic innervation of bronchial muscle. In *Proceedings of the Tenth Aspen Emphysema Conference* held in Aspen, Colorado, June 7-10, 1967. Public Health Service Publication 1787, Washington, D.C., U.S. Government Printing Office, 1967, pp. 257-266.
65. Widdicombe, J. G., Regulation of tracheobronchial smooth muscle, *Physiol. Rev.,* **43**:1-37 (1963).
66. Bando, T., N. Shindo, and Y. Shimo, Non-adrenergic inhibitory nerves in tracheal smooth muscle of guinea pig, *J. Physiol. Soc. Jpn.,* **35**:508-509 (1973).
67. Coleman, R. A., Evidence for a non-adrenergic inhibitory nervous pathway in guinea pig trachea, *Br. J. Pharmacol.,* **48**:360-361 (1973).
68. Richardson, J. B., and T. Bouchard, Demonstration of a nonadrenergic inhibitory nervous system in the trachea of the guinea pig, *J. Allergy Clin. Immunol.,* **56**:473-480 (1975).
69. Gershon, M. D., and E. B. Thompson, The maturation of neuromuscular function in a multiply innervated structure: Development of the longitudinal smooth muscle of the foetal mammalian gut and its cholinergic excitatory, adrenergic inhibitory and nonadrenergic inhibitory innervation, *J. Physiol. (Lond.),* **234**:257-277 (1973).
70. Kuchii, M., J. T. Miyahara, and S. Shibata, ($^3$H)-Adenine nucleotide and

($^3$H)-noradrenaline release evoked by electrical field stimulation perivascular nerve stimulation and nicotine from the taenia of the guinea-pig caecum, *Br. J. Pharmacol.,* **49**:258-267 (1973).

71. Weisenthal, L. M., C. C. Hug, Jr., N. W. Weibrodt, and P. Bass, Adrenergic mechanism in the relaxation of the guinea-pig taenia in vitro, *J. Pharmacol. Exp. Ther.,* **178**(3):497-508 (1971).
72. Richardson, J. B., and J. Béland, Non-adrenergic inhibitory nerves in human airways, *J. Appl. Physiol.,* **41**:764-771 (1976).
73. Richardson, J. B., and C. C. Ferguson, The fine structure of the ganglia in human lung, *J. Cell Biol.,* **70**:48a (1976).
74. Gabella, G., Fine structure of the myenteric plexus in the guinea-pig ileum, *J. Anat.,* **111**:69-97 (1972).
75. Wood, J. D., Electrical activity from single neurons in Auerbach's plexus, *Am. J. Physiol.,* **219**:159-169 (1970).
76. Hirst, G. D. S., and H. C. McKirdy, A nervous mechanism for descending inhibition in guinea-pig small intestine, *J. Physiol. (Lond.),* **238**:129-143 (1974).
77. Widdicombe, J. G., Reflex control of tracheobronchial smooth muscle in experimental and human asthma. In *Asthma: Physiology, Immunopharmacology and Treatment.* Edited by L. M. Lichtenstein and K. F. Austen. New York, Academic, 1977.
78. Vanpeperstraete, F., The cartilaginous skeleton of the bronchial tree, *Adv. Anat. Embryol. Cell Biol.,* **48**(3):1-80 (1973).
79. Reid, L., Visceral cartilage, *J. Anat.,* **122**(2):349-355 (1976).
80. Bucher, U., and L. Reid, Development of the mucus-secreting elements in human lung, *Thorax,* **16**:219-225 (1961).
81. Bienenstock, J., N. Johnston, and D. Y. E. Perey, Bronchial tissue. II. Functional characteristics, *Lab. Invest.,* **28**:693-698 (1973).
82. Bienenstock, J., R. L. Clancy, and D. Y. E. Perey, Bronchus associated lymphoid tissue (BALT): Its relationship to mucosal immunity. In *Immunologic and Infectious Reactions in the Lung.* Edited by C. Kirkpatrick and H. Y. Reynolds. New York, Marcel Dekker, 1976.
83. Emery, J. L., and F. Dinsdale, The post-natal development of lymphoreticular aggregates and lymph nodes in infant's lungs, *J. Clin. Pathol.,* **26**:539-545 (1973).
84. Lauweryns, J. M., and L. Boussauw, The ultrastructure of pulmonary lymphatic capillaries of newborn rabbits and of human infants, *Lymphology,* **2**(3):108-129 (1969). New York, Marcel Dekker, 1977.
85. Leak, L. V., Pulmonary lymphatics and their role in the removal of interstitial fluids and particular matter. In *Respiratory Defense Mechanisms Part II.* Edited by J. Brain, D. Proctor, and L. Reid. New York, Marcel Dekker, 1977, pp. 631-685.
86. Monkhouse, W. S., and W. P. Whimster, An account of the longitudinal

mucosal corrugations of the human tracheo-bronchial tree, with observa tions on those of some animals, *J. Anat.*, **122**(3):681-695 (1976).
87. Ferguson, C. C., and J. B. Richardson, A simple technique for the utilization of post-mortem tracheal and bronchial tissues for ultrastructural studies, *Hum. Pathol.*, **9**(4):463-470 (1978).

# 2

# Ultrastructure, Biophysics, and Biochemistry of Airway Smooth Muscle

*NEWMAN L. STEPHENS and EDWIN A. KROEGER*

University of Manitoba
Winnipeg, Manitoba, Canada

Two recent symposia on lung cells [1,2] indicate the opening up of new directions in respiratory research. As in every other area of research, understanding is being sought at cellular and subcellular levels. From this knowledge, better methods of diagnosis and treatment will develop. The phase of phenomenological description, using classic methods at whole-organ levels, is now being complemented by research directed at understanding mechanisms at molecular levels.

The realization that airways are not passive conduits has created considerable interest in airway smooth muscle control mechanisms. From this has developed the recent interest in studying the biophysics and biochemistry of this muscle. It is hoped that such studies will, for example, help us understand better how regional distribution of ventilation is controlled. The increasing incidence or recognition of asthma has also served to focus attention on airway smooth muscle.

---

The research described in this chapter was supported by funds from the Medical Research Council of Canada, the Canadian Heart Foundation, the Canadian Tuberculosis and Respiratory Disease Association, and the Richardson Foundation of Winnipeg.

It is very difficult to study airway smooth muscle cells in vivo in the human subject, and hence the physiological information we seek is not available to us. In studying the isolated muscle one is bedeviled by the fact that the muscle chosen, generally because of ease in handling, may not be the best model for that particular, in vivo, airway smooth muscle for which understanding is sought. This is akin to the situation in the circulatory system where studies of carotid artery or aortic strips tell us, in a qualitative way only, what the behavior of the resistance arterioles is.

In spite of the above, airway smooth muscle may be, within limits, an adequate model for smooth muscle throughout the body, and data derived from it could help us understand the physiology of intestinal, uterine, and vascular smooth muscles.

Finally, we must point out that most of the material in this chapter deals with canine tracheal smooth muscle. Our reason for focusing on this muscle is that it appears to be the model of airway smooth muscle on which the most work has been done. Furthermore, it has those properties which make it eminently suited to valid study of its biophysical properties. We are aware that this muscle is not very important in controlling distribution of ventilation; however, other investigators have shown that tracheal smooth muscle, in the intact human and dog [3,4], responds to agonists and nerve stimulation in the same way as the muscle in those small airways where the bulk of the resistance to airflow resides, and this is our justification for the use of the former as a model for the latter.

## I. Structure and Ultrastructure

### A. Musculature

*Tracheal Smooth Muscle*

While this chapter purports to deal with airway smooth muscle in general, major attention is paid to canine tracheal smooth muscle. This deliberate bias stems from the fact that our own experience has been mainly with this muscle, and our feeling is that it is a good model for airway smooth muscle down to the sixth generation of bronchi. This view is based partly on histologic survey, which shows that bronchial smooth muscle, structurally, closely resembles that of the trachea; and partly in the great similarity in pharmacologic and mechanical properties of the two muscles, as judged by comparison of their dose-response, length-tension, and stimulus-response curves. Hence, we feel that studies of tracheal smooth muscle provide insight into the more important (from the point of view of controlling airflow) bronchial smooth muscle. This is an echo of Permutt's

[3] statement: "I doubt that the increase in resistance to airflow resulting from changes in the large airways is of much significance, other than providing us with a sensitive indicator of changes that are likely to correlate with changes in the smaller airways."

**Macroscopic Characteristics**

In the dog, as in the human, the cartilaginous rings of the trachea are incomplete posteriorly. The gap is closed by a sheet of muscle and another of fibrous tissue. It is important to remember that while the muscle is ventral to the fibrous layer in the human, guinea pig, and hedge hog, this order is reversed in the dog, cat, and rabbit.

Tracheal rings can be cut transversely very easily. If the cartilage is divided vertically and the cut ends are everted, the muscular layer and the fibrous spring apart as shown in Figure 1. The muscle can be quickly and cleanly dissected out and provides an excellent preparation for mechanical studies. For electrophysiological studies, more carefully microdissection is needed to remove collagen and elastic tissue, after which impalement with microelectrodes is very easy. We must iterate that unless the adherent connective tissue is removed, impalement is extremely difficult. For biochemical studies, the tissue is suitable, at least with respect to the fact that more than 75% of it is muscle; however, the quantity of muscle available from the entire trachea is so little that to obtain adequate material for a single experiment, three or four dogs have to be killed.

The *musculus transversus trachea* consists of a unified layer of thick bundles of smooth muscle which branch little and are transverse in direction. In the canine trachea, the sheet is about 30 cells thick. The muscle bundles are fastened by elastic tendons to the external perichondrium of the tracheal cartilage (near the dorsal ends of the cartilages) and the annular ligaments. This type of insertion is seen in the dog. In the human the insertion is on the internal perichondrium. Luschka [5] has indicated that bundles of muscle extend from the trachealis and insert into the ventral wall of the esophagus. The nutrient blood supply to tracheal and bronchial smooth muscle is the bronchial artery; however, airway smooth muscle may also obtain oxygen directly from the gas in the lumen.

**Light Microscope Characteristics**

The trachealis, in common with smooth muscle elsewhere, is made up of fusiform muscle cells with a centrally located, cigar-shaped nucleus. Many nuclei are seen in Figure 2. From their parallel orientation, it is inferred that the cells are arranged parallel to each other. This is confirmed directly on electron microscopy, where the cell outlines are clearly delineated.

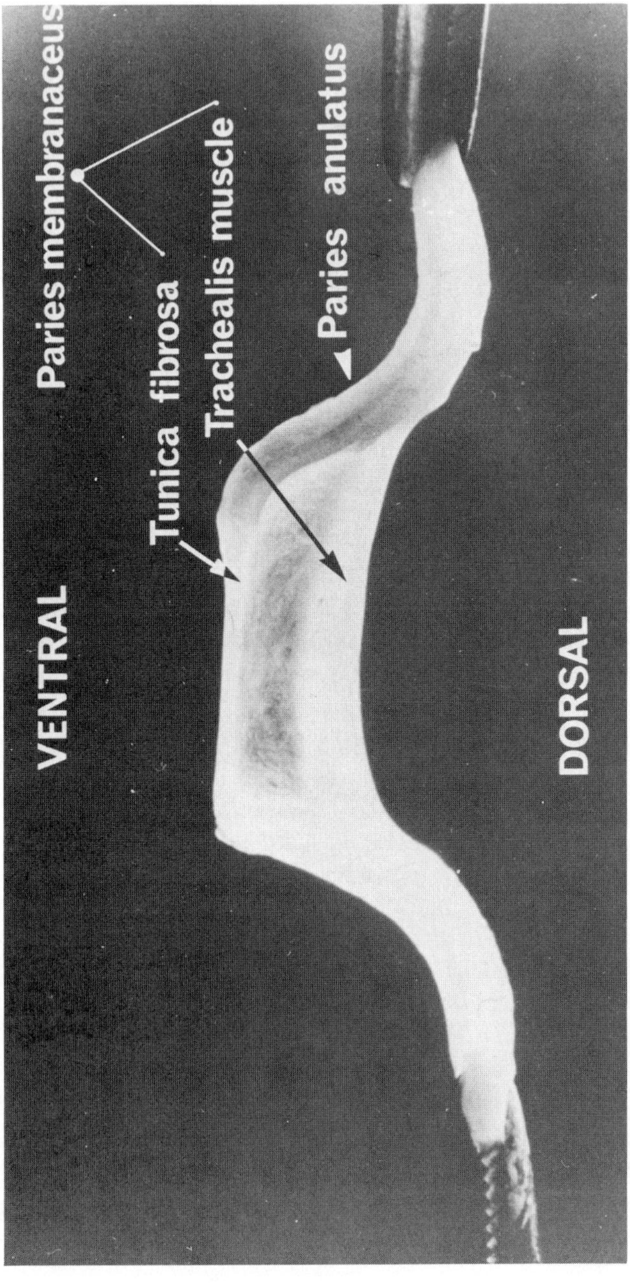


**FIGURE 1** Photograph of canine tracheal ring cut and everted to display the muscle. (From Ref. [93].)

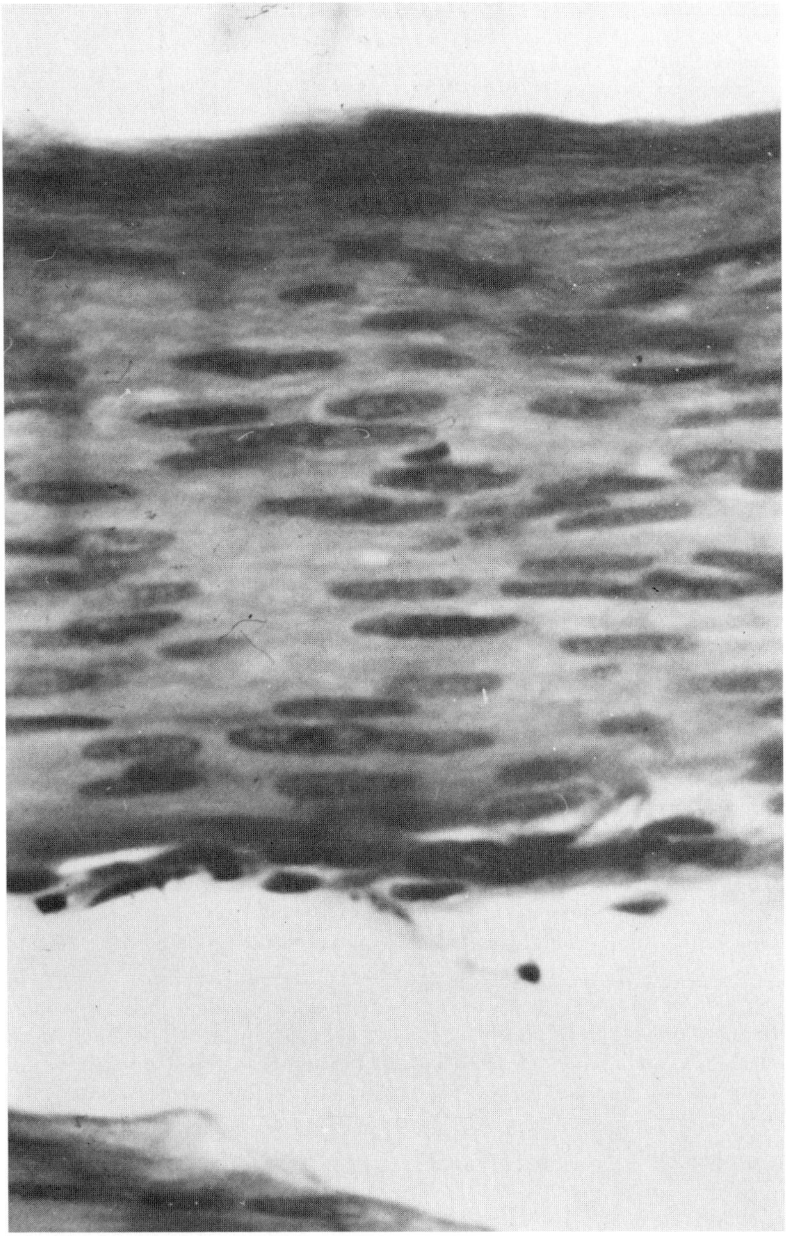

**FIGURE 2** Light microscopy of canine tracheal smooth muscle. Section stained with hematoxylin and eosin (×800).

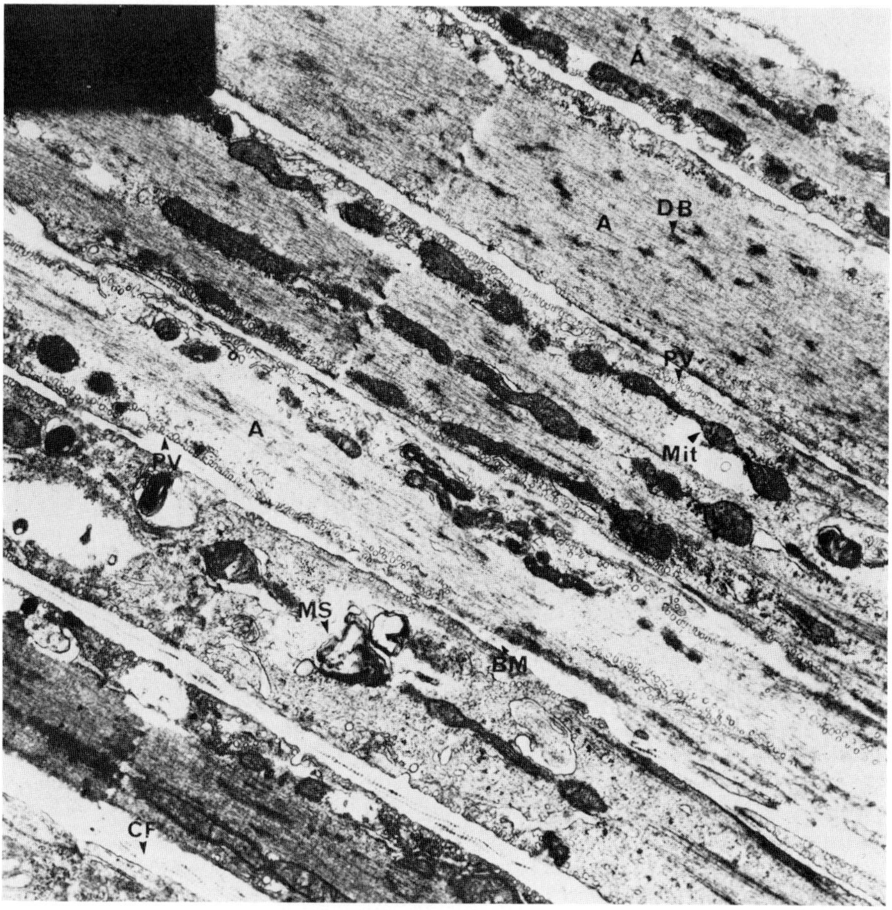


**FIGURE 3** Electron micrograph of a longitudinal section of canine tracheal smooth muscle. A, actin filaments; BM, basement membrane; Mit, mitochondria, these are long and serpiginous; CF, collagen fibrils; PV, pinocytotic vesicles. Myelin swirls (MS) and dense bodies (DB) are also seen (×16,500).

In the canine trachealis, the amount of tissue that is not muscle is less than 25%. As pointed out before, this is an advantage in biochemical studies, since in most other smooth muscles the amount is greater and one is not sure then how much of what one measures really refers to muscle cells.

## Electron Microscope Characteristics

In Figure 3, a longitudinal section of the resting trachealis is seen. Conventional methods of preparation were employed using glutaraldehyde, osmium tetroxide, uranylacetate, and lead nitrate.

The cells are very long and thin. Suzuki et al. [6] reported that the dog tracheal muscle cell has a diameter of 3.3 ± 0.5 μm (SD) and exceeds 1 mm in length. We have confirmed this.

The trachealis muscle tendon junction in the cat [7] shows some regions of direct contact between the elastica and the plasma membrane of the smooth muscle cell as well as regions in which the plasma membrane is separated from the elastica by a basement membrane.

**The Plasma Membrane, or Sarcolemma, and Pinocytotic Vesicles** The plasma membrane is well defined and, in the resting state, quite smooth. In the isotonically contracted state, the sarcolemma shows considerable undulation (Fig. 4). Basement membrane is visible in Figure 3, as are collagen fibrils between the cells. In Figure 5, a transverse section, arcuate, darkened segments (indicated by arrow) are seen alternating with clear stretches of the cell membrane. The dark segments probably represent dense bodies which are sites for attachment of actin filaments. Very few organelles are seen subjacent to the dark segments, while the clear zones contain pinocytotic vesicles.

In Figure 6, in which the muscle has been fixed during isotonic shortening of greater degree, the pinocytotic vesicles containing relatively clear outpouchings (OP) are clearly seen. Again, the alternation between dark and light segments along the sarcolemma is evident. Fay et al. [8] have shown that isolated smooth muscle cells from the stomach of *Bufo marinus* shorten by well beyond 70% of their rest length. During this, the entire sarcolemma becomes sacculated with outpouchings which make the cell look like a cluster of grapes. We believe that the outpouchings seen in our isotonic preparations represent the same phenomenon. They are not as well developed in our muscle strip preparation because the individual cells have not shortened to the same degree as in the isolated cell.

Fay's explanation, that the folding of the sarcolemma results from shortening of the cell, probably also applies to the trachealis. The sarcolemmal dense bodies have actin filaments attached to them, as mentioned before. During contraction, the pull exerted draws the dark segment in, forming bays.

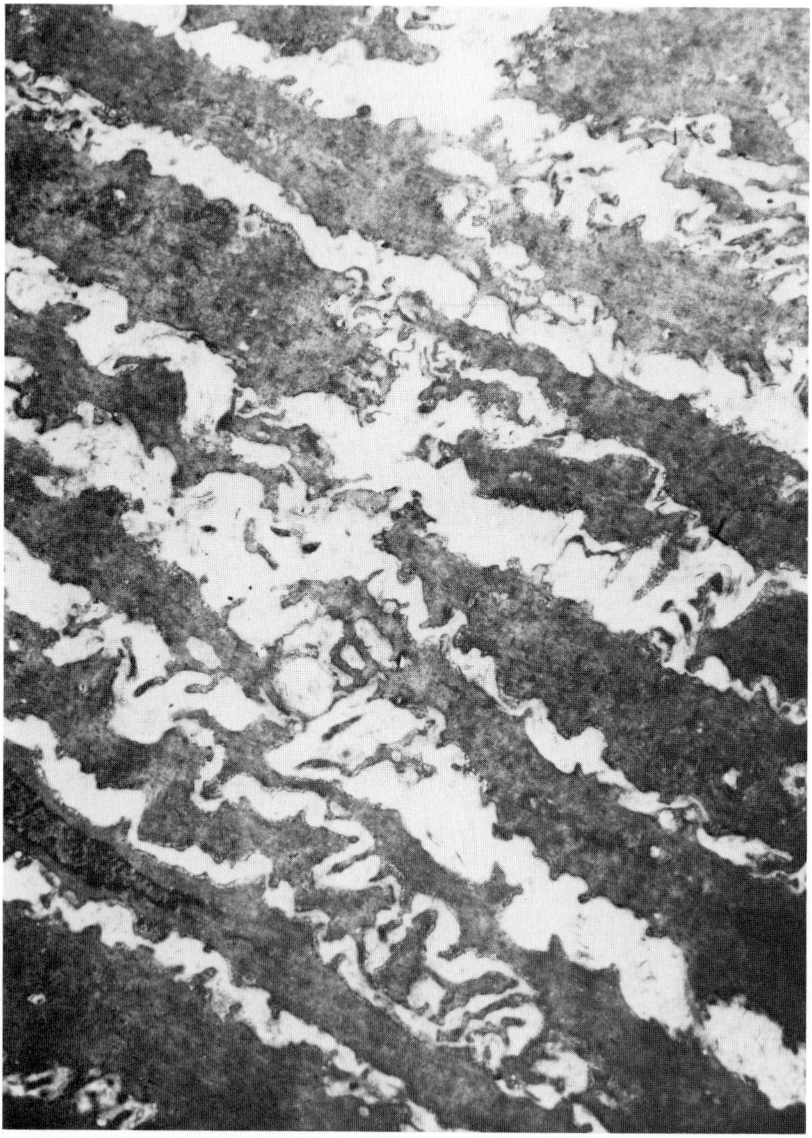

**FIGURE 4** Electron micrograph of a longitudinal section of canine tracheal smooth muscle fixed at maximum shortening during an isotonic contraction. Though the picture is of poor quality, the undulation of the sarcolemma is well seen (X1100).

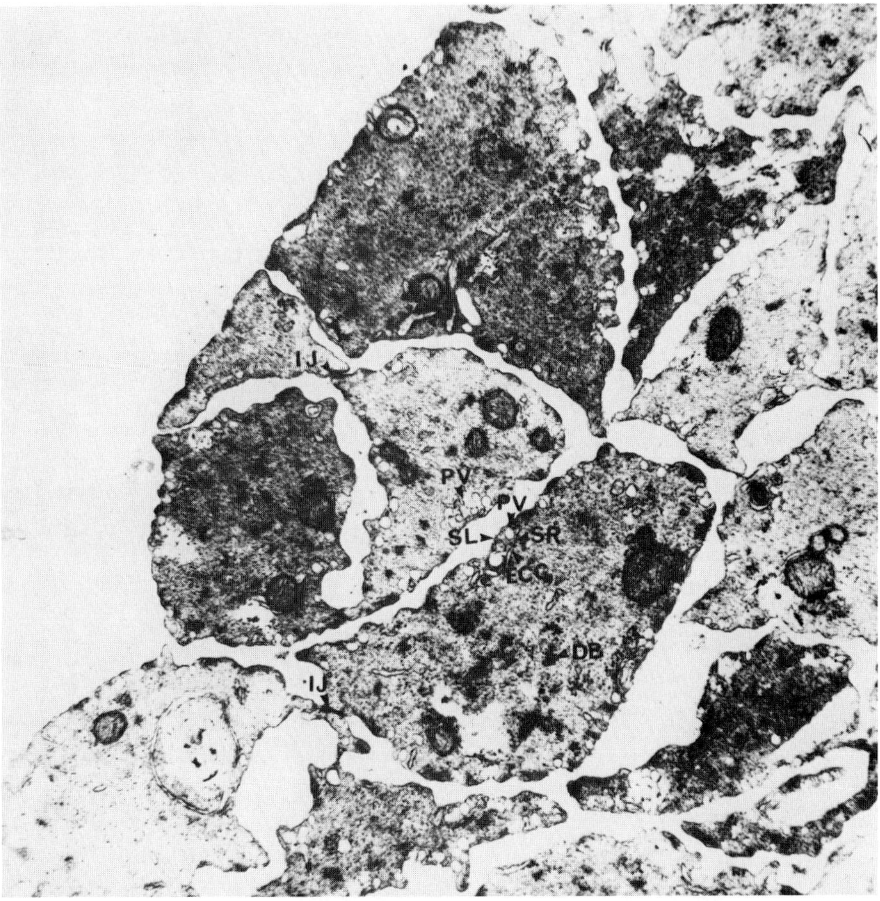


**FIGURE 5** Electron micrograph of a transverse section of canine tracheal smooth muscle. Arrows indicate dense bodies (DB), pinocytotic vesicles (PV), and a tentative excitation-contraction coupling apparatus (ECC) consisting of sarcolemma (SL), pinocytotic vesicle (PV), and sarcoplasmic reticulum (SR). Several intermediate junctions (IJ) are seen (X29,570).

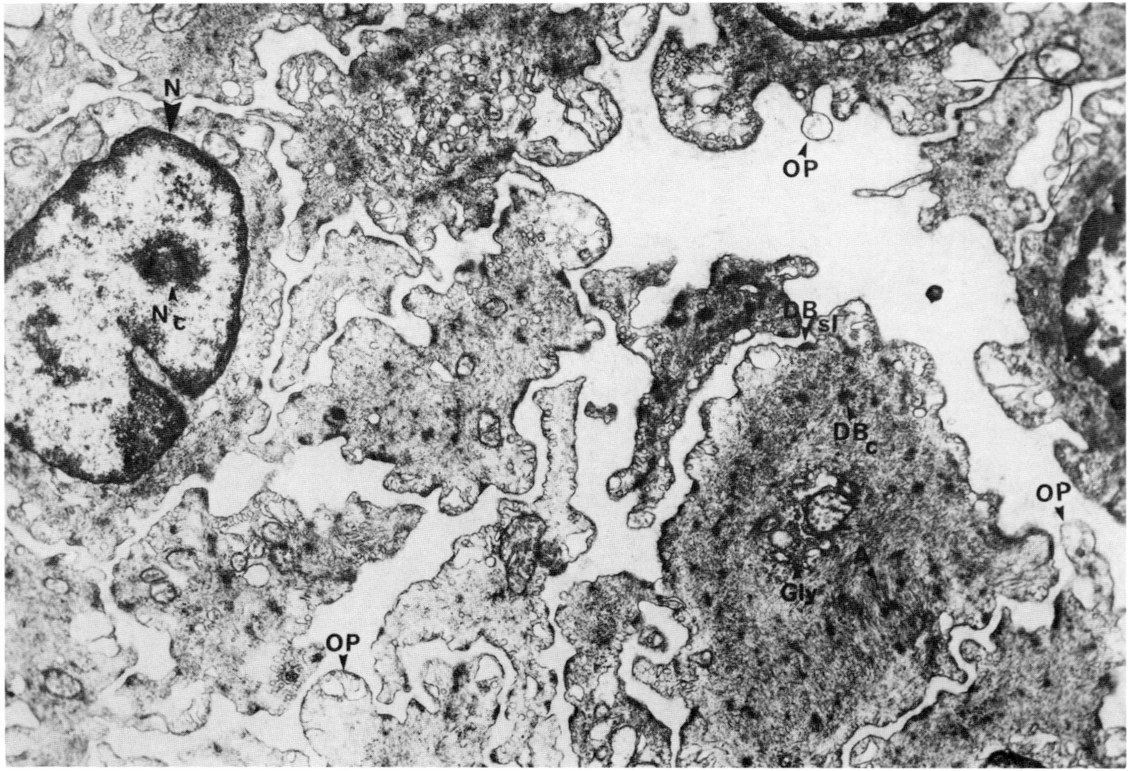


**FIGURE 6** Electron micrograph of a transverse section of canine tracheal smooth muscle. The muscle was fixed in isotonic shortening. Outpouchings (OP) containing pinocytotic vesicles but relatively free of other organelles are seen. Numerous dense bodies are seen scattered throughout the cytoplasm ($DB_c$) and on the sarcolemma ($DB_{sl}$). Portions of several nuclei (N) are visible. The largest nucleus shows an indentation which is probably resulting from the shortening of the muscle cell; within this nucleus a nucleolus is seen (Nc). An undulating band of actin filaments (A) cut tangentially is also seen. Glycogen (Gly) granules are also present (×29,570).

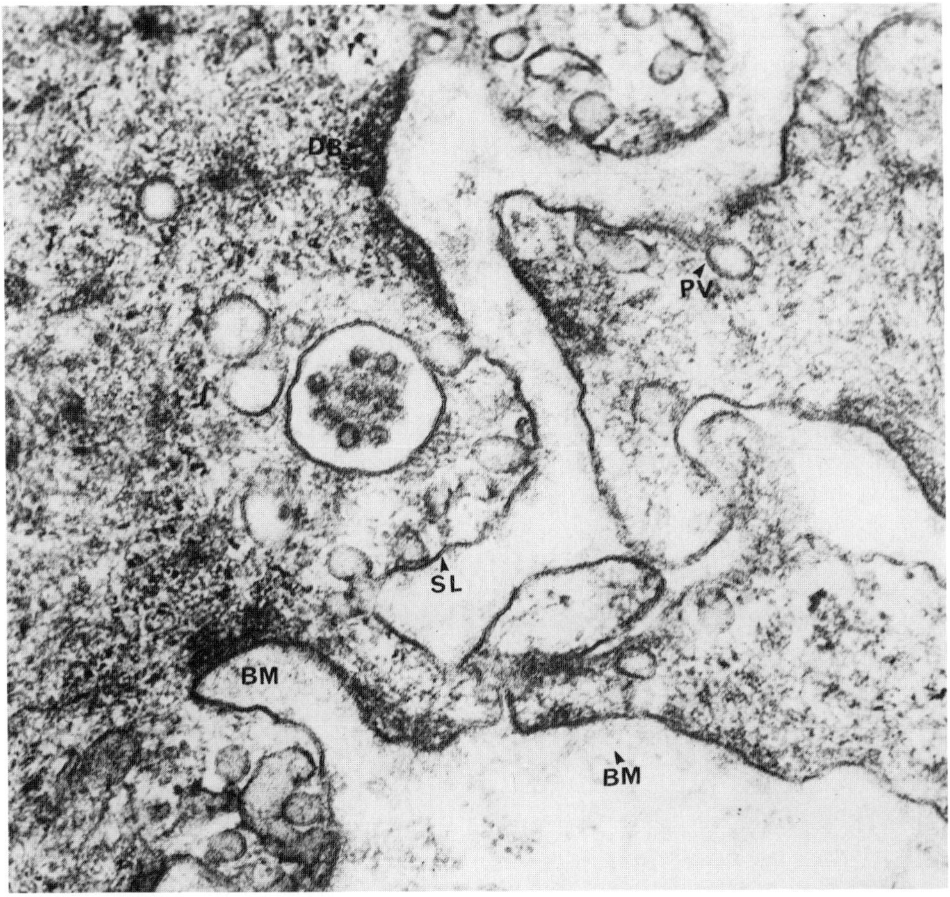


**FIGURE 7** Electron micrograph of transverse section of canine tracheal smooth muscle. The lacy basement membrane (BM) and the "railway track" membranes of the sarcolemma (SL) and pinocytotic vesicles (PV) are clearly seen. Sarcolemmal dense bodies ($DB_{sl}$) are present (X75,000).

Note that In Figure 5, a transverse section fixed at rest, and in Figure 3, the cell membrane is relatively smooth.

Subjacent to the sarcolemma and in many cases directly opening onto the plasma membrane, numerous pinocytotic vesicles are seen (Figs. 3-5). They appear to have the same membranous structure as the sarcolemma and those that open to the outside of the cell also appear to be lined with basement membrane material. This is clearly seen in Figure 7. The "railway track" outlines of both the sarcolemma and the pinocytotic vesicles are seen. There are two darkly osmophilic layers separated by a dark layer. The basement membrane is distributed irregularly and is separated from the plasma membrane by an irregular, clear interspace.

The function of pinocytotic vesicles is not well understood at this time. It has been suggested that they are a mechanism for increasing the area of membrane available for exchange of nutrients, ions, and fluid across the cell membrane. In conjunction with the sarcolemma, sarcoplasmic reticulum, and mitochondria, another role has been suggested for these pinocytotic vesicles by Somlyo [9], namely the mediation of excitation-contraction coupling. In Figure 5, pinocytotic vesicles (PV) are seen in close contact with the sarcolemma on their outer aspect and with tubular sarcoplasmic reticulum (SR) on their inner aspect. (This is seen even better in Figure 11.) These juxtaposed structures could serve as an excitation-contraction coupling apparatus in smooth muscle, where the highly organized sarcoplasmic reticular and T-tubule systems typical of skeletal muscle are not seen. On occasion, mitochondria may be seen as intercalated structures in the apparatus just described. Since they contain calcium, they could participate in excitation-contraction coupling. As to whether these structures act as sources or sinks for calcium, or both, has not yet been decided. Langer and Frank [10] and Hajdu and Leonard [11] have suggested that in heart muscle, while sarcolemma, sarcoplasmic reticulum, and mitochondria act as calcium sinks and thus control relaxation, it is likely that the calcium for contraction comes from a source external to the sarcolemma, possibly the basement membrane.

**Cell-to-Cell Junctions** The next structures of interest are the cell-to-cell junctions. These are said to be pathways of low impedance which facilitate current transmission. Electrical activity initiated in one cell can readily spread to others by way of these connections. If these are present in adequate numbers and involve every cell, then the muscle tissue, for example, uterus at term or tenia coli, behaves as a functional syncytium. Such tissues are spontaneously and rhythmically contractile, demonstrate a myogenic response, are characterized by conducted action potentials, and have sparse nerve supplies. The latter may be the result of the large number of cell-to-cell connections which, since they facilitate current transmission, eliminate the need for discrete innervation of each cell. Such smooth muscle are of the so-called single-unit type.

Smooth muscles, such as those of the larger arteries and the urinary bladder, are of the so-called multiunit type. These have no spontaneous rhythmic contractile activity, may not have action potentials (such as in the pulmonary artery), may not possess a myogenic response, and have very few cell-to-cell connections. Because of poor cell-to-cell conduction, each individual muscle cell has to be separately innervated, and a rich network of nerve fillaments is thus present.

Tracheal smooth muscle of the dog does not seem to fall into either of these two categories. This is not unique, since Burnstock [12] reports that the vas deferens of the guinea pig may show features of both types.

Tracheal smooth muscle under in vitro control conditions shows no spontaneous rhythmic contractile activity, no myogenic response, and no action potentials. On this basis, it should be a multiunit type of smooth muscle. However, neither a dense innervation is seen (this will be discussed below), nor are the intracellular connections sparse. While such connections are visible in Figures 3, 5, and 6, they are maximum in the transverse sections of Figures 5 and 11. Practically every cell has at least one connection and about 30% have two connections. There must be many more connections involving any single cell, if the entire extent of the cell is considered and not just that part in the plane of the micrograph. The presence of this relatively large number of junctions suggests that the muscle should be of the single-unit type. It appears that tracheal smooth muscle falls into an intermediate group.

The junctions seen in Figure 5 are of the following types.

**Tight Junctions or Nexuses and Gap Junctions** First, projections of one cell into another (intrusions) are said to be more dominant in smooth muscle from cat and guinea pig intestine, but it is evident that canine tracheal smooth muscle has them also (Figs. 5, 8, and 13). These are also known as peg-and-socket (PS) junctions. Burnstock noted that when contraction was suppressed, projection-type nexus were seen more often than in muscle tissues undergoing contraction. Although we have not made a systematic study of the problem, our material shows essentially the same phenomenon. In the vas deferens, the cytoplasm beneath the membranes at the junctions usually does not contain organelles and appears less electron dense than the rest of the cell. This is seen in the PS-labeled area in Figure 13. The sarcolemmal membranes of the two contiguous cells are evident. Although the membranes are fairly close together, they are not as close as described by Burnstock. While at the coapted area a clear space is visible between the component membranes, at places the coaptation is much closer and the membrane appears much darker. It must be pointed out that in the absence of views of the junction area in multiple axes (such pictures are obtained using a tilt-stage microscope), our interpretation is only tentative. As determined from Figures 8 and 13, these peg-and-socket junctions are very variable in size and shape, some seeming to mushroom into a cell, others forming narrow, finger-like projections.

Second, simple abutment of adjacent cells are said to act as a mechanical tie between contracted cells, whereas projections are more likely to be involved in electrical coupling. The tightness of coupling is variable. Several such abutments, or gap junctions (GJ), are seen in Figures 5, 8, and 11. Unfortunately, because of the low magnification, detail is obscured. These abutments appear not to be areas of true fusion of membrane, but rather gap junctions with separation of opposing membranes.

**Intermediate Junctions** Intercellular junctions (IJ) are seen in Figure 5. In these, a narrow intracellular space is occupied by a homogenous and amorphous material of moderate density. The strictly parallel plasma membranes which make up the junction show increased density of subjacent cytoplasm. Such intermediate junctions have also been described in rat intestine [13] and in rabbit colon [14]. These structures should be distinguished from the desmosome. They have been termed as intermediate junctions (IJ) or zonula adherens in other tissues by Sjostrand and Elfvin [15] and Farquhar and Palade [16].

Our description of the types of intracellular connection we have seen in canine tracheal smooth muscle is qualitative. We have been struck by the great variability in the numbers, size, and shape of these junctions. No systematic quantitative study has been undertaken up to this time. Hence, we cannot say with any confidence whether junctions, for example in a canine tracheal smooth muscle, are consistently few or many. However, on occasion, we have seen sections which show numerous junctions (Fig. 8).

**Dense Bodies and Intermediate Filaments** Dense bodies are darkly staining areas distributed throughout the cytoplasm of the tracheal smooth muscle and are seen incorporated into the sarcolemma also. Gabella [17], Pease and Molinari [18], and Devine and Somlyo [19], had suggested, on the basis of conventional transmission microscopy, that these were the attachment sites for actin filaments. More recently, Somlyo et al. [20] reported that their stereoelectron microscope study revealed unequivocal evidence of thin filament insertion on cytoplasmic dense bodies. The current view is that they are analogous to the Z lines which define the sarcomeres in striated muscle and to which actin filaments are attached.

In connection with dense bodies, two other topics need to be mentioned briefly. The first deals with so-called intermediate filaments which are approximately 10 nm in diameter. These are not to be confused with the thin, or actin, filaments. The intermediate filaments were believed to be within the core of myosin filaments originally. However, using 200-kV accelerating voltage electron microscopy, Somlyo and Somlyo [9] disproved this. These filaments are frequently associated with the dense bodies, often forming bundles extending for several nanometers. They are said to be analogous to the cytoskeleton of obliquely striated muscles [21]. Nonomura and Ebashi [22], have shown that intermediate filaments remain associated with dense bodies even after fractionation of

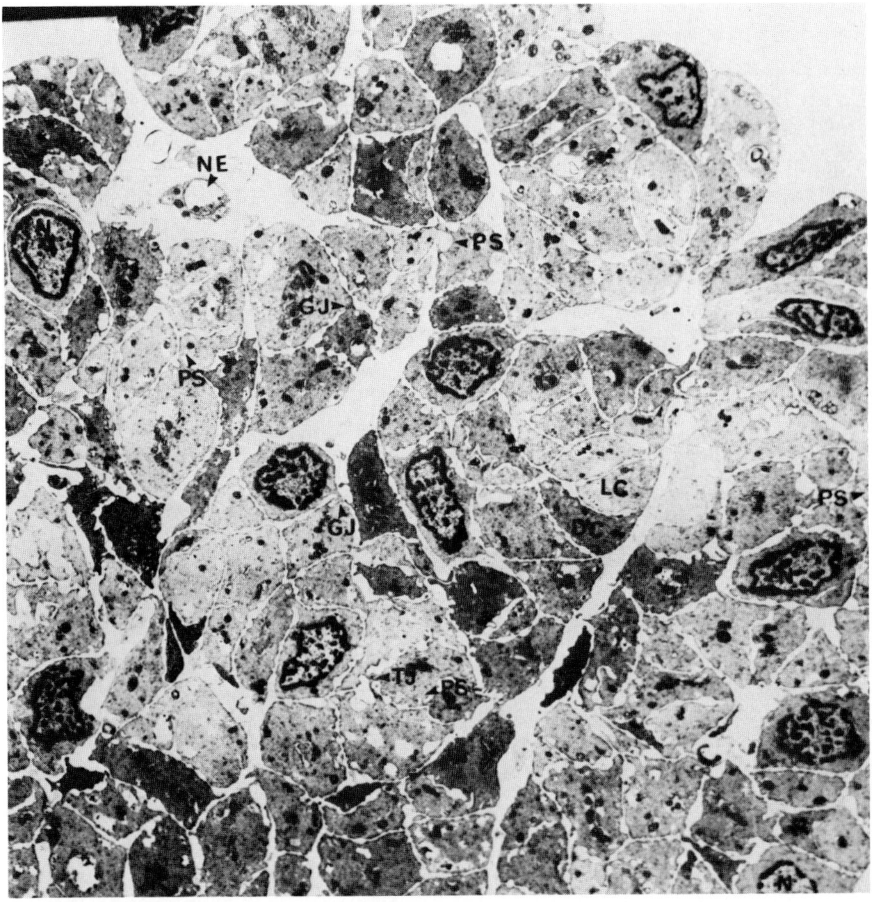


**FIGURE 8** Electron micrograph of a transverse section of canine tracheal smooth muscle. The muscle was fixed during the early phase of isotonic shortening. Several nuclei (N) are clearly seen, as also are cell membranes. The latter show some undulation. Both light (LC) and dark cells (DC) are seen. In between the muscle bundles, nerve elements (NE) are seen. Within the bundle and between the cells, nerve filaments are occasionally seen; their paucity is striking. The cell-to-cell connections are perhaps the most remarkable feature of this picture. Practically every cell forms at least one, if not more connections with neighboring cells. Close oppositions (GJ) are present. Many peg-and-socket (PS) junctions of the type described before are also seen. TJ represents a triple junction, each component of which appears to be of an intermediate junction (IJ) type. The magnification, however, is insufficient to positively identify these at IJ (×6270).

the cells. A recent and exciting finding has been reported by Lazarides and Hubbard [23] in connection with the intermediate filaments of smooth muscle. They have isolated a protein from these which they have termed desmin, which may eventually turn out to be one of the main building blocks of the animal cell, since it has also been found in heart and skeletal muscle cells.

While only the dense bodies have been identified in airway smooth muscle, it is probable that intermediate filaments are also present. Moreover, the same relation of thin and intermediate filaments to dense bodies probably also holds in airway smooth muscle.

The second point deals with the finding that α-actin is also present in smooth muscle dense bodies [24]. Since α-actin is present in the Z-line material from skeletal muscle, this strengthens the argument that dense bodies are analoges of the Z line.

The main reason for the above speculation is that as more and more data are elicited, they seem to justify the view that the ultrastructural organization of the contractile unit for smooth muscle will be the same as for striated muscle. Therefore, the sliding filament model of contraction may also apply to smooth muscle.

**Mitochondria** Previously we reported oxidative phosphorylation parameters for canine tracheal smooth muscle mitochondria and shown that the ADP:O ratio and respiratory control ratio are the same as for mitochondria from skeletal muscle [25]. Also, we have estimated that the content of mitochondrial protein present in a gram of wet canine tracheal smooth muscle is much less than that of skeletal muscle. From these data we computed that the amount of ATP synthesized oxidatively in smooth muscle is about 10% of that in skeletal muscle. Several mitochondria are visible in Figure 3. While they are often found located near both poles of the nucleus, this is not invariable. They may be scattered throughout the cytoplasm, sometimes in rows as in this figure or in a clump as shown in Figure 9. Glycogen granules (Gly) are evident in proximity to the mitochondria. These granules are distinguished from ribosomes by their nonlinear arrangement. Tracheal smooth muscle mitochondria are of varying shape and size. Figure 3 shows considerably elongated ones. These are occasionally formed by the abutment of two or more mitochondria. Figures 3 and 9 both show that the mitochondria have clearly defined, continuous, outer and inner membranes. From the inner membrane, cristae project into the mitochondrion. Their number is few compared to those in heart or skeletal muscle mitochondria. All the mitochondria seen in these figures are in the "orthodox" configuration, as described by Hackenbrock [26]. In this state they are not transporting electrons. This very likely is due to the tissues becoming hypoxic during preparation. When steps are taken to ensure oxygenation during the preliminary preparative steps the mitochondria are seen to be in a "condensed" form [26] in which they are actively transporting electrons.

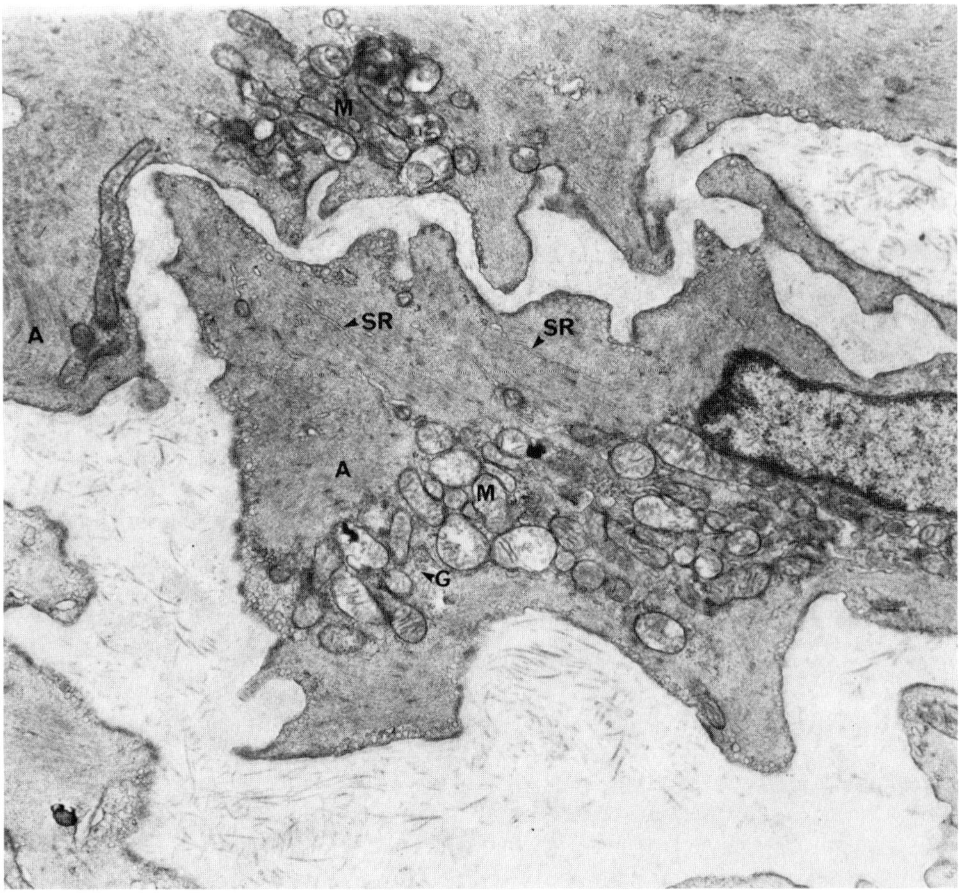


**FIGURE 9** Electron micrograph of a longitudinal section of canine tracheal smooth muscle. Mitochondria (M) are seen arranged in clumps. Tubular sarcoplasmic reticular (SR) elements are seen clearly also. The cell is isotonically contracted and undulating bundles of actin filaments (A) are seen. Glycogen (G) granules are present (×8100).

The role of mitochondria in excitation-contraction coupling has been referred to above. Carsten [27], Hurwitz et al. [28], and Somlyo et al. [20] have carried out considerable work in this area. The present position is that mitochondria are a sink for calcium, and take it up during or after mechanical relaxation of the smooth muscle. A similar role has been assigned them in striating muscle. Whether they are part of the calcium source (other components of which are the sarcolemma, extracellular space, and the sarcoplasmic reticulum)

**Golgi Bodies and Lysosomes** In Figure 10, which is a transverse section of canine tracheal smooth muscle, the large cell shows a mitochondrion just below the nucleus. Above and to the left of the mitochondrion, and in contact with the perinuclear membrane, a structure made up of a series of vacuoles is adjacent to some parallel membranes and smaller vacuoles. This is a fairly well defined Golgi body. These must exist in every muscle cell but are hard to demonstrate.

Lysosomes have not been identified by us in number in normal, acutely hypoxic, or acidotic canine tracheal smooth muscle cells. However, one is seen in Figure 11 and is labeled (L). Burnstock [12] reports that few structures resembling lysosomes have been described in smooth muscle cells. However, since that report, De Duve showed that active smooth muscle cells can be transformed into foam cells, and postulated that this is a consequence of a relative inefficiency of some lysosomal enzymes [29]. Paul et al. [30] have conducted studies on piglet aortic smooth muscle cells exposed to hypoxia for 5 days and shown the development of considerable numbers of lysosomes or phagosomes, and of membranous swirls or myelin figures.

While we ourselves have made no systematic study of lysosomal enzymatic activity in airway smooth muscle, we believe that some of the impairment of contractile activity seen during hypoxia [31,32] is due to activation of lysosomal enzymes. In Figure 3, the third cell from the bottom shows some myelin swirls. The tissue was taken from a healthy mongrel dog. Whether the swirl resulted from tissue hypoxia and activation of lysosomal enzymes is hard to say.

**Sarcotubular System, Rough Endoplasmic Reticulum** The sarcoplasmic reticulum system in airway smooth muscle appears very poorly developed, although it must be pointed out that no thorough study has been conducted. Sarcoplasmic reticular structures (SR) are seen in Figures 5 and 9. They are very variable and disordered in their distribution. Yamauchi [33] has described the existence of a fairly organized, longitudinal smooth sarcoplasmic reticular system in intestinal smooth muscle. Rogers [34] also claimed to be able to demonstrate transverse tubular structures (akin to the T tubules of striated muscle) in guinea pig ureter. However, we have not yet been able to identify organized sarcoplasmic reticulum or T tubule-like structures in airway smooth

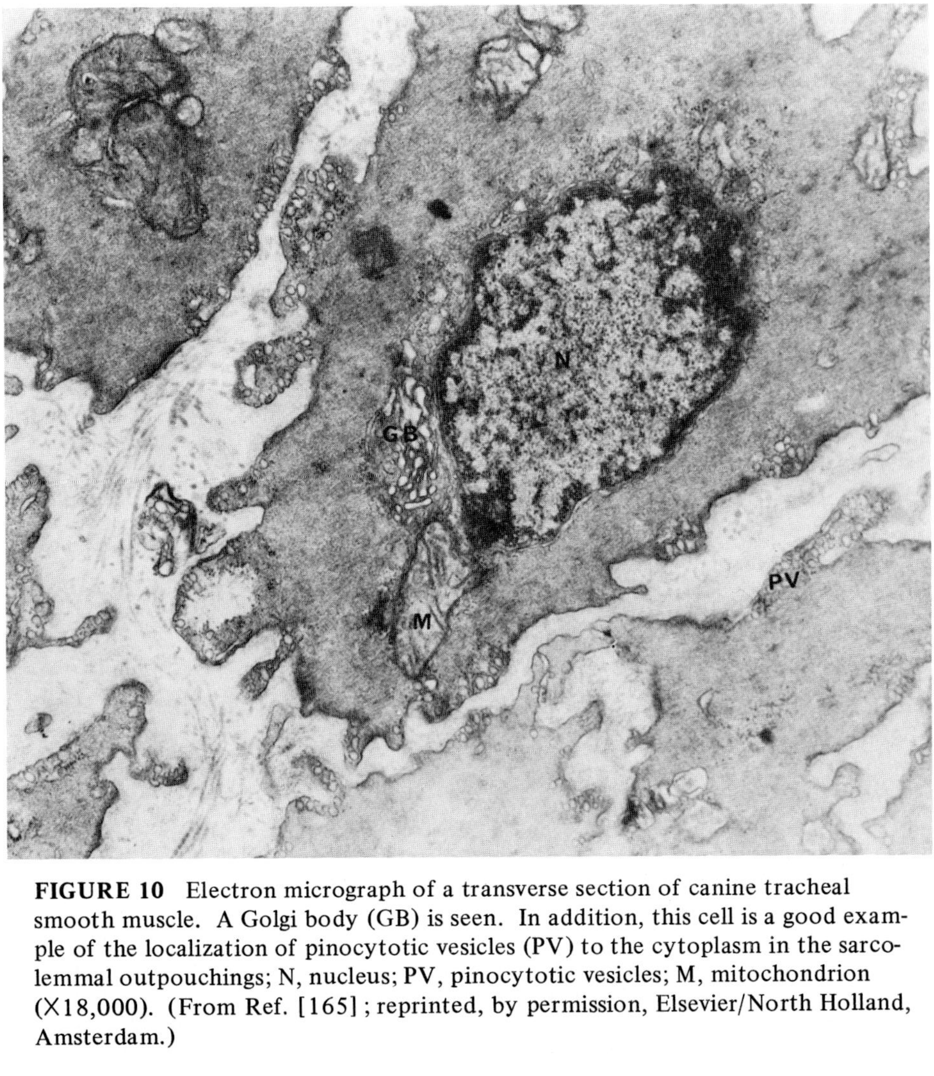


**FIGURE 10** Electron micrograph of a transverse section of canine tracheal smooth muscle. A Golgi body (GB) is seen. In addition, this cell is a good example of the localization of pinocytotic vesicles (PV) to the cytoplasm in the sarcolemmal outpouchings; N, nucleus; PV, pinocytotic vesicles; M, mitochondrion (X18,000). (From Ref. [165] ; reprinted, by permission, Elsevier/North Holland, Amsterdam.)

muscle. Somlyo et al. [35] have shown that these are involved in the intracellular translocation of calcium. Carsten [27] has also estimated that there are enough sarcoplasmic reticulum and mitochondria within the cell to suffice for the needs of contraction and relaxation. However, it must be remembered that since smooth muscle cells are very small, diffusion distances are small, and surface:volume ratios are large, extracellular calcium could easily satisfy the calcium needs of the smooth muscle cell for contraction. The pumps in the sarcolemma would suffice to extrude calcium out in adequate amounts to ensure relaxation.

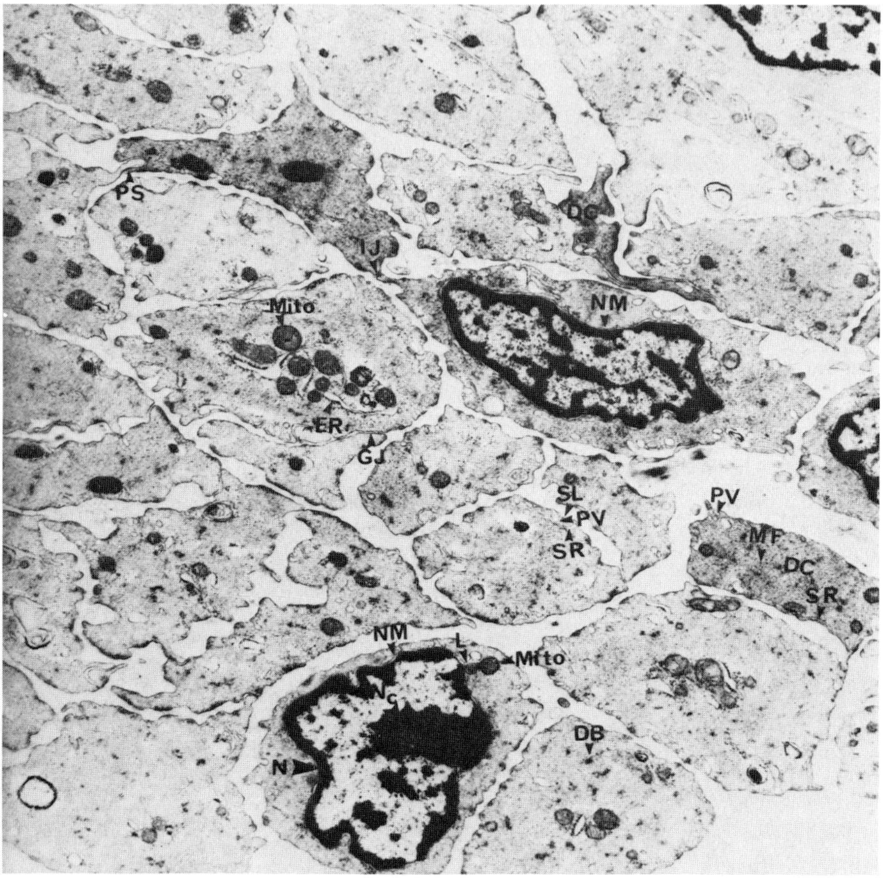


**FIGURE 11** Electron micrograph of a transverse section of canine tracheal smooth muscle. An excitation-contraction coupling apparatus of the type described in Figure 5 is shown in this picture also and is delineated by the three closely grouped arrows labeled SL (sarcolemma), PV (pinocytotic vesicle), and SR (sarcoplasmic reticulum, which appears tubular). Many cells show closely apposed junctions, for example, the dark cell in the top right quadrant of the figure: In addition, intermediate cell junctions (IJ) are seen. Peg-and-socket junction (PS) are also seen. The participating membranes of this type of junction are in close opposition (with increased electrodensity) only for limited extents of the junction. The cell at the bottom shows a nucleus (N) with a nucleolus (Nc). Close to the perinuclear membranes (NM), a small, circular structure is seen with homogeneous gray contents. This may be a lysosome (L). It is in contact with a mitochondrion (Mito). Rough endoplasmic reticulum (ER) is also seen. Several dark cells (DC) are seen. In all of them, what appear

Rough reticulum is visible in tracheal smooth muscle and is distinguished from glycogen in having its granules arranged linearly. It does not occur in any abundance in cells from mature dogs. However, Yamauchi and Burnstock [36] have shown that it is particularly prominent in developing smooth muscle.

**Mosaicism in Airway Smooth Muscle Cells** Studies to demonstrate mosaicism, stemming from differences in fiber types, and of the type existing in skeletal muscle, have not been reported for smooth muscle. We have carried out histochemical studies in which canine tracheal smooth muscle cells were stained with NADH oxidase, succinic dehydrogenase, and ATPase stains. The cells in the tissue stained uniformly, suggesting that mosaicism did not exist. However, the cellular content of these enzymes is small, and hence cell-to-cell differences may be hard to demonstrate. We do have some mechanical data—to be described more fully below—which suggest that as the strength of a contractile stimulus is progressively increased the active response increases. This increase is achieved by recruitment, at least in functional terms, of fibers which have homogeneous contractile properties. This is consonant with the histochemical data.

**Light and Dark Cells** Almost everybody who studies the ultrastructure of smooth muscle cells has come across light and dark cells in the same section. Their causation is not understood at this time. In tracheal smooth muscle, we see two types of dark cell. The first is seen in tissues fixed when considerably shortened. In these, the cytoplasm around the nucleus appears darker than that near the cell membrane. In the second kind, the cell, when dark, is uniformly so across its entire cross section. Dark and light cells are seen in Figures 5, 6, and 8. As seen in Figure 5, in which tissue was fixed under isometric conditions and in which the cell membrane is relatively smooth, dark cells are present. At low magnification, where more cells can be inspected, the same holds. However, in muscle strips which have shortened considerably under isotonic conditions, a larger number of dark cells are seen. Gansler [37] and Conti et al. [38] have reported similar findings. This has led to the development of one hypothesis that smooth muscle contraction depends on syneresis of the contractile proteins. Dark cells are believed to be highly contracted, having lost water and shrunk. There are other reports which suggest that under some circumstances

---

**FIGURE 11** (continued)
to be thick filaments (MF) cut in transverse section are seen. This cell also shows pinocytotic vesicles (PV) and a long tubular sarcoplasmic reticulum (SR) situated just beneath the sarcolemma. Dense bodies (DB) are also visible (×15,890).

the abnormal cells may be the light ones; they appear light because of the increased content of water.

**Nucleus** Under the light microscope, study of a specimen of tracheal smooth muscle shows the typical cigar-shaped nuclei of smooth muscle in general. The nucleus is centrally placed and there is only one nucleus to each cell. This is quite unlike skeletal muscle where the nuclei are many and are situated just under the sarcolemma. Mitochondria and Golgi bodies are generally present close to the nucleus, the former at the nuclear poles. However, this location of mitochondria is not invariable and they may be found, as pointed out before, relatively far away from the nucleus.

With electron microscopy, nuclear detail is better seen (Figs. 6, 8, and 10-12). In Figures 11 and 12, the double-layered nuclear membrane is well defined; it is perforated by a few nuclear pores. A clear space is present between the two layers. In the resting muscle, the nucleus has smooth margins, but in the considerably shortened cell, the nucleus twists to a marked degree. An indentation produced in this way is seen in the nucleus of a cell in Figure 6. Cytoplasmic material flows into the cleft. Darkly staining chromatin material is seen in all the nuclei of Figures 6, 8, 10, 11, and 12. It is aggregated mainly around the rim of the nucleus.

One or two nucleoli per nucleus have been reported in other smooth muscle cells. In Figure 6, the indented nucleus (N) appears to contain a nucleolus (Nc). The nucleolus in other tissues has been shown to contain a fair amount of RNA. We have not carried out the appropriate cytochemistry and cannot unequivocally say that what we report as a nucleolus in Figure 6 is indeed a nucleolus. Structurally, the nucleolus is felt to be an essential link in the communication pathway between nucleus and cytoplasm. Granules within the nucleolonema of the nucleolus may be newly synthesized ribosomal subunits.

**Contractile Apparatus** Smooth muscle has been so named because of the absence of the striation pattern typical of skeletal and cardiac muscle. No repeating sarcomeric units have been demonstrated to date. Actin filaments cut longitudinally or transversely are seen in Figures 3, 5, 9, and 11 and form the major portion of the greyish cytoplasmic background of the cell. In the relaxed canine tracheal smooth muscle cell, the filaments run in parallel array from one end of the cell to the other. They pass thorugh dense bodies, and this is seen in Figure 13. Their attachment to such bodies on the cell membrane is not seen clearly. However, the bays formed during contraction (Figs. 6, 9, and 10) are said to result from the inward pull of the actin filaments attached to the dense bodies on the sarcolemma in these areas. Why the cell should contract in this way is not known. Skeletal and cardiac muscles do not produce such undulations of their sarcolemma. This, however, may be related to the fact that they

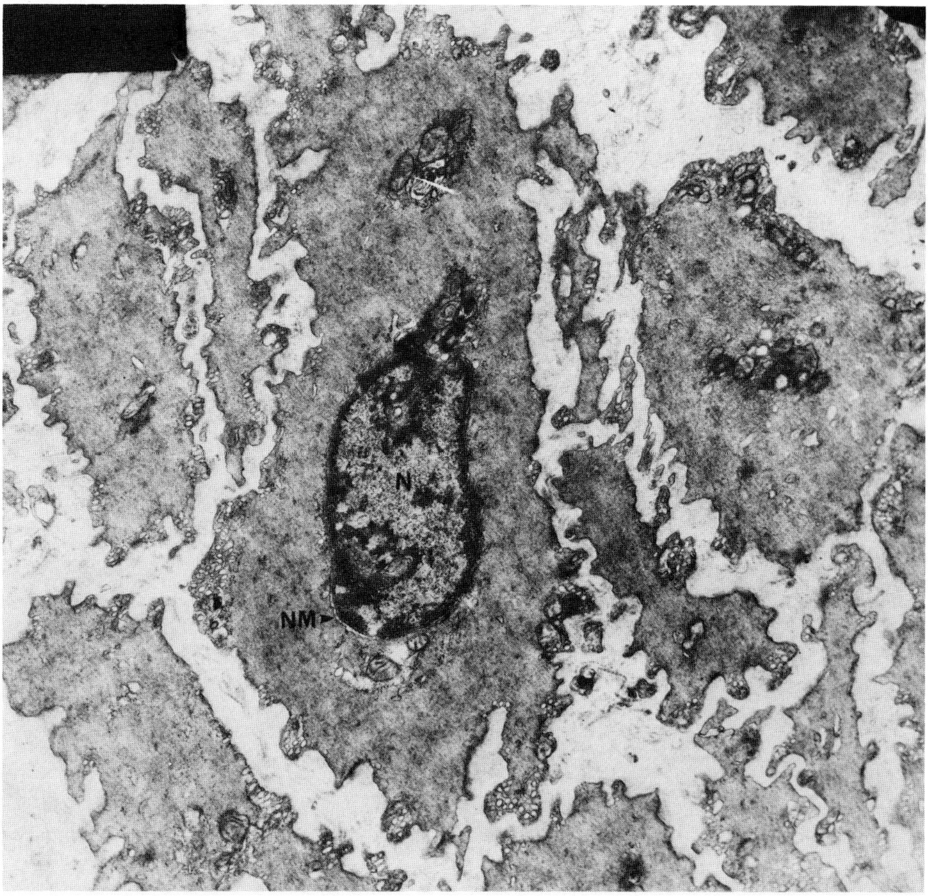


**FIGURE 12** Electron micrograph of a transverse section of a partially contracted tracheal smooth muscle cell. N, nucleus; NM, nuclear membrane (×18,000).

are only capable of a maximal shortening of 35% of their rest length under in vitro conditions. In vivo, they probably shorten only 10%, and this is not sufficient to throw the sarcolemma into folds. Smooth muscle, as we will show later, is a "supercontractor" and can shorten by almost 80% of its rest length.

While myosin has been shown by biochemical means to be present in smooth muscle cells, until recently it has been very difficult to demonstrate its occurrence in the thick filaments so typical of striated muscle. The feeling

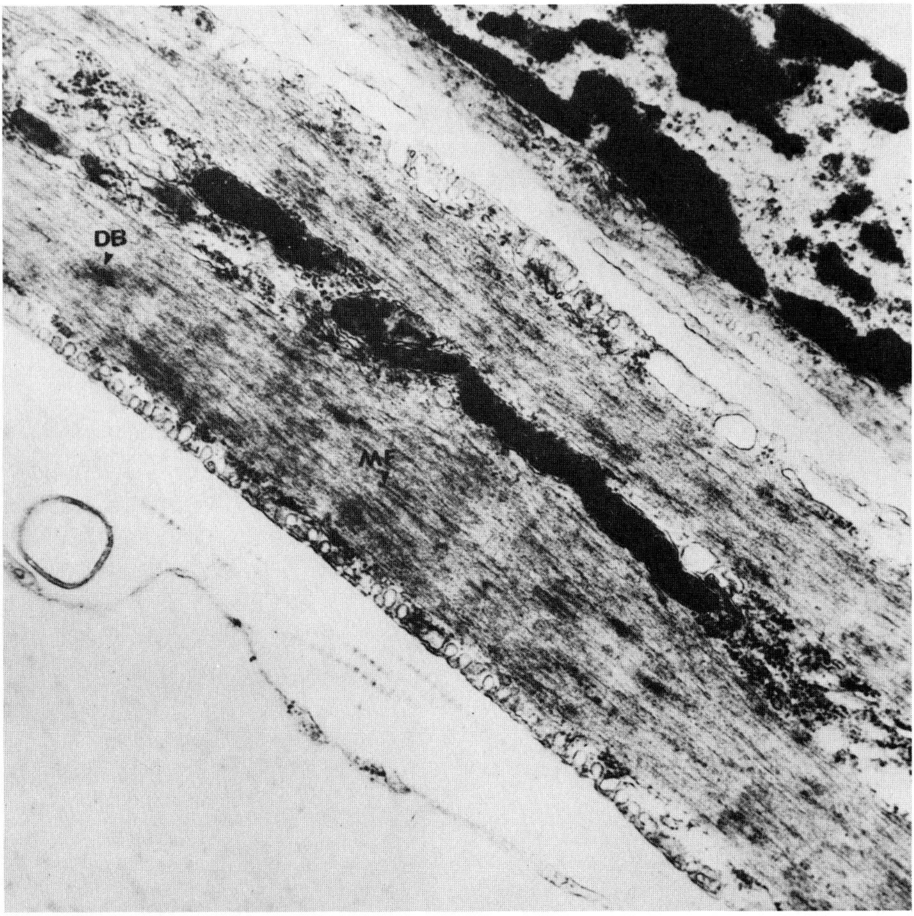


**FIGURE 13** Electron micrograph of a longitudinal section of canine tracheal smooth muscle. DB, dense body with thin filaments passing through it; MF, myosin filament (X40,600).

has been that myosin probably does exist in filaments in the contracting cell, but that in preparation for microscopy the filamentous organization is lost. However, in chicken gizzard, Choi [39] noted thick filaments about 6 nm in diameter; these were distributed among thin filaments 3 nm in diameter. Subsequently, Needham and Shoenberg [40], Yamauchi and Burnstock [36], and Conti et al. [38] demonstrated thick filaments in a variety of smooth muscle. Perhaps the most thorough studies in this area have been conducted by Somlyo et al. [35], Small [41], and Sobieszek [42].

The demonstration of a third set of filaments, the so-called 100-Å filaments, has been alluded to already in describing the dense bodies. These, with the dense bodies, probably form a cellular cytoskeleton.

Regulatory protein filaments, such as tropomyosin, and the $Ca^{2+}$-sensitizing troponin system, will be described below when the biochemistry of contractile and regulatory proteins is discussed.

**Contractile Apparatus Filaments in Tracheal Smooth Muscle**

*Actin Filaments* These are seen and constitute the bulk of the greyish cytoplasm in electron micrographs of both longitudinal (Figs. 3 and 12) and transverse sections (Figs. 5, 6, and 12). In Figure 6, part of a cell shows actin filaments (A) cut tangentially. These form a wave across the cell which, as judged from its undulating sarcolemma, has shortened actively. No measurements of the length of the actin filaments have yet been reported for airway smooth muscle.

Judging by the constancy of actin filaments in the contractile apparatus in a variety of cells (nerve, endothelial, and epithelial cells) from a variety of animals (both vertebrate and invertebrate), it is probable that actin from airway smooth muscle will conform to pattern. In other smooth muscles [35], as in striated smooth muscle, thin filaments are 5 to 8 nm in diameter. In sectioned material, the substructure of actin filaments is not preserved. In vertebrate smooth muscle, the ratio of thin to thick filaments is 15:1 [9]. No hexagonal array of the type existing in striated muscle has been reported in smooth muscle; however, on the basis of optical diffraction studies, Rice et al. [43] have shown a quasirectangular pattern with the spacing of the thick filaments being 38 nm. This has been reported for the rat portal-anterior mesenteric vein preparation only.

*Myosin Filaments* Until relatively recently, these were not demonstrable in micrographs of smooth muscle. However, in the last 7 or 8 years, they have been demonstrated. X-ray diffraction patterns from living-smooth muscle cells (tenia coli of guinea pig), recorded by Lowy et al. [44,45], demonstrated meridional reflections at a spacing typical for longitudinally ordered aggregates of myosin. This suggested that, in smooth muscle, myosin was present in filaments. The average length of myosin filaments is $2.2 \pm 0.14$ $\mu$m SD, as reported by Somlyo et al. [35] for vascular smooth muscle, and the filaments taper at either end.

No study of airway smooth muscle filaments has been reported to date. Using conventional techniques and working at a pH of 6.2, we have been able to demonstrate myosin filaments in canine tracheal smooth muscle. These have not been seen with the regularity of arrangement that Somlyo's picture for rat portal-anterior mesenteric vein show. In Figure 14, which is a longitu-

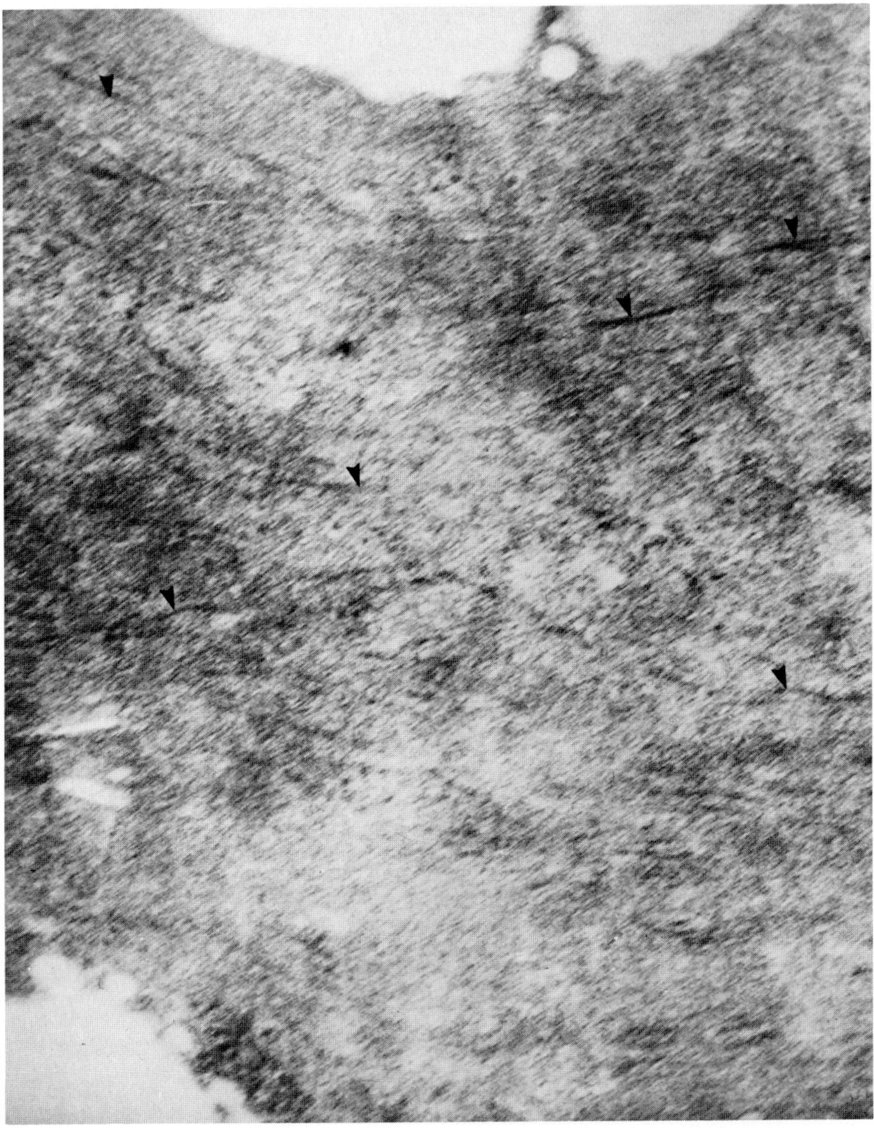

**FIGURE 14** Electron micrograph of a longitudinal section of canine tracheal smooth muscle. Arrowheads indicate thick (myosin) filaments (×75,000).

dinal section of a relaxed muscle, parallel myosin filaments (indicated by arrowheads) are seen. No measurements of their dimensions have been made as yet.

**Intermediate Filaments and Microtubules** These have been demonstrated in several types of smooth muscle cells [46], but as yet no search for them has been conducted in airway smooth muscle.

**The Structural Correlates of the Sliding Filament Model** The demonstration of cross bridges, so crucial to this theory of contraction, are not easy to demonstrate in smooth muscle because of the large thick-filament spacing. However, Somlyo et al. [35] have produced fairly convincing evidence for their existence in smooth muscle. Similar studies for airway smooth muscle have not yet been attempted.

**Summary** Data from a variety of smooth muscle cells suggest that ultrastructural organization of a contractile apparatus consisting of thin filaments attached to dense bodies with interdigitating thick filaments is consistent with a sliding filament model of contraction in mammalian smooth muscle. While dense bodies, actin filaments, and myosin filaments have been demonstrated in airway smooth muscle, a considerable amount of ultrastructural work needs to be done before the sliding filament model can be conclusively applied to this muscle.

### *Bronchial, Bronchiolar, Parenchymal, and Interstitial Smooth Muscle*

The structure and ultrastructure of smooth muscle from the bronchi and bronchioles have not been studied in recent times, interest having shifted to study of the innervation of the airways. Contractile interstitial cells have been described recently by Kapanci et al. [47] and could be important in the regulation of regional ventilation perfusion.

### Bronchial and Bronchiolar Smooth Muscle

This has been described well by von Hayek [48] for human airways. At light microscope levels, there seems to be no difference between smooth muscle cells in the bronchioles, bronchi, and trachea. Differences are mainly in orientation at different levels and in numbers of cells present. As quoted by von Hayek [48], Michelassi and Franzeschi pointed out the especially high glycogen content of these cells.

In the larger bronchi, the thick musclebundles run nearly transversely. In humans, while the muscle is attached to the dorsal ends of the cartilages in the trachea, in the bronchi it is inserted onto the perichondrium of the inner surface of the large cartilages by means of well-defined tendons. (In the dog, nothing is known about the disposition of smooth muscle in the bronchi; in the trachea, as already stated, it is inserted on the external aspect of the cartilage.) In human airways, as one proceeds from the large bronchi to those of medium size, the insertion becomes displaced more ventrally until, eventually, the muscles form almost a completely closed sheet with a few slips extending to the cartilages for insertion.

In the small bronchi, muscle bundles are helically arranged. The same arrangement exists in bronchioles except that the pitch becomes steeper and the thickness of the muscle layer increases. In the terminal bronchioles, the ratio of muscle layer to total wall thickness is larger than in any of the other airways.

### Parenchymal Muscle

Baltisberger [49] made a very careful study of human parenchymal muscle in a single case. This stimulated other investigators, notably von Hayek [48]. From the evidence they collected, the following locations for parenchymal smooth muscle were described.

1. The presence of muscle in the *subpleural* location is debated. von Hayek confirmed Baltisberger's report of its existence, but found it was present at only a few places.
2. Baltisberger described *interstitial* aggregation of smooth muscle cells in irregular polygonal bodies consisting of tissue. However, it is believed that these collections stemmed from nothing more than a tangential section of a bronchiole or of an alveolar duct. The muscular alveolar entrance rings are really continuations of muscle from the bronchioles; not all alveoli have muscular entrance rings, in particular those situated subpleurally.

In addition to this pseudointerstitial muscle, there are isolated muscle bundles which fan outward from the bronchi and traverse the surface of four or five alveoli.

### Interstitial Smooth Muscle Cells

Finally, very recently, interest in interstitial cells has been rekindled. Kapanci et al. [47] have described interstitial cells with contractile properties in the lungs of humans, rats, cows, and monkeys. Using smooth muscle antiactin antibodies from sera of patients with chronic progressive hepatitis, they were able to demonstrate the presence of actin in pulmonary parenchymal cells. These were located in the alveolar septa and around precapillary and postcapillary vessels. Antimyosin antibodies also stained many septal cells. Thus, their evidence, while not conclusive, strongly suggests that contractile cells exist in pulmonary interstitial tissue. These cells resembled fibroblasts, but differed in having microfilaments organized in places, with smooth bundles scattered through the cytoplasm. Kapanci et al. [47] have described these cells in considerable detail. Using isolated strips of lung parenchyma, they showed that these contracted quite markedly under hypoxia. The reactions of vascular and bronchial muscle strips were reportedly quite different. However, this evidence, which was presented in support of the argument that the interstitial cells have unique contractile properties, is not conclusive. A further criticism the authors have to contend with is that of von Hayek [48], who suggested these cells are offshoots from bronchial muscle.

### *Function of Airway Smooth Muscle*

At this time, the role of airway smooth muscle is still understood poorly. All we will do is enumerate the various proposals offered by investigators. The key question of how the mechanical properties of airway smooth muscle affect the mechanical properties of the lung in which they are contained still awaits investigation.

1. von Hayek [48] postulates that, because of its long contraction time, airway smooth muscle can be involved only in changes which take place more slowly than the normal respiratory rhythm. The retraction of lung tissue in open-chested animals or humans during surgery, on the application of a contact stimulus, has been cited as the most compelling evidence supporting the contractile function of pulmonary interstitial muscle cells. This retraction has been termed a partial contraction atelectasis. Whether it is purely the effect of interstitial cell contraction, or results from bronchial muscle cell contraction disturbing the interstitium directly or indirectly, is hard to decide. Such retraction is clearly and most easily demonstrable only in the open chest. In the closed thorax, the contraction may be obscured by stretching of adjacent alveolar walls.

von Hayek [48] further feels that "contraction of parts of the lung musculature could make possible the formation of reserve atelectasis . . . , so that we can imagine that parts of the lung work alternately, as is well known to be the case, for instance, in the glomeruli of the kidney, when that organ is not extremely taxed."

2. Widdicombe and Nadel [50] point out that airway smooth muscle contraction would optimize the relation between anatomical dead space and airway resistance to minimize the work of breathing. However, the predominance of nasal breathing patterns makes one wonder what the practical significance of the optimization referred to really is.

3. Olsen et al. [51] concluded from studies of rapidly frozen trachea in situ, with and without tone, that contraction of muscle pulled cartilages into overlapping opposition in both trachea and bronchi. This, they felt, could increase the ability of these airways to withstand compressive narrowing. This stability would result in a more efficient cough.

4. Macklem and Engel [52] studied the influence of isoproterenol and methacholine on regional distribution of inspired boluses of $^{133}$xenon. They differed from Olsen et al. and concluded that their findings are incompatible with tone-improving stability. Their interpretation of their own findings is that "tone is irregularly distributed throughout the lung leading to a broad range of critical and opening pressures." Abnormal degrees of tone probably render the lung anisotropic from a mechanical point of view and thus more prone to damage by unequal stress distribution. Minimal degrees of tone would minimize the inequality of these stresses. The usefulness of these mechanisms must await evaluation until the magnitude of normal tone present in vivo, and measured by noninvasive techniques, can be assessed.

5. Regional increments in tone could influence regional distribution of ventilation and help in adjusting ventilation:perfusion ratios locally.

6. It has been shown in guinea pig airways and in human material obtained either postmortem or at surgery that airway smooth muscle may be spontaneously, rhythmically contractile. We have not observed this in isolated canine tracheal or bronchial smooth muscle under control conditions, and feel that rhythmicity develops under abnormal circumstances (see the discussion given below, which deals with the action of tetraethylammonium on airway smooth muscle). Be that as it may, it has been suggested by Hakansson and Toremalm [53] that this rhythmic activity may be involved in emptying mucous glands of their contents.

7. Kapanci et al. [47] believe that the contractile interstitial cells they have demonstrated are the most likely candidates for regulating capillary blood flow and thereby exert a fine control over regional ventilation:perfusion ratios. They feel that the alveolus should be conceived no longer as a passive air sac, but as an "active organ."

## B. Innervation

### *Cholinergic and Adrenergic Nervous Systems*

With the rapidly developing interest in the role of airway smooth muscle in controlling the distribution of ventilation to the lung, and in contributing to its mechanical properties, the status of the innervation of this muscle has assumed importance. While studies of innervation have been made in airways of various animals, the significant fact is that there are considerable species differences, and, therefore, extrapolations from one species to another are hazardous. A cogent example of this is in the field of research in asthma, where definitive information is needed for the human patient, but where the favorite experimental, model animal is the guinea pig; the innervation of the lungs of these two species is different.

**General Autonomic Innervation**

von Hayek [48] has described the general autonomic innervation to thoracic structures. However, he does not deal in any great detail with the innervation at different levels of the tracheobronchial tree. Krahl [54] has described the course of the autonomic nerves in the mediastinum and then through the lungs. The trachea and esophagus are supplied by branches from the right vagus and its recurrent laryngeal branch. Branches from both vagi and the sympathetic nerves (from the second, third, and fourth ganglia of the thoracic sympathetic chain) form pulmonary plexus which supply branches to the bronchi and blood vessels.

In those airways containing cartilage, the nerves form suprachondral and subchondral plexus. In the terminal, cartilage-free airways, however, the plexus unite to form a single, delicate plexus. The suprachondral plexus contains myelinated and nonmyelinated fibers and vagal ganglion cells. It is the unmyelinated ribers arising from multipolar ganglion cells which innervate the helical bands of bronchial smooth muscle. Larsell and Dow [55] have followed the unmyelinated fibers to smooth muscle of all divisions of the bronchial tree as far as the terminations of the alveolar ducts. These are probably the vagal branches responsible for the contraction of bronchial and bronchiolar smooth muscle. Nerve branches from the ganglion also supply the bronchial glands.

These earlier studies were predominantly structural and it was only the availability of histochemical techniques that has enabled identification of adrenergic and cholinergic nerves. Hebb [56], using acetylcholinesterase stains, demonstrated a dense cholinergic innervation of bronchi in all the species he studied. Widdicombe and Nadel [50,57], Olsen et al. [51], and Karczewski et al. [58] have employed wither vagal resection or atropine block and confirmed this in dogs, cats, rabbits, and healthy humans. It is interesting that, while what appear to be motor vagal nerves have been demonstrated to them, terminal bronchioles and alveolar ducts are unaffected by reflex bronchoconstriction.

Suzuki et al. [6] showed that in canine tracheal smooth muscle acetylcholinesterase stained diffusely between the muscle cells and also on the surface of the muscle membranes. Catecholamines, identified by photofluorescence, were distributed mainly in the perivascular regions and close to cartilage, and only minor fluorescence was detected between the muscle cells. They also reported that they were unable to find any evidence of a nonadrenergic-noncholinergic inhibitory nervous system in the canine tracheal smooth muscle. Obviously, species differences are present, since Coburn and Tomita [59] have reported the presence of such a system in the guinea pig tracheal muscle. In the dog, relaxation seems to be by way of β-adrenoceptor responses.

We have conducted electron microscope studies which show nerve fibers lying on the surface of muscle bundles, but penetration and ramification within the bundle to any considerable extent were not evident. Figure 15 demonstrates this. Cameron and Kirkpatrick [60] reported similar findings for bovine tracheal smooth muscle. The absence of innervation to every cell was a surprise since,

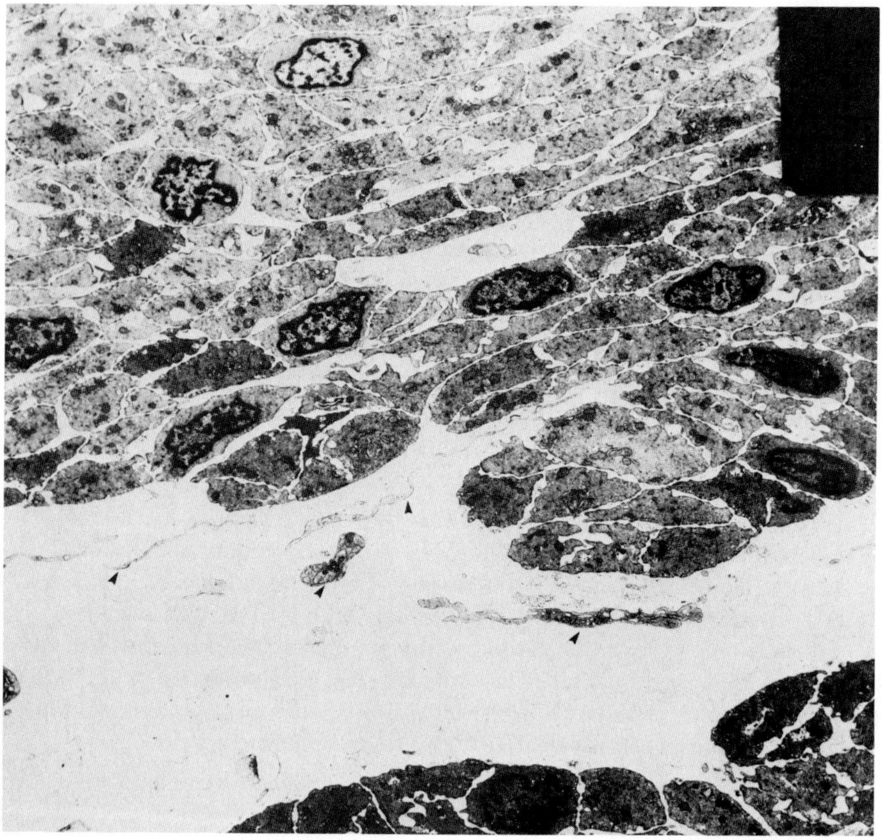

**FIGURE 15** Electron micrograph of a tangential section of canine tracheal smooth muscle. Arrowheads indicate nerve fibers (×6000).

from its mechanical and electrical properties, we expected the muscle to be of a multiunit type. In this type of muscle, cell-to-cell junctions are few and innervation is rich, with each cell receiving a nerve filament. We have yet not made a systematic study of the problem, and it is possible that each cell in our preparation has its nerve but our search has not been extensive enough to detect it. There is also a paucity of nerves in Figure 11. We plan to conduct fluorescence studies in the future.

Mann [61] studied the innervation of the bronchial tree in rabbit, sheep, bull, piglet, and goat. He confirmed the presence of two nerve plexus. The suprachondral plexus consisted of preganglionic and postganglionic fibers in large nerve trunks interrupted by ganglia, and the subchondral consisted mainly of postganglionic fibers which supplied bronchial and vascular smooth muscle. Both plexus stained strongly for acetylcholinesterase and probably contain the cholinergic, parasympathetic fibers that innervate the bronchial muscle of the species tested.

With respect to the adrenergic system, only in the rabbit was there found to be almost no evidence for an adrenergic nerve supply to bronchial muscle. Some fibers are seen in its tracheal muscle and a few may have supplied the muscle of the larger bronchi, but in the smaller bronchi and bronchioles, the adrenergic fibers seen supplied only bronchial and bronchiolar blood vessels. Golla and Symes [62] found that, in rabbits, epinephrine produced a graded response from dilating the trachea to constricting the terminal bronchioles. This suggests inhibitory receptors are paramount in the trachea while excitatory receptors predominate in the bronchioles.

In all the examined species, no adrenergic fibers were seen in bronchiolar muscle; however, cholinergic fibers supplied the muscle of the terminal bronchioles. No evidence for innervation of respiratory bronchioles was found except in the cat and dog, as reported by Daly and Hebb [63].

The situation in the cat appears to differ somewhat. Silva and Ross [7], on the basis of a very careful histochemical study, showed that the tracheobronchial muscle of the cat receives a rich autonomic nerve supply. The dense nerve plexus on the surface of the tracheal, bronchial, and bronchiolar muscle reported by others was also observed. From this plexus, adrenergic fasciculi passed between bundles of smooth muscle, as well as into the bundle and between the muscle cells. Cholinergic nerves accompanied the adrenergic nerves.

### *Intraneuronal Vesicles*

In feline tracheobronchial muscle, Silva and Ross [7] reported that small (300-600 Å) and large granular vesicles with specific green fluorescence, indicative of catecholamines, were seen in nerves identified as adrenergic. After sympatholysis with 6-hydroxydopamine, no fluorescent nerves were seen and the surviving nerves were probably all cholinergic. Electron microscopy showed that these only contained agranular vesicles and considerably fewer large granular vesicles (700-1200 Å). No large, oval, cored granules were seen.

In canine tracheal smooth muscle, Suzuki et al. [6] reported three different kinds of vesicles within the nerve fibers: agranular vesicles with a diameter ranging from 500 to 700 Å, small granular vesicles with diameters ranging from 600 to 800 Å, and large granular vesicles with diameters ranging from 1000 to 1500 Å. The small granular vesicles contained a cored granule and the large granular vesicles contained diffuse granular material. The fibers containing agranular vesicles were present in larger numbers than those containing granular vesicles.

### *Nonadrenergic Inhibitory Nervous System*

With recent ferment in research activity directed at asthma, the role of nervous control of airway smooth muscle has assumed considerable importance. If a nonadrenergic inhibitory system normally existed and was hypoactive, it would play a major part in the pathogenesis of the bronchospasm of asthma.

As mentioned above, Coburn and Tomita [59] have suggested such a system exists in the trachea of the guinea pig. Suzuki et al. [6], however, conclude that in canine tracheal smooth muscle, such a system does not exist. The most significant contribution in this area is probably that of Richardson and Beland [64] since they have investigated human tissue from surgical operations and recent autopsies. They demonstrated that the airway nervous system, from the middle of the trachea to the distal bronchi, showed some of the characteristics of the nonadrenergic inhibitory system of the gastrointestinal tract and of the guinea pig tracheal smooth muscle just alluded to. Furthermore, since they found no evidence of adrenergic inhibitory fibers in the bronchial muscle with either pharmacological or histochemical techniques, they concluded that the nonadrenergic inhibitory system is the principal inhibitory system for the smooth muscle of human airways. However, isoproterenol and epinephrine are certainly very effective bronchodilators in human disease and, even though adrenergic nerves may not exist, $\beta$ receptors must be present. The problem, then, is to determine the relative roles of the adrenergic and the nonadrenergic inhibitory systems.

Much of the insight into the role of the nonadrenergic inhibitory system has been derived from work done in the prototype system which exists in the gastrointestinal tract. In that system, Burnstock [12] has suggested that this is a "purinergic" system and the putative inhibitory transmitter is adenosine triphosphate or one of its breakdown products.

In concluding this section, it is evident that there are exciting new developments in control mechanisms for airway smooth muscle. These are probably going to be very important with respect to the applied physiology of airway smooth muscle in conditions such as asthma and emphysema.

## II. Biophysics of Airway Smooth Muscle

### A. Electrophysiology

The electrophysiological characteristics of respiratory airway smooth muscle have not been systematically investigated as they have in many other smooth muscle systems. The presence of cartilage and the relative paucity of smooth muscle in the lower airways constitute serious difficulties for careful electrophysiological studies. The smooth muscle of the cervical trachea, which contains the most accessible smooth muscle, has thus become the experimental model on which most of our understanding of airway electrophysiology is based.

Consistent with its tonic, multiunit mechanical behavior in vitro, the membrane potential of canine and bovine tracheal smooth muscle does not show spontaneity; indeed, no evidence of phasic activity is seen even on depolarization with acetylcholine (Fig. 16) or with increased $[K^+]_o$ [32]. Upon stepwise exposure to increased $[K^+]_o$, the membrane potential shows graded depolarization with a mechanical threshold at about 27 mM $[K^+]_o$ [89]. As the $[K^+]_o$ is further increased, both electrical and mechanical records show graded responses without any phasic component. These observations are consistent with a characterization of the muscle as being of the multiunit type.

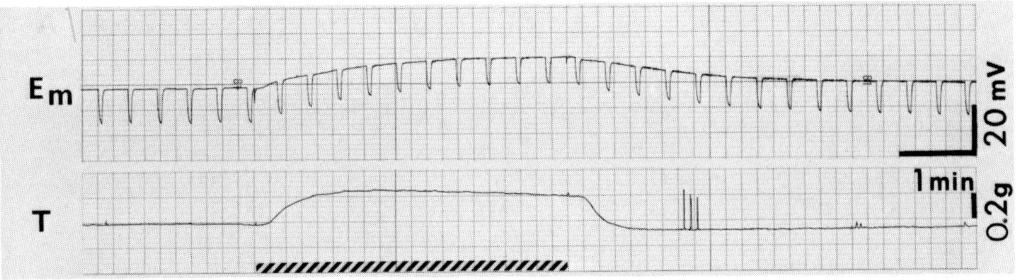


**FIGURE 16** Effect of carbamylcholine ($10^{-7}$ M), indicated by hatched line, on electrical (upper trace) and mechanical (lower trace) properties of canine tracheal smooth muscle. Hyperpolarizing potentials in the electrical recording result from the application of constant-current pulses in the double sucrose gap and indicate membrane resistance. (Unpublished data of Dr. H. Yamaguchi, 1977.)

The reports of phasic electrical activity of airway smooth muscle in certain conditions in vivo [65,66], as well as during metabolic inhibition and exposure to histamine in vitro [67,68], suggest that the possibility of multiunit-single-unit interconversions be thoroughly evaluated with reference to the physiology of airway smooth muscle. In addition to tonic responses upon stimulation, multiunit muscles have been characterized as (1) lacking pacemaker activity, being activated primarily by a dense innervation; (2) having a high membrane resistance ($R_m$); and (3) being poorly interconnected electrically with adjacent cells (through nexus and tight junctions [69-72]. With reference to these criteria, we have observed that electrical field stimulation of tracheal smooth muscle is mediated largely by cholinergic neural elements in the preparation. In the presence of atropine, such stimulation is quite ineffective [71]. Evidence regarding intercellular connection, however, has indicated that, both from ultrastructural and functional viewpoints, the smooth muscle cells are connected. The presence of a variety of ultrastructural correlates of intercellular connections has been demonstrated repeatedly, and these are rapidly influenced by conditions which affect the contractile properties of the preparation [73,74]. The functional presence of such connections is also demonstrated in electrophysiological studies of the passive (cable) spread of hyperpolarizing potentials (Fig. 17) [68,75]. If these cells were electrically isolated, the spread of these potentials would be limited almost completely to one cell length; the observation of an exponential decline of these electronic potentials with distance (up to 6 mm; length constant, 1.6 mm) thus argues strongly for the functional importance of intercellular electrical connections.

In view of the electrical continuity of airway smooth muscle, conclusions with reference to its possible single-unit characteristics require detailed information concerning the excitability of the muscle membrane. In normal Krebs-Ringer solution, the strong membrane rectification (without any active compo-

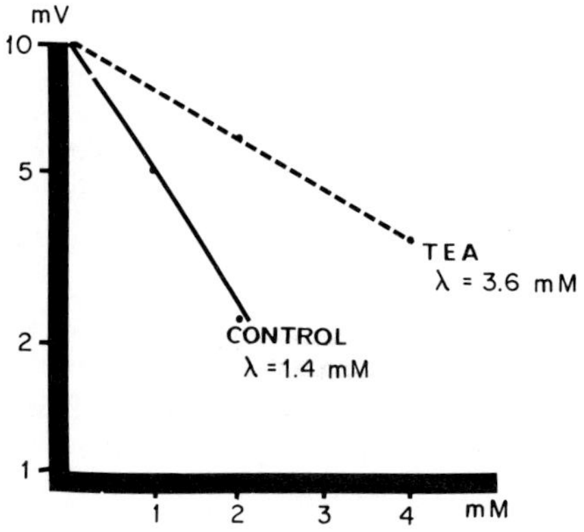


**FIGURE 17** Effect of TEA (33 mM) and distance from the stimulus on the magnitude of hyperpolarizing electronic potentials. Stimuli of constant strength were delivered by extracellular electrodes. (From Ref. [75].)

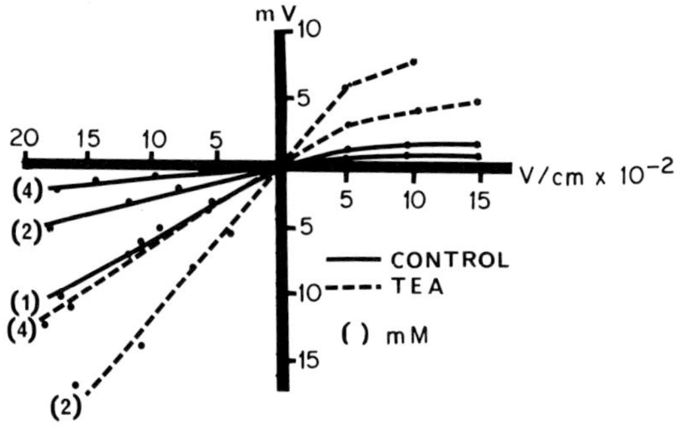


**FIGURE 18** Effect of the strength of extracellularly applied stimuli on the magnitude of the electronic potentials at the distances indicated in brackets. Note the increase in apparent membrane resistance in the presence of TEA (33 mM). (From Ref. [75].)

nent) seen in the depolarizing region of the current-voltage realtion (Fig. 18) [68,75] argues against the possibility of spontaneous electrical activity in this muscle. Experimental conditions, such as exposure to increased $[K^+]_0$ or $BaCl_2$, which have been used to elicit spontaneity in other smooth muscles, are ineffective in tracheal smooth muscle [76]. The response to histamine, however, is accompanied by slow electrical waves [68] and increased permeability to chloride, and it has also been shown that in severe metabolic inhibition, phasic membrane electrical activity is produced [67]. These in vivo findings contrast with recent reports [65,66] in which extracellular recordings from bronchial smooth muscle have shown phasic electrical activity associated with wheezing sounds in asthmatic attacks of both dogs and humans in vivo. Preliminary investigations have also shown phasic electrical and mechanical responses of tracheal smooth muscle to an as yet unidentified low molecular weight factor in serum (Kroeger, unpublished, 1979). One agent, which is of special interest in that it appears to unmask excitable properties in airway smooth muscle, is tetraethylammonium chloride (TEA). In the presence of TEA, the muscle exhibits "single-unit" characteristics, responding with an unfused tetanus, phasic electrical activity (Fig. 19), and a myogenic response to stretch [68,75]. The membrane depolarization produced (from a normal $E_M$ of -47 to -34 mV) is accompanied by increased electronic conduction (Fig. 3), indicating a decreased $K^+$ conductance and possibly an increase in the number of close contacts between cells in the presence of TEA.

In view of the number of smooth muscles which appear to be activated by "Ca-spikes" [77], the ion species responsible for action potentials in airway smooth muscle is of interest. The observations that (1) the effect of TEA has an absolute requirement for extracellular $Ca^{2+}$ [78,79], in contrast to other stimulatory agents such as histamine and acetylcholine [68,76], (2) the effect of TEA is antagonized by D-600, a calcium antagonist [76]; and (3) the rate of rise (dv/dt) and amplitude of these action potentials are increased with increased

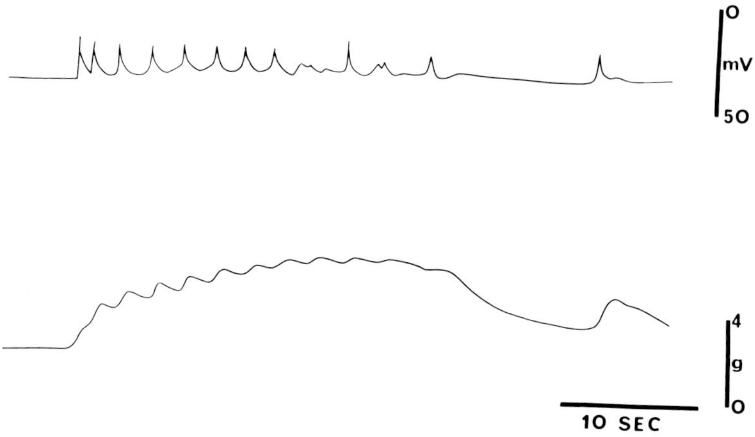


**FIGURE 19** Electrical and mechanical activity of tracheal smooth muscle in the presence of TEA (33 mM). Electrical activity was measured intracellularly. (From Ref. [75].)

$[Ca^{2+}]_0$ (6 mM; Kroeger and Simmons, unpublished, 1977) suggest an important role for $Ca^{2+}$ in the action potential of this muscle.

The source of activator $Ca^{2+}$ in smooth muscle appears to vary both with the ultrastructure (presence of sarcoplasmic reticulum) and the nature of the stimulus applied. As has been discussed above, the activation of contraction by membrane electrical activity (TEA) and simple depolarization (high $[K^+]_0$) are rapidly abolished by Ca-deficient solutions and thus appear to utilize only extracellular $Ca^{2+}$ for the activation of the contractile apparatus. It should be noted that the myogenic response to stretch, which also required the production of an action potential, similarly is dependent on extracellular $Ca^{2+}$. Tracheal muscle does contain substantial stores of tightly bound $Ca^{2+}$, however, and it appears that these may be mobilized by some stimulatory agonists through pharmacomechanical coupling, a membrane-independent process [35,68].

### B. Mechanics

Ventilation is determined, to a considerable extent, by the physical properties of the lung and its conducting airways. However, overall alveolar ventilation can be modified by the caliber of the airway, which in turn is controlled by airway smooth muscle. Furthermore, the regional distribution of ventilation is also controlled by contraction of this same muscle. An understanding of the mechanisms which underlie disorders of pulmonary mechanics involves an understanding of the biophysical and biochemical properties of airway smooth muscle.

The fundamental information is at subcellular and molecular levels. This established the primary position of biochemistry in the analysis of muscle function.

The classic methods of investigation of skeletal muscle have elucidated operative mechanisms, both biophysical and biochemical, for the muscle cell. Even though the models tested have not been physiologic, to the extent that they were not in the intact animal, whatever is known about muscle function in vivo has become explicable on the basis of mechanisms elucidated from such models.

It is not unexpected, then, that smooth muscle research has been patterned in the skeletal muscle mold. The format we will follow as we deal with the mechanics of airway smooth muscle contraction will consist of describing and discussing what we know about its stimulus-response, length-tension, and force-velocity properties. This will involve describing the physical properties of the so-called contractile element and the series-elastic component of the muscle.

What follows deals exclusively with tracheal smooth muscle. We have attempted previously to justify that this muscle is a good model for airways down to the sixth bronchial generation. We have obtained evidence in the past (unpublished observations, 1969) that the stimulus-response and length-tension properties of sixth-generation bronchial muscle are very similar to those of the tracheal muscle. We have also found that the force-velocity characteristics of muscle from the upper trachea are very similar to those from the lower parts of the trachea, above the carina.

### *Methods*

For studying the stimulus-response, length-tension, and force-velocity relationships, the apparatus shown in Figure 20 is employed. The upper end of the muscle strip is securely tied by a 1.5-cm length of size 000, braided, surgical silk. The lower end of the muscle may be tied similarly, but stray compliance is reduced if this end is tightly held by a spring-loaded Lucite clamp firmly connected to a metal rod which traverses the mercury seal shown. This rod is connected to a Grass FT.03 force gauge or a Statham UC2 gauge. The Grass gauge is provided with springs which determine sensitivity and also the magnitude of displacement of the sensing plate of the gauge. The springs should be chosen to optimize these parameters. We have also employed an RCA 5734 valve since it has the least compliance.

The upper ligature is tied to a 5-cm length of annealed wire which is connected to the long arm of the magnesium lever shown. Afterload stops are provided. The lever rotates on jewelled bearings to minimize friction. From the short arm of the lever, loads are hung by an elastic band which minimizes inertial effects. The lever arm ratio is 20:1.

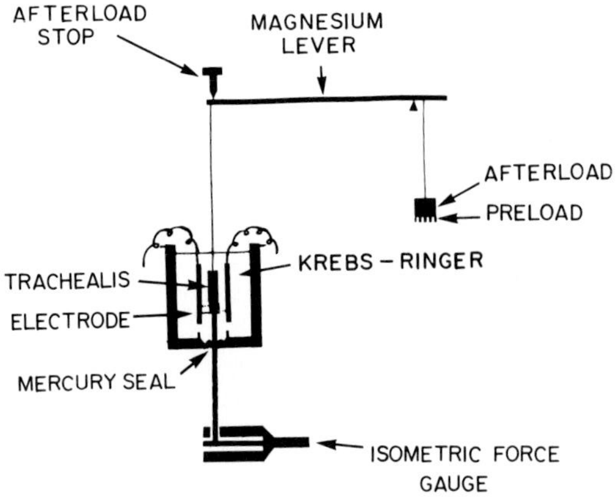


**FIGURE 20** Schematic diagram of apparatus used for the study of mechanical properties of smooth muscle. (From Ref. [100].)

The chamber is circulated with mammalian Krebs-Henseleit solution at 37°C. The inflow medium is preequilibrated with appropriate gases such that the medium in the bath chamber itself has a $Po_2$ of 600 mmHg, a $Pco_2$ of 40 mmHg, and a pH of 7.40.

The muscle strip, when obtained from a 20-kg dog, has a length of about 0.7 to 0.8 cm. After mounting, it is equilibrated for 1 hr, which we have determined is the optimal period. From previous experience, we have found that for such a strip, $l_o$, or the optimal length, which is the length at which maximum active tetanic tension develops isometrically, is about 1.0 cm. During the hour's equilibration, the muscle should be stimulated tetanically at 5-min intervals. The predetermined supramaximal stimulus is applied using platinum plate electrodes with a constant, mean-voltage, 60-cycle ac source. Each tetanus is of about 12 to 15 sec in duration. This regimen yields a very stable preparation on which a 5- to 6-hr experiment can be conducted easily. Furthermore, the results show smaller interexperimental variation when this procedure is followed. Storage overnight in a refrigerator also helps reduce variability.

The signals from the tension transductor and the lever are recorded on a storage oscilloscope. Isotonic shortening is assessed as lever displacement, using a Sanborn 7DCDT displacement gauge (not shown). Differentiation of the shortening trace with respect to time yields the velocity trace.

The apparatus described above enables one to study the properties of the contractile element of the muscle by measuring force-velocity curves. Conventional quick-release techniques that we have described before [80] enable study of the series-elastic component.

**Stimulus-Response Relationship of Tracheal Smooth Muscle**

The upper left-hand panel of Figure 21 shows isometric tetanic myograms from tracheal smooth muscle hels at optimal length ($l_o$). With increasing voltage, the maximal response increases. Beyond 13 V, no further increase is seen. If the plateau values developed at the different voltages are plotted against voltage, the sigmoid, graded response curve of the upper right-hand panel is obtained. This

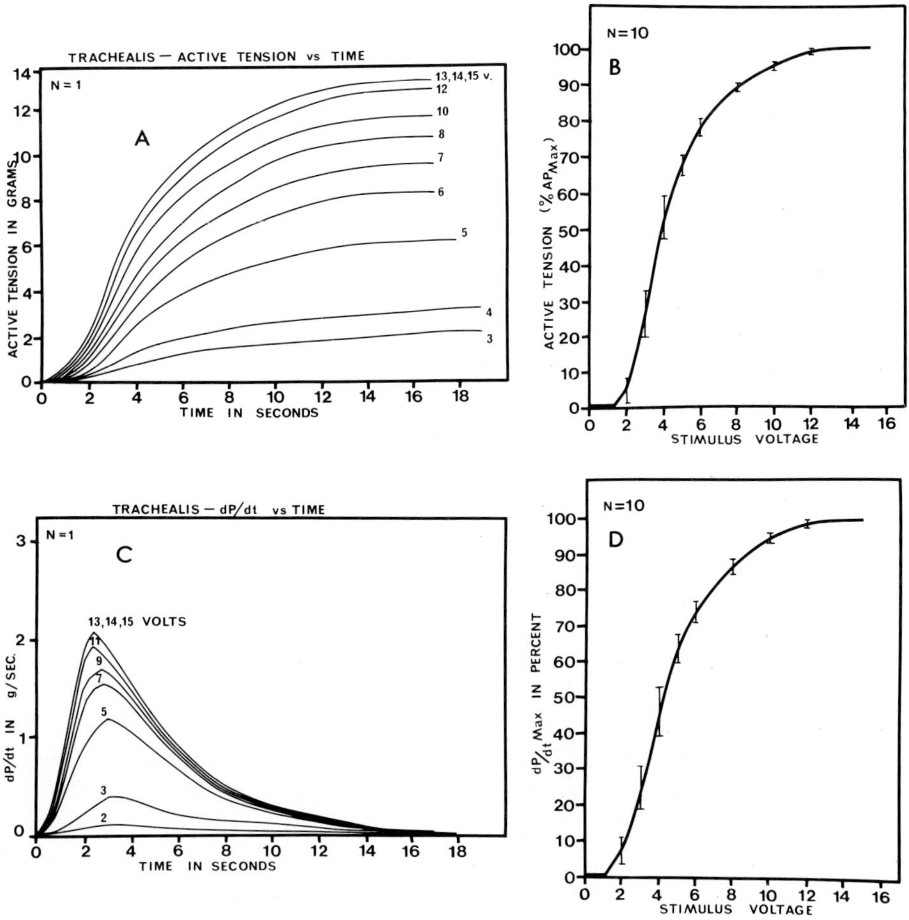


**FIGURE 21** Stimulus-response characteristics of canine tracheal smooth muscle. (From Ref. [25].)

enables one to determine the voltage for the maximal stimulus. Stimuli of greater strength are supramaximal. In conducting mechanical studies of any type, we first determine the maximal voltage and then use a stimulus which is 2 V greater. This is to try to ensure that if the excitability of the muscle decreases in the course of the experiment, the muscle will still be maximally stimulated and the active state of the muscle will be held invariant. A doubling of the maximal voltage would be better insurance, but smooth muscle does not remain stable under such relatively strong stimulation.

It must be pointed out that the isometric tetanic myogram does not show a sustained plateau with continued electrical stimulation. The fall-off in developed tension from the peak value is very rapid and is probably due to depletion of acetylcholine from the nerve terminals. The fall-off is also quite considerable, there being a decrement of almost 75%. With carbamylcholine, a sustained plateau develops which decreases by less than 15% over a 4-hr period. This suggests that processes distal to and at the postsynaptic membrane are not involved in the fall-off seen with electrical stimulation. We do not think the fall-off is due to inhibition by stimulation of any $\beta$-adrenergic system since it is totally unaffected by $\beta$ blockade. Blocking of any histamine ($H_2$) receptors with burimamide or metiamide does not affect the fall-off either. Finally, in the dog, we have no evidence that a nonadrenergic inhibitory system exists of the type described in guinea pig or human tracheal smooth muscle.

The curve in the upper right-hand panel demonstrates that with respect to mechanical response, tracheal smooth muscle is not an all-or-none type of muscle like the cardiac muscle. No data exist to determine whether the graded response in tracheal smooth muscle is produced in the same way as in skeletal muscle, where each contractile unit, namely, the cell, responds in an all-or-none manner. The grading results from the different units having different excitabilities. At lower voltages only those cells close to the electrode or with higher excitabilities are activated; with increasing voltages those further afield and those with lower excitabilities are recruited. The all-or-none response depends on a very rapid cell-to-cell conduction of electrical activity. This is facilitated by the presence of relatively large numbers of low-impedance, intracellular connections in cardiac muscle. In tracheal smooth muscle, these connections are not present to the same degree.

The lower left-hand panel is a plot of the instantaneous slopes (dP/dt) of the curves of the panel directly above it versus time. The point of interest—apart from the fact that maximum dP/dt at each voltage increases with increasing voltage—is that all the curves start, peak, and finish at the same time. This suggests that the contractile units recruited by increasingly stronger stimuli are functionally homogeneous. This is somewhat surprising, since in skeletal muscle, where direct visualization of sarcomeres is possible, nonhomogeneity exists. The nonhomogeneity is contributed to partly by processes of deactivation which affect the centrally located sarcomeres [25]. We have no explanation for the homogeneity that we see in tracheal smooth muscle. ATPase, cytochrome oxidase, and succinic dehydrogenase histochemical stains fail to reveal any mosaicism in the tracheal smooth muscle. This finding could be used to explain the contractile homogeneity seen. What the status of intracellular inhomogeneity in sarcomeric level is in smooth muscle is difficult to assess since sarcomeres have not been clearly demonstrated in this type of muscle.

The lower right-hand panel merely confirms that maximum dP/dt values (i.e., peak dP/dt values from the curves of the panel directly above it) are a graded function of stimulus strength.

While 60-cycle ac is a very effective stimulus for smooth muscle and allows easy maximal stimulation of the muscle, it does not permit a study of the relationship between stimulus parameters and contractile response. To study these, rectangular pulses are easier to work with. The ordinary Grass types of stimulator, which are so effective for nerve and striated muscle, are ineffective for smooth muscle, the chief problem being inability to deliver adequate current. With suitable current-boosting devices, however, this problem can be overcome. Using appropriate equipment which provided adequate current density for the smooth muscle cell, we [80] have shown that at $l_o$ the maximal contractile response was seen at a pulse width of almost 0.5 msec. Between 0.2 and 1 msec there is a very slight decrease in contractile response, but on either side of these values, the response rapidly declines. At the 0.5-msec optimal pulse width, stimulation evidently is occurring by way of the cholinergic nerves in the tissue, since Suzuki et al. [6] have shown that tetrodotoxin will completely eliminate the response to a 0.5-msec stimulus. It is known that tetrodotoxin only acts on nerve cell membranes and not on muscle cell membranes. The muscle cell membrane can be directly stimulated by a pulse whose width is between 5 and 10 msec.

With respect to the influence of cycling frequency on contractile response, the maximal response (for a pulse 0.5 msec in duration) is seen at 80 Hz. Between 50 and 150 Hz the response is reduced very little; however, outside this range the response falls rapidly [80]. The frequency range of 50 to 150 Hz also includes the 60-cycle ac frequency and may partly explain why the ordinary house current is such a good stimulus for smooth muscle. It is possible that because of the alternation, the stimulus frequency actually applied is not 60 but 120 Hz.

## Length-Tension Relationships of Tracheal Smooth Muscle

Conventional length-tension curves for tracheal smooth muscle are seen in Figure 22. These were elicited using supramaximal electrical stimulation of a muscle

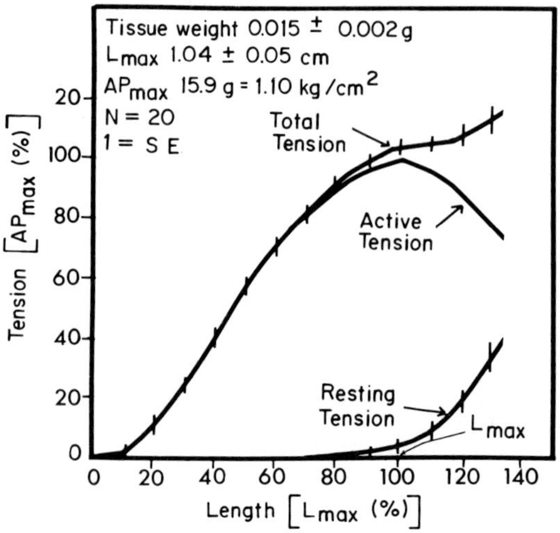


**FIGURE 22** Length-tension curves for canine tracheal smooth muscle. (From Ref. [93].)

which had been equilibrated in the manner already described. Increments in length were made very slowly, and at lengths approaching $l_o$ and beyond (since a considerable amount of stress-relaxation occurred), 5 to 8 min had to elapse before a relatively steady state emerged, when the stimulus could be applied.

To obtain valid length-tension curves, a 1-cm length of muscle tissue should weigh between 10 and 15 mg. Above 15 mg, studies (to be described below) showed that the tissue was hypoxic.

The resting tension curve is nonlinear; its initial slope indicates the resting muscle is fairly compliant. At $l_o$ or $L_{max}$ or the optimal length (so called because it is there at $P_o$ or $AP_{max}$ or the maximum active tension develops) the resting tension is very small (about 5% of $P_o$. In this, tracheal smooth muscle resembles skeletal muscle (frog sartorius), but differs markedly from other smooth muscles and cardiac muscle in which resting tension is quite high at $l_o$. A high resting tension is a drawback since it limits the range of loads over which the force-velocity curve can be measured.

It must be pointed out that, quite inaccurately, but sanctioned by custom, the terms force, load, and tension are used interchangeably. The other point worth mentioning is that $l_o$ does not carry the same connotation it does in the frog sartorius muscle. In the latter, $l_o$ is the point at which the maximum contraction is seen. It is also the length the muscle is set at in situ, and thus in situ and presumably in vivo skeletal muscles operate at the peak of their active tension curves. In smooth muscle, while $l_o$ is the length at which maximum contraction is seen, no studies have been done to determine whether it also represents the in situ length of the muscle. For this reason, $l_o$ is sometimes referred to as $L_{max}$, as in cardiac muscle [81].

The total tension curve shows a small plateau at lengths just a little greater than $l_o$. Occasional curves will shown an actual dip in place of the plateau. This resembles what is seen in length-tension curves obtained from frog sartorius muscle and is due to the particular compliance of the resting muscle at this length. In cardiac muscle and most other smooth muscles, neither the plateau nor the dip are seen, primarily because the resting tissue is much less compliant than the resting sartorius or the tracheal smooth muscle.

The active tension curve, obtained by subtracting the measured total tensions from the resting tensions, demonstrates that the Frank-Starling relation holds for the tracheal smooth muscle. This provides tentative evidence that the sliding filament model of contraction [82,83] applies to this muscle also.

The maximum tension developed at $l_o$, which is termed $P_o$, is about 1 kg/cm$^2$ of muscle cross-sectional area. This is in the same range as other smooth and striated muscles. It is obviously only an indirect index of muscle strength, since the cross-sectional area referred to also contains noncontractile structures, such as collagen, elastin, membranes, nuclei, and mitochondria.

The descending limb of the active tension is not seen in its entirety in Figure 22. We have, however, measured it (unpublished observation, 1975) to a length where the active tension response was about 5% of $P_o$, the corresponding length being 1.4 $l_o$. It descends much more sharply than the ascending limb, producing a much more asymmetrical curve when compared to that of the striated muscle. We have no data to explain this finding and speculate that deactivation is occurring. Increasing the calcium concentration in the bath does not increase the contractile response at lengths greater than $l_o$; evidently, increased stretch does not impair calcium influx from extracellular sites or release from intracellular depots. It is not clear whether this asymmetry of the descending limb is due to a time-dependent artefact, and this question must be excluded.

Taylor [84] has shown in striated muscle that at lengths less than $l_o$, due to increasing muscle diameter and tension on the T tubules, there is decreased calcium release with resultant muscle deactivation. This results in a depressed active tension curve. Whether such a phenomenon operates in smooth muscle is not known and awaits delineation of length-tension curves for single smooth muscle cells in the presence of increased amounts of $Ca^{2+}$ in the bathing medium. Fay et al. [8] have reported techniques for measuring developed tensions in single smooth muscle cells, and it soon may be possible to determine whether deactivation of the active state of the smooth muscle does occur at short lengths.

Inspection of the length-tension curves of Figure 22 shows one other interesting finding. Since a finite degree of active tension is seen at a muscle length of about 10% of $l_o$, it suggests the muscle can shorten from $l_o$ (which represents the 100% optimal length point) to 10% of $l_o$. Since striated muscles can shorten to only 65%, this places tracheal smooth muscle in the category of muscles that can supercontract, other examples of which are seen in muscles from the water bug [85] and *Gouldfingia goldii* [86]. Most smooth muscles from vertebrates show this ability to supercontract to varying degrees. The inability of striated muscle to supercontract stems from the delimitation of further sliding by well-organized Z bands. These prevent the thick filaments from passing through the bands and permit increased shortening. Such a mechanism has been reported in the literature [85]. In tracheal smooth muscle, organized sarcomeres do not exist, nor are there any discrete Z bands; hence, the hindrance to sliding of the myosin filaments does not exist. A further mechanism stems from the fact that smooth muscle myosin filaments do not have a central bare area free of jutting bridges as seen in striated muscles. The presence of bridges along the entire length of the thick filament facilitates supercontraction. Supercontraction is seen directly in isotonic shortening, where it is dramatically demonstrable. The shortening is not, however, down to 10% of $P_o$, but to about 20% of $l_o$. This difference probably results from the loss of energy due to frictional and inertial losses, which sets a limit on shortening.

The usefulness of the ability of tracheal smooth muscle to supercontract is open to speculation and further study. The magnitude of airway smooth muscle supercontraction enables a considerably greater control of airway lumen than in any other hollow viscus.

The slope of each of the length-tension curves of Figure 22 delineates the elasticity of the muscle tissue. Because of the difficulty in restoring a muscle to its initial length after any sizeable stretch, elasticity, as strictly defined, cannot be used to define the physical properties of this tissue. However, an index of stiffness [87] has been evolved which is represented by the change in muscle tension ($\Delta P$), divided by the corresponding change in length ($\Delta L$). No attempt is made to relate $\Delta l$ to initial muscle length since the latter is hard to determine. Stiffness ($\Delta P/\Delta l$) is essentially an operational parameter.

The area under the active tension represents the work done by the muscle as it shortens under different loads. It is an overestimate, since it is based on quasistatic measurements and does not account for viscous and inertial forces. At any rate, the work derived from the active tension curve constitutes a first-order approximation of work actually done and could profitably be used when chemomechanical relationships are studied.

Just how the curves we report could be associated with critical closure of the type envisaged by Burton [88] is not easy to see. Active tension does not become independent of length (such that the active tension curve lies parallel to the length axis), as would be required for critical closure to occur. At the very low lengths to which the muscle can shorten, active tension is perhaps inadequate to effect complete closure of the airways. The closure could, however, result from folding of the endothelial cells. It must be borne in mind that the failure of tracheal smooth muscle to demonstrate critical closure is perhaps not very conclusive. In situ and in vivo, critical closure is probably occurring in airways much smaller and narrower than the tracheal. The length-tension curves may be different in muscles from those locations.

A question that has intrigued investigators of cardiac and skeletal muscle is whether the active tension developed by a muscle depends on the mode in which it contracts. In skeletal muscle, for example [89], it is claimed that active tension is independent of the mode of contraction. However, Rosenblueth et al. [90] have presented evidence to the contrary.

Figure 23 is a schematic diagram detailing the various possible modes of contraction by which shortening occurs. In A, the muscle first shortens isometrically until it develops a force equivalent to the preload on the muscle which holds it at $l_o$. At this point, the muscle shortens isotonically, as confirmed by tracings from the displacement gauge. This is the mode which applies to conventional force-velocity studies. In mode B, the muscle, which is set at $l_o$ by a suitable preload, is not constrained by a stop, and is, in essence, free loaded. After it has shortened a given distance, further shortening is arrested by a stop and the consequent isometric tension developed is measured. In mode C, weights are applied to the muscle, which is free loaded. On stimulation, the muscle is allowed to shorten to its maximal extent and the shortening is measured. The fourth mode studied is the standard isometric. The isometric tetanic curve acts as the reference curve for tetanic curves elicited in modes A, B, and C.

Mean results are depicted in Figure 24. They show that the isotonic curves (modes A, B, and C) differ quite significantly and considerably from the isometric tetanic. Among the isotonic curves, those elicited in modes A and B are similar; they both differ from the curve elicited by mode C. For these studies, the mus-

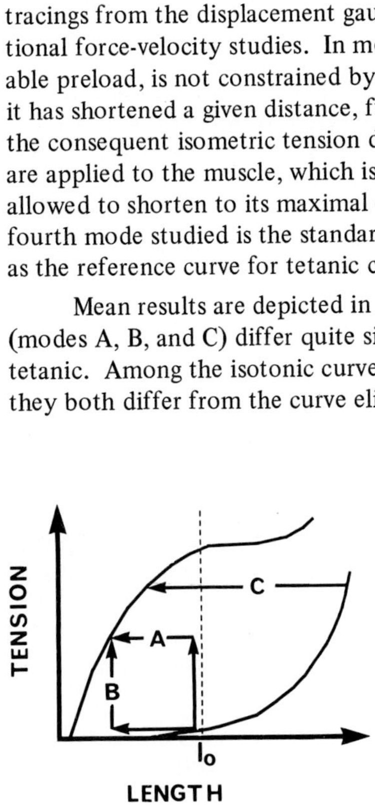


**FIGURE 23** Schematic diagram showing length-tension curves derived by different modes of contraction.

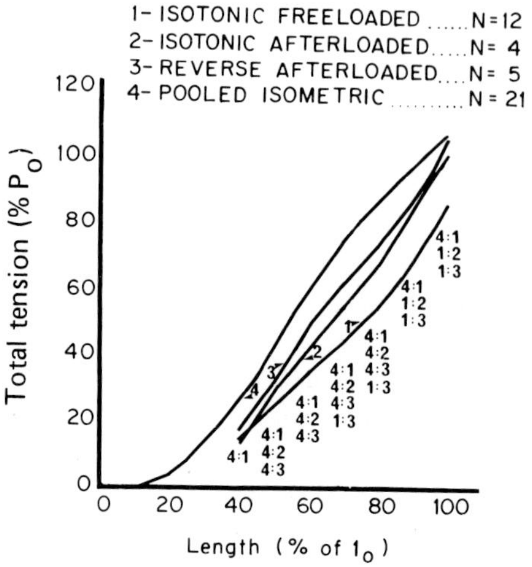


**FIGURE 24** Mean total tension-length curves for the isometric preparations shown. The free-loaded curve (1) differs from the after-loaded (2) at lengths greater than 60% of $l_o$. All comparisons were made using Duncan's new multiple range test (1955) with $\alpha = 0.05$. The test used the error mean square derived from a factorial analysis of variance with unequal replications per cell, applied to the raw data for all the four curves. The comparisons of curves (e.g., 4:1, 40%; 4:1/1:2/1:3, 100%) represent those comparisons found to be statistically significant for lengths of 40, 50, 60, 70, 80, 90, and 100% of $l_o$ from left to right, respectively. (From Ref. [164]. Reproduced by permission of the *Canadian Journal of Physiology and Pharmacology,* Vol. 55, 1977, pp. 833-838.)

cles were stimulated electrically. Essentially, similarly related curves are elicited when carbachol is used to stimulate the muscles.

The physiological significance of these curves could be that if regional distribution of ventilation is to be controlled by the magnitude of developed tone (isometric tension), then it will depend on the mode by which the final diameter of the lumen of the airway is attained.

When considering stimulus-response curves elicited isometrically, it was shown (see Fig. 21) that at any given stimulus strength, maximum dP/dt developed very early in the contraction. Furthermore, the maximum value of dP/dt increased with increasing voltage. Finally, from the similar time course of the dP/dt curves at different voltages, inferences were made about the homogeneity of voltage-recruited contractile units.

Similar relationships are shown for length, tension, and dP/dt in Figure 25. The plot was derived from a representative experiment. The dP/dt curves have been related to the active tension curve and, hence, all commence at the abscissa. A supramaximal electrical stimulus was used throughout. It is evident that dP/dt shows a peak at each length. This peak occurs early in the tension change experienced by the muscle. Plots of dP/dt versus time at different lengths (see Fig. 26) also revealed that maximum dP/dt developed very early in the shortening (within the first second). The influence of time and tension (or load imposed on the muscle's contractile element) on maximum dP/dt at $l_o$, represents optimal interaction between developed active state intensity and load.

The dP/dt versus time plots at different lengths (Fig. 26) also show that the different curves peak at the same time. Analysis of the dP/dt versus length and dP/dt versus stimulus strength (Fig. 21) curves thus reveals the homogeneity of contractile units, regardless of their mode of recruitment.

Therefore, we can conclude that tracheal smooth muscle qualitatively resembles skeletal muscle with respect to its length-tension properties, and in demonstrating a Frank-Starling relationship. It differs, however, in two respects,

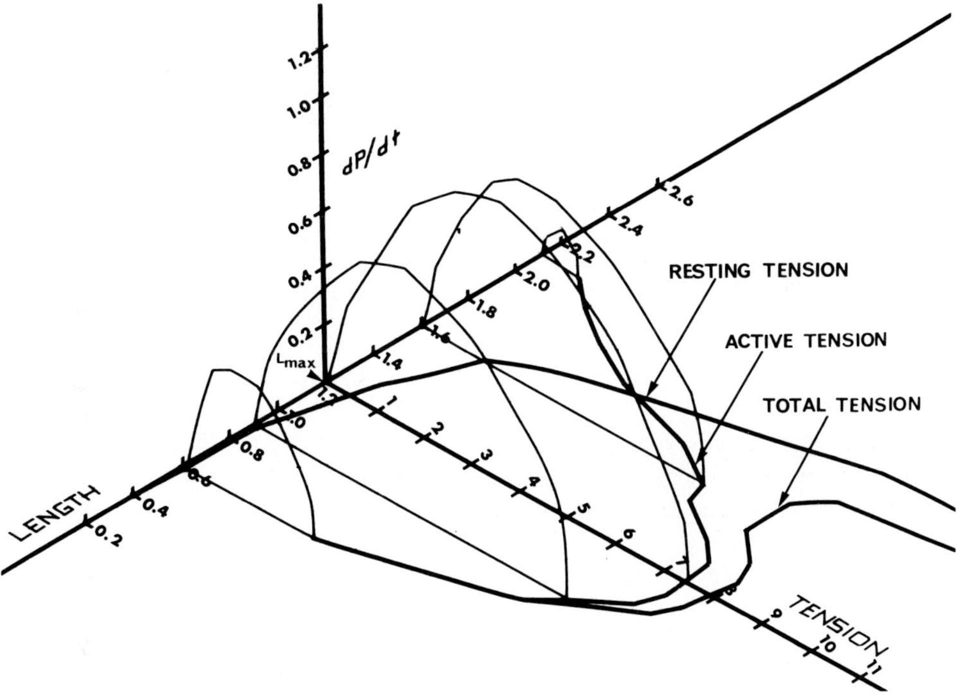


**FIGURE 25** Plot of length versus tension versus dP/dt for canine tracheal smooth muscle.

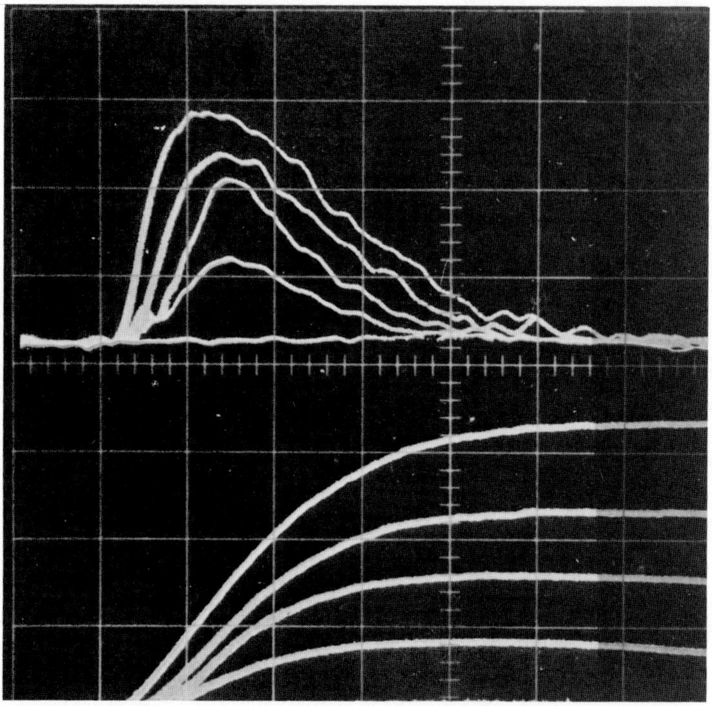

**FIGURE 26** Direct osilloscope recording of isometric tetanic tension versus time records at different muscle lengths (lower panel). The highest tension developed is that for the muscle set at longest length (in this case, $l_o$). Each square represent 2 sec along its abscissa and 4 g along its ordinate. Each of the curves is differentiated electronically and displayed in the upper panel as a function of time.

one being its ability to supercontract, and the other the considerable asymmetry of its active tension curve. Quantitatively, normalized $P_o$ values have the same order of magnitude in the two muscles.

## Force-Velocity Relationships of Tracheal Smooth Muscle

Study of the force-velocity relationships in muscle represents a powerful analytical tool in both basic and applied research. Fundamentally this is so because it permits delineation of the properties of the contractile element (CE) of the muscle. The same model used by striated muscle physiologists is invoked for smooth muscle. This consists of a contractile element (in which ATP hydrolysis occurs and the liberated energy is coupled to either tension development or shortening) in series with a series-elastic component (SEC). Huxley and Simmons [91] have produced evidence in single frog skeletal muscle cells which shows that the series-elastic component is not an inert, relatively undamped structure as was generally believed, but in fact is itself active. The in-series CE and SEC exist in parallel with a parallel elastic component (PEC) which supports the muscle at rest. Whether the series-elastic component in TSM is an active or inert structure has not been decided.

Force-velocity curves have not been reported for as many types of smooth muscle as one would expect. The reason for this is that the muscles themselves are not suited to such studies. The criteria to be met before valid force-velocity curves can be elicited are as follows:

1. The muscle should have low resting tension at $l_o$, since this is the best length for conducting such studies. Both active tension production and shortening are maximal at this length. The load required to hold the muscle at this length is termed the preload and is exactly equal to resting tension at $l_o$. If this preload is high, then only velocities at high loads can be studied, and that part of the curve where velocity is higher and more accurately measurable cannot be studied. Most smooth muscles have high resting tension at $l_o$ and so cannot be studied.
2. The active state of the muscle should be held at a steady maximum during the duration of the muscle shortening, otherwise the relationship between load and velocity will be obscured by the varying active state. As a simplification, active state could be biochemically represented as a steady maximal rate of energy utilization by the contractile machinery, the energy source being ATP. Maintenance of active state at steady maximal levels is most conveniently achieved by tetanizing the muscle. This, until recently [92], was a considerable problem in measuring force-velocity relationships in cardiac muscle, which could not be tetanized. In tracheal smooth muscle, however, tetanization is easy.
3. All the cells in the tissue should be muscle, and excessive amounts of connective tissue should not be present. Fortunately, tracheal smooth muscle has very little collagen and elastin (less than 25%) and its cells are oriented parallel to each other.
4. The change in active tension as the muscle passes from $l_o$ to $0.90\ l_o$ should not be significant. If it were, then it would invalidate measurements of force-velocity, since the velocity point generally measured

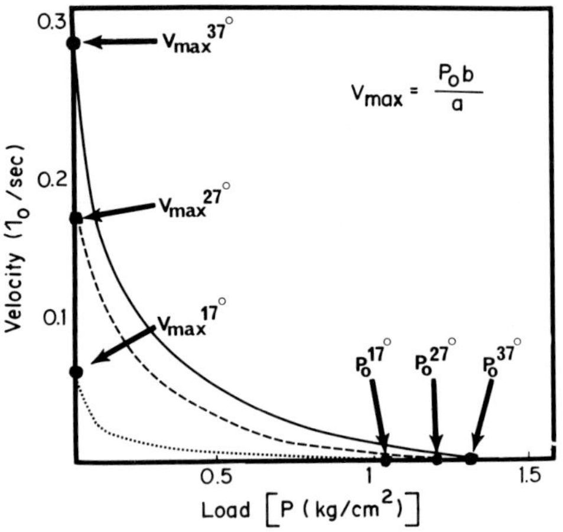


**FIGURE 27** Force-velocity curves for tracheal smooth muscle. Load and velocity are expressed in normalized units. (From Ref. [163].)

occurs not at the very onset of shortening but shortly thereafter when the muscle has shortened by about 5 to 10% of $l_o$. Again, in tracheal smooth muscle, there is no significant change in active tension over this range.

Figure 27 shows force-velocity curves for tracheal smooth muscle at three different temperatures. The effect of temperature will be discussed later. For present purposes we will focus on the curve elicited at 37°C. Mean curves derived from data obtained in 32 experiments have the same shape as the one shown. The standard error at each data point is less than 10% of the mean value. We have shown [93] that the curve is a rectangular hyperbola. It thus displays the same relation between load and shortening as does the classic frog sartorius muscle. Therefore, the equation developed by Hill [94] can also be used for tracheal smooth muscle:

$$(P + a)(V + b) = (P_o + a)b$$

where P = load.

$P_o$ = load that muscle is just unable to lift; it corresponds to isometric tetanic tension at the given muscle length.

V = velocity of shortening.

$a$ = asymptote value of the hyperbola; it has units of force.

$b$ = asymptote value of the hyperbola; it has unit of velocity.

The linear transformation of this equation is:

**TABLE 1 Dynamic Muscle Constants**

| Constants | Muscle: Frog satrorius[a] 0°C | Cat heart papillary muscle[b] 22°C | Hog artery[c] 37°C | Dog trachealis[d] 37°C |
|---|---|---|---|---|
| $a$, g/cm$^2$ | 399 | 175 | – | 244 |
| $a/P_o$ | 0.26 | 0.22 | 0.18 | 0.21 |
| $b$, lengths/sec | 0.337 | 0.27 | 0.02 | 0.06 |
| $P_o$, kg/cm$^2$ | 2.0 | 0.80 | 1.80 | 1.39 |
| $V_{max}$, lengths/sec ($= P_o\, b/a$) | 1.29 | 1.24 | 0.12 | 0.29 |

[a]From Hill [94].
[b]From Sonnenblick [81].
[c]From Murphy [154].
[d]From Stephens et al. [93].

$$\frac{P_o - P}{V} = \frac{P}{b} + \frac{a}{b}$$

When $(P_o - P)/V$ is plotted against P, the data points can be fitted to a linear equation as proven by a goodness of fit test. From the slope $(1/b)$ and the intercept $(a/b)$ the values of the asymptotes can be calculated.

Mean values for force-velocity parameters are shown in Table 1. From the table, it is evident that $P_o$ and $a$ are not greatly different for all the muscles shown. According to Hill [94], the $a$ constant is an index of the numbers of force-generating sites present in the cross section of the muscle. Hence, muscles having large $P_o$ values would necessarily have large $a$ values. If one assumes that all the force-generating sites (or the actomyosin bridges as these are now identified) are homogeneous, then this could lead to the conclusion that the same numbers of bridges are present per unit cross-sectional area of the various muscles.

This interpretation of the significance of the $a$ value is based on $a$ being independent of length. In fact, Hill [95] obtained data to show that some part of $a$ is length dependent and, hence, the interpretation has to be somewhat modified. Since the relationship between $a$ and length has not been studied in smooth muscle, the position is unclear.

One result of the similarity in the behavior of $a$ and $P_o$ is that the ratio $a/P_o$ is constant and for most striated and smooth muscle ranges between 0.20 and

0.30. The lower the value of $a/P_o$ the more curved is the force-velocity hyperbola. Woledge has shown values much less than 0.2 for tortoise muscle [96]. He has suggested that this is associated with increased efficiency of the muscle.

$V_{max}$ is the maximum velocity of shortening at zero load. It is obtained by solving for V when P = 0, and under that condition V is equal to $P_o b/a$. To enable comparison between different muscles, $V_{max}$ is expressed in $l_o$/sec. If one assumes a value of 3 for $Q_{10}$ of the frog sartorius, as suggested by Hill [94], then calculation shows that tracheal smooth muscle is more than 100 times slower than the frog sartorius if both are compared at 37°C. From this, it is evident that while airway smooth muscle shortening can control the size of the airways on a relatively long-term basis (15 sec or more), it cannot achieve any breath-by-breath control.

Integration of the force-velocity curve yields the power curve. A plot of power versus load (Fig. 28) shows that peak power develops at a load which is one-third of $P_o$. This is very similar to what occurs in skeletal muscle.

The *b* constant is an index of the rate at which energy is liberated in the muscle. If $V_{max} = P_o\ b/a$, and if $P_o/a$ is generally constant for practically all muscles, it is evident that differences in the velocity of shortening of different muscles (skeletal, cardiac, and smooth) must be due to differences in the energy-liberating reaction rates. The process involved is said to be the hydrolysis of ATP by actomyosin ATPase. Barany [97] has confirmed this by measuring ATPase activity and $V_{max}$ for a variety of muscles with a wide range of shortening velocities, and has shown a positive, linear relationship between the two for practically all muscles.

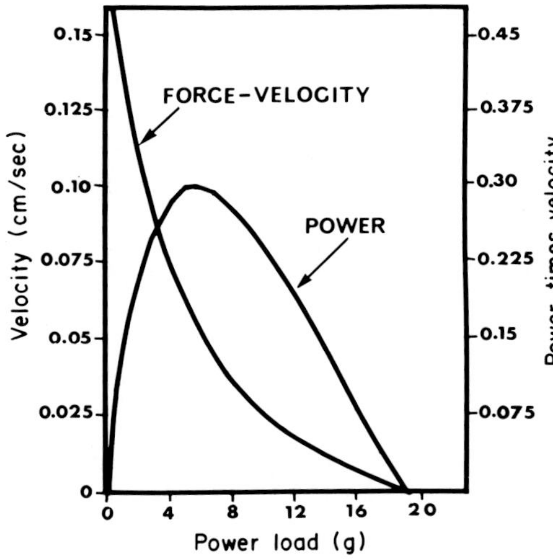


**FIGURE 28** Power curves (derived by integration of the force-velocity curve shown) for canine tracheal smooth muscle. (From Ref. [93].)

The slowness of smooth muscles compared to striated is thus due to a difference in ATPase activities. It has been shown (on the basis of ultracentrifugation studies) that in striated muscle the ATPase activity resides in a single light chain present in subfragment I of the heavy meromyosin moiety of the myosin molecule. Heavy meromyosin is itself obtained by appropriate enzymatic digestion. The cause for the difference in shortening velocities among various muscles is then to be sought in the physical properties of the light chain. In studying tracheal smooth muscle strips from antigen-sensitized pups and comparing these to control strips, we have found a considerably increased $V_{max}$ in the former [98]. We propose, in the near future, to study the properties of the actomyosin and myosin ATPases of the two muscles and, eventually, the physical properties of the light chains. We have already confirmed the presence of a light chain in tracheal smooth muscle actomyosin on the basis of SDS-polyacrylamide gel electrophoresis. This is discussed in Section III.

In concluding this section, we reiterate that any study of smooth muscle function under normal or abnormal (disease-simulated) conditions must be based on delineation of force-velocity relationships. First, it enables both muscle functions (stiffening and shortening) to be studied, and, second, evaluation of the various muscle constants allows speculation about possible mechanisms involved. On the basis of these, further experiments can be designed.

**Physical Properties of the Series-Elastic Component of Tracheal Smooth Muscle**

Quick-stretch and quick-release studies carried out by Hill [95] and Abbott and Wilke [89] have shown that, in the active muscle, the contractile element which utilizes energy and develops force or shortening is in series with another inert, undamped component termed the series-elastic component. It is this which transduces shortening of the contractile element to the outside world and results in the smooth movements of locomotion, for example. In an isometric contraction, however, the series-elastic component has to be stretched out first before external force is manifested by the muscle. If this element is very long or highly compliant, then the contraction would be very uneconomical in terms of energy consumption. The series-elastic component has been measured in a large number of muscles, generally using the quick-release method. We have described the application of this method to tracheal smooth muscle elsewhere [100]. Smooth muscles are reported to have the longest series-elastic components, as shown in Table 2, in which the amount this element is stretched while the muscle develops maximum isometric tetanic tensions is given.

The table shows that the series-elastic component of tracheal smooth muscle is shorter than that in all smooth muscle except the hog carotid. We have shown that in hypoxia the series-elastic component becomes stiffer, which suggests that it may not be an inert structure [79]. In the inserts of Figure 29,

**TABLE 2** Series-Elastic Component in Different Muscles

| Muscle | Percentage |
|---|---|
| Whole skeletal muscle [69] | 3.0 |
| Cat heart papillary muscle [158] | 7 |
| Cat intestinal muscle [159] | 25 |
| Rabbit tenia coli [160] | 20 |
| Hog carotid artery [161] | 7.2 |
| Rat portal vein [162] | 15 |
| Tracheal smooth muscle [100] | 7.5 |

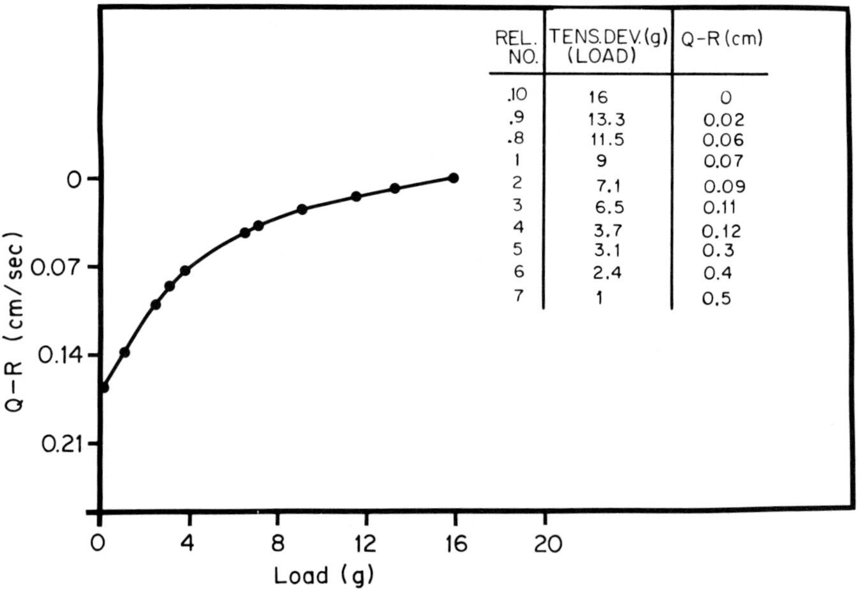


**FIGURE 29** Length-tension data obtained by quick-release methods, for series-elastic component of canine tracheal smooth muscle. (From Ref. [100].)

quick-release data for tracheal smooth muscle released at the peak of isometric tetanic tension development are shown. The muscle was set at $l_o$, which in this case was 2.0 cm. The length-tension curve for the series-elastic components is plotted also. The actual quick releases, which were applied at a velocity 10 times faster than the maximum velocity of the contractile element, showed a very rapid linear response of the series-elastic component, which demonstrates that in tracheal smooth muscle this structure is also relatively undamped. Conventional curve-fitting techniques showed that the curve could be described by a single experimental function.

### Effects of Temperature on the Contractile and Series-Elastic Component

The change in temperature that occurs between sickness and health in the human organism is fortunately not very great but, nevertheless, is great enough to affect biochemical reactions (in airway smooth muscle, for example) sufficiently to alter its mechanical properties. This is, therefore, one reason for determining the effects of temperature on smooth muscle mechanics. The second is that the force-velocity parameters we obtained are derived from mechanical studies. From these, conclusions are made about thermodynamic processes. This is really only valid when heat or quantitative mechanochemical measurements are made on contracting muscles. Such measurements have been made by Hill [94], for example. They have been carried out to a very limited extent in airway smooth muscle and are reported below in Section III. We have also measured $Q_{10}$ values for several mechanical constants in airway smooth muscle in an attempt to show that those parameters which we feel derive from active processes, for example, $V_{max}$ and *b*, are indeed active and have high $Q_{10}$ values (unpublished, 1977). Table 3 incorporates $Q_{10}$ data for isometrically, tetanically contracting tracheal smooth muscle. The mean values and standard errors were computed from five experiments. The parameter $t_{P_o}$ signifies contraction time.

The interesting observation here is that $P_o$ seems to be independent of temperature. The lowered dP/dt and increased $t_{P_o}$ can be envisaged as stemming

**TABLE 3 $Q_{10}$ Values from the Isometric Myogram**

| | Temperature (0°C) | $P_o$ (kg/cm$^2$) | dP/dt (kg cm$^{-2}$ sec$^{-1}$) | $t_{P_o}$ (sec) | *N* |
|---|---|---|---|---|---|
| Mean ± SE | 27 | 1.28 ± 0.11 | 1.41 ± 0.12 | 18 ± 0.8 | 5 |
| | 37 | 1.39 ± 0.10 | 3.04 ± 0.26 | 10 ± 1.3 | 5 |
| $Q_{10}$ | | 1.1 | 2.16 | 0.55 | |

from a drop in the intensity of the active state of the muscle and in a prolongation of its duration [10]. The constancy of $P_o$ is due to dP/dt and $tp_o$ varying in opposite directions. It is well known that dP/dt and $tp_o$ depend on active processes, yet the former has a $Q_{10}$ of 2.16 and the latter 0.55, which does not fit the $Q_{10}$ interpretation for active processes. An explanation for this seeming paradox is that on stimulation of the muscle, $Ca^{2+}$ is released and $Ca^{2+}$ pumps are turned on to resequester $Ca^{2+}$. These are not sequential processes with a rate-limiting step but additive processes (net free $Ca^{2+}$ is determined by the difference between the influx and efflux rates). With cooling, the active pump ($Q_{10}$ about 2) slows down while the passive influx ($Q_{10}$ about 1) changes little. Thus, cooling causes net intracellular $Ca^{2+}$ concentration to stay higher for a longer period of time, thus increasing $tp_o$. The measured $Q_{10}$ of 0.55 does not necessarily mean that active processes are not involved, but that both active and passive processes could be acting in opposition to each other.

Table 4 shows $Q_{10}$ values derived from force-velocity measurements of the type shown in Figure 23.

These measurements show that the *a* constant was unchanged, there being no statistically significant difference between the values at the temperatures shown. This could suggest, on the basis of Hill's interpretation of the *a* constant [94], that the numbers of force-generating sites in the muscle do not change with temperature. On the other hand, the constancy of *a* may have been brought about by the same factors that resulted in the stability of $P_o$ and does not permit any statements regarding constancy of numbers of force-generating sites. For the same reason, the low $Q_{10}$ value does not mean that *a* is not dependent on chemical energy.

The parameter $a/P_o$, which is almost a universal muscle constant, did not change significantly with temperature, mainly because *a* and $P_o$ did not change.

The *b* constant and $V_{max}$ should have $Q_{10}$ values close to 2.0. This suggests that these two parameters are derived from processes which consume chemical energy. Since $V_{max}$ (= $P_o$ $b/a$) and $P_o/a$ are unchanged as the temperature increases from 27 to 37°C, it is evident that the increased shortening velocity seen is due to an increase in the rate at which energy-liberating reactions (most likely ATP hydrolysis are occurring.

Table 5 shows the effect of temperature on the series-elastic component of tracheal smooth muscle. The experiments were carried out using conventional quick-release techniques. This table reveals that between 27 and 37°C there seem to be no differences in the stiffness of the SEC. Statistical analysis confirmed this. The $Q_{10}$ value indicates that the SEC is only influenced passively, which is surprising in view of the recent idea [91] that it is contributed to partly by active processes at the actomyosin bridges. One explanation is that, of the

**TABLE 4 $Q_{10}$ Values Derived from Force-Velocity Measurements**

| | Temperature (°C) | $a$ (g/cm²) | $b$ ($l_o$/sec) | $V_{max}$ ($l_o$/sec) | $a/P_o$ | $N$ |
|---|---|---|---|---|---|---|
| Mean ± SE | 27 | 242 ± 50 | 0.03 ± 0.002 | 0.17 ± 0.02 | 0.20 | 5 |
| | 37 | 262 ± 30 | 0.06 ± 0.006 | 0.29 ± 0.03 | 0.24 | 5 |
| $Q_{10}$ | | 1.1 | 2.1 | 1.9 | 1.2 | |

**TABLE 5 SEC Parameters**

| | Temperature (°C) | dP/dL (g/cm) | $N$ |
|---|---|---|---|
| Mean ± SE | 27 | 11 ± 1.3 | 5 |
| | 37 | 9 ± 1.0 | 5 |
| $Q_{10}$ | | 0.82 | |

total length of the SEC, perhaps only a very small fraction originates from active processes and the bulk of it resides in inert structures in smooth muscle. We have shown [101] that the SEC is about 7% of $l_o$ at $P_o$. If 1% came from active processes and 6% from passive, then any increase in the stiffness of the active component would be masked by that in the passive. Finally, the fact that the properties of the SEC do not change as the temperature drops from 37 to 27°C must mean that the reduced dP/dt seen is due to changes in the shortening ability of the muscle, since $dP/dt = (dP/dl)_{SEC} \times (dl/dt)_{CE}$.

## The Active State of Tracheal Smooth Muscle

The active state, as originally defined [102], was characterized by a change in the stiffness of the muscle after it was stimulated. This alteration had a well-defined onset, plateau, and decay which could be delineated by quickly stretching the electrically activated muscle and measuring the change in tension at different points in the contraction cycle. The magnitude of stretch was held constant. The attractiveness of the concept lay in the fact that the quick stretch, by eliminating the damping effect of the series-elastic component, enabled study of the contractlie component.

No studies of the active state have been made as yet in tracheal smooth muscle. As mentioned before, the ability to tetanize tracheal muscle enables one to maintain a maximal steady value of the active state which facilitates carrying out other mechanical studies.

It is possible that the active state of airway smooth muscle will resemble that of other smooth muscles in having a rather short onset, an ill-sustained plateau, and a prolonged decay phase. All these phases are present in skeletal muscle where they have a considerably faster time course; the plateau phase is maintained better in skeletal muscle.

Quick stretching or quick releasing the muscle to measure its active-state curve itself alters the active state. This fact has detracted from the usefulness of these methods.

To summarize this section on the mechanical properties of airway smooth muscle, it may be said that tracheal smooth muscle lends itself to analysis along the classic pathways developed for the frog sartorius muscle. Because of the marked similarity in the length-tension, stimulus-response, and force-velocity curves of the two muscles, it is very likely that the sliding filament model of contraction [83] will apply to tracheal smooth muscle as well. One of the crucial questions still awaiting an answer is: How do the static and dynamic properties of airway smooth muscle affect the mechanical properties of the lung? These two areas of pulmonary research have developed independently and are still some distance removed from each other. The shortcomings lie (1) in the slow development of airway smooth muscle research, which lagged far behind lung research; and (2) from the relatively late recognition that the airways can no longer be regarded as passive conduits.

## III. Biochemistry of Airway Smooth Muscle

### A. Introduction

Perhaps the major objective of a biochemical study of airway smooth muscle is to delineate that facet of it which helps us to understand the structure, physiology, and pathophysiology of the muscle. From this point of view, bioenergetics, or mechanochemistry, and the contractile and regulatory proteins are proper subjects for study.

Unfortunately, smooth muscle is extremely difficult to work with because it is present in very small amounts and contains a considerable admixture of tissue which is not muscle. It is predominantly as a measure of expediency that much of the protein biochemistry of smooth muscle has been worked out from the chicken gizzard muscle. Some hesitation arises in attempting to use those data to explain what happens in airway smooth muscle. Nevertheless, it is from unusual muscles like frog sartorius and rabbit psoas that so much of our insight into the physiology of striated muscle has been gained, so the situation is not hopeless. Having said that, we must now point out that the chief difficulty in attempting biochemical analysis of tracheal smooth muscle is the small amount of muscle available. In studying oxidative phosphorylation (see Sec. III.B), we have to kill three to four dogs to obtain an adequate amount of muscle providing enough mitochondria to study relevant parameters. For the present, however, we do not wish to look for another biochemical model since we wish to use the same animal model for biochemical studies that we employed for biophysical studies, namely, the canine tracheal smooth muscle.

### B. Carbohydrate Metabolism Bioenergetics

In studying any machine, the question uppermost is: How efficient is it? To assess this, the relation between the work done and the energy consumed has to be measured. In studying muscle, the same considerations apply. The application of tcchniques to study the mechanochemistry of smooth muscle in the same manner as in striated muscle has been initiated by Paul et al. [103] and the Lundholms [104]. The approach has been mainly to assess energy utilization by measuring rates of oxygen uptake and lactate production.

#### Oxygen Uptake Measurements

As far as airway smooth muscle is concerned, whatever work has been done has come from the Lundholms' laboratory [105] and ours [106].

We have published the oxygen uptake characteristics of canine tracheal smooth muscle previously [98]. The method utilizes a Clarke type of oxygen electrode incorporated into a Gilson oxygraph [106]. Using this, the oxygen uptake of a strip of canine tracheal smooth muscle set at $l_o$ has been measured. Values were obtained during a resting steady state, during the development of isometric tonic contraction elicited by maximal doses of acetylcholine, and at the plateau of maximum developed tension. It is important to point out that acetylcholine is degraded very slowly in our experimental setup, where the muscle strip is suspended in Krebs-Henseleit solution. One index of this is that such a muscle maintains a plateau of developed tone for about 3 hr.

From several series of experiments, we were able to conclude that optimal oxygen uptakes in tracheal smooth muscle, as in skeletal muscle, depend critically on muscle thickness. It seems that a muscle more than 0.5 mm thick is almost certainly diffusion limited to oxygen. Muscle thickness is a notoriously difficult thing to measure and in practical terms, in our laboratory at least, a 1-cm length of muscle which is more than 10 mg in weight is probably hypoxic in its core. Hence, all studies on canine tracheal smooth muscle should be conducted on strips weighing 10 mg or less. The lower limit seemed to be about 4 mg. Below that the proportion of damaged cells is probably intolerably high, and the $Q_{O_2}$ values obtained are unreliable.

**TABLE 6 $Q_{10}$ Values for Canine Tracheal Smooth Muscle[a]**

| | Resting | During development of tension | At plateau of developed tension | After ACh washout |
|---|---|---|---|---|
| Oxygen uptake | | | | |
| $\mu$mol $hr^{-1}$ $g^{-1}$ wet weight | 45 ± 3 | 68 ± 4 | 52 ± 4 | 45 ± 6 |
| $\mu$l $hr^{-1}$ $g^{-1}$ wet weight | 1017 ± 71 | 1517 ± 98 | 1175 ± 90 | 1010 ± 137 |
| $\mu$mol $hr^{-1}$ $g^{-1}$ dry weight | 172 ± 14 | 258 ± 21 | 205 ± 19 | 155 ± 26 |
| $\mu$l $hr^{-1}$ $g^{-1}$ dry weight | 3852 ± 302 | 5772 ± 469 | 4582 ± 432 | 3476 ± 575 |
| Mechanical tension in $g/cm^2$ of muscle cross-sectional area | 54 ± 3 | — | 740 ± 183 | 57 ± 3 |

[a]Oxygen uptake in tracheal smooth muscle (mean and standard errors) after treatment with acetylcholine (ACh, $10^{-4}$ g/ml). TSM parameters: $l_o$ = 0.63 ± 0.04; wet weight, 0.005 ± 0.0003 g; dry weight, 0.00013 ± 0.00001 g; cross-sectional area, 0.0083 ± 0.0001 $cm^2$. From the average cross-sectional area and assuming the tissue to be cylindrical, the averaged diameter of the strips was computed to be 0.102 cm. $N$ = 10 strips from five animals for all values given. All these observations were made at 37°C.

In Table 6, $Q_{O_2}$ data for canine tracheal smooth muscle are provided. Noteworthy points are: (1) that the $Q_{O_2}$ values of the equilibrated, resting tracheal muscle are almost the same as that for the resting frog sartorius. Several adjustments have to be made since the temperatures under which the two preparations are studied differ almost fourfold; the comparison was achieved by converting microliters of oxygen to millicalories of heat from the data of Hill [94]; (2) that smooth and striated muscles differ remarkably in their oxygen uptake rates during activity. The increase in $Q_{O_2}$ for the striated muscle is 40 times greater than that for the smooth. This suggests that either the smooth muscle is much more efficient (this has already been suggested for other slowly contracting muscles by Woledge [96]) or that it relies more heavily on the lactate pathway as an energy source. It is likely that a combination of both these mechanisms operates in tracheal smooth muscle.

**Muscle Heat Measurements**

Apart from our own extremely limited observations, we are unaware of any work in the area of heat measurement in airway smooth muscle. The method we use is an adaptation of Hill's technique [94]. It incorporates a conventional thermopile of the type described by Woledge [107] and Clinch [108]. The heat measurements were carried out in collaboration with Clinch.

The principle of the method utilizes the fact that when the temperature of the muscle is steady, the rate of heat production is equal to the rate of heat loss and is proportional to the temperature difference between the hot and cold thermopile junctions. The rate of heat production is given by

$$h = \frac{(60\,yck)}{\mathrm{u}}$$

where $h$ is the rate of heat production in cal $g^{-1}$ $deg^{-1}$, $k$ is the cooling constant in $sec^{-1}$, $c$ is the specific heat of the muscle in cal $g^{-1}$ $deg^{-1}$, $y$ is the output from the thermopile in $\mu$V, and u is the temperature sensitivity of the thermopile in $\mu$V/mdeg. The specific heat of tracheal smooth muscle has been taken to be 0.88 cal $g^{-1}$ $deg^{-1}$ at all temperatures. This figure is slightly incorrect since we do not know the muscle's total solid content; this is required to make the correction.

For a muscle strip at 28°C, weighing 0.07 g and 1.5 cm long ($l_o$), the resting heat turned out to be 9.2 mcal $g^{-1}$ $min^{-1}$. The resting heat for frog sartorius at 0°C is 2.5 mcal $g^{-1}$ $min^{-1}$. After applying a correction in which an assumed $Q_{10}$ of 3 is used, the resting heat for the smooth muscle turns out to be 1 mcal $g^{-1}$ $min^{-1}$. Hence, the two muscles appear to have the same order of heats. Since the smooth muscle cell is many times smaller than the skeletal, for the same size of muscle there must be a greater area of surface membrane in the smooth muscle.

If one assumes that the bulk of the resting heat stems from ion pump activities, then either the density of these pumps is much less in smooth muscle or the pumps in the membranes of the two muscles have greatly dissimilar energy requirements.

The maintenance heat, which is the increment over the resting heat when the muscle was stimulated with a maximal dose of acetylcholine as in the $Q_{O_2}$ studies, was on the average 4.9 mcal $g^{-1}$ $min^{-1}$ at 28°C. After adjusting for temperature, this maintenance heat rate is about 1/30 of that for frog sartorius. This compares favorably with the 1/40 value we obtained on the basis of $Q_{O_2}$ measurements. The difference (1/120) may represent the extent to which the lactate pathway supplies energy for contraction in the smooth muscle. Since the lactate pathway supplies relatively little energy for maintenance of active processes, we are left with the conclusion that tracheal smooth muscle is very efficient.

**Oxidative Phosphorylation**

The key question with respect to the bioenergetics of normoxic tracheal smooth muscle contraction is: To what extent does the muscle utilize energy derived from oxidative processes in relation to that from anaerobic glycolysis? In skeletal and cardiac muscles, oxidative phosphorylation supplies about 95% of the energy required for contractile purposes. In smooth muscle, the situation is more like that occurring in so-called white muscles, where mitochondrial content is low and anaerobic glycolysis plays a major role.

Various authors have stated that as much as 80 to 90% of the smooth muscle cell's glycogen is metabolized through the lactic acid pathways [109]. As far as we know, studies to determine what fraction of cell glycogen is metabolized through the lactate pathway have not been carried out in airway smooth muscle. Our own studies [25] have provided indirect evidence that this pathway must also be the more important energy source for airway smooth muscle. The evidence itself is that the amount of mitochondrial protein present in tracheal smooth muscle is very small compared to that in striated red muscle.

We isolated mitochondria [25] from the dog tracheal smooth muscle using a procedure modified from that of Chance and Hagihara [110]. The yield of mitochondrial protein we obtained in seven experiments was 0.43 ± 0.05 (SE) mg/g wet weight of muscle.

Oxidative phosphorylation was studied polarographically with an Oxygraph (G.M.E., Madison) fitted with a Clark type of electrode.

Under the electron microscope, the mitochondria resemble those seen in skeletal muscle. They demonstrate a typical double membrane, the inner layer of which is invaginated to form the cristae. The numbers of cristae present in a

**TABLE 7 Oxidative Phosphorylation Parameters**

| | $O_2$ uptake rate ($\mu$mol $O_2$/min per g mitochondrial protein) | Respiratory control ratio (RCR) | ADP/O | Phosphorylation rate |
|---|---|---|---|---|
| *N* | 8 | 14 | 14 | 8 |
| Mean ± SE | 94 ± 5 | 4.5 ± 0.2 | 2.30 ± 0.03 | 393 ± 21 |

mitochondrion are less than those seen in cardiac and skeletal muscle. When fixed for electron microscopy in State 3, during which mitochondria are taking up oxygen maximally and phosphorylating ADP to ATP, they appear to be in the conformationally "condensed" form. At rest, in State 4, they appear to be in the "orthodox" form wherein they are more uniformly gray. These forms have been described by Hackenbrock [26].

With respect to oxidative phosphorylation and response to standard inhibitors and uncouplers, tracheal smooth muscle mitochondria behave very much like those from striated muscle.

Mean oxidative phosphorylation parameters are given in Table 7. The substrate used for the above experiments was 5 mM pyruvate and 1 mM L-malate (P/M).

The ADP:O ratio, which is a measure of the efficiency of phosphorylation with respect to respiration, was obtained by dividing the amount of ADP added to the Oxygraph cuvette by the gram-atoms of oxygen consumed. The average value we obtained was within low normal limits for hamster skeletal muscle mitochondria studied in our laboratory.

A more sensitive index for assessing the tightness of coupling of phosphorylation to respiration was obtained from the RCR (respiratory control rate) which is the ratio of State 3 respiration to that of respiration in State 4. The values shown in Table 6 are within normal limits for hamster skeletal muscle mitochondria.

Tracheal smooth muscle mitochondria are able to use substrates other than P/M as is shown in Table 8. We dound that palmityl carnitine is oxidized at about 65%, acetyl carnitine at about 85%, and succinate at about 86% of the rate obtained with P/M in the same experiments. As expected, we obtained an ADP:O ratio of less than 2.0 with succinate. The ability to use fatty acid as a substrate demonstrates that smooth muscle resembles skeletal muscle in this regard. One still unsettled question for smooth muscle is whether it resembles skeletal in

**TABLE 8 Oxidative Phosphorylation in Tracheal Smooth Muscle Mitochondria[a]**

| Substrate | $O_2$ uptake rate ($\mu$mol $O_2$/min, per g mitochondrial protein) | RCR | ADP/O |
|---|---|---|---|
| Palmityl-L-carnitine | 64 | 3.3 | 1.9 |
| Acetyl-L-carnitine | 84 | 3.9 | 2.2 |
| Pyruvate/malate | 94 | 4.5 | 2.3 |

[a]Oxidative phosphorylation parameters for pyruvate/malate as substrate are given for the sake of comparison.

*Source:* Reproduced by permission of *Am. J. Physiol.*

utilizing fatty acids as a preferred energy source between "feasts," and carbohydrates at meal times [111]. Whatever the final answers, at least our study shows that tracheal smooth muscle mitochondria can successfully metabolize fatty acids.

The response of oxidative phosphorylation in tracheal smooth muscle to standard inhibitors and uncouplers such as oligomycin, dinitrophenol, rotenone, antimycin, and sodium cyanide is the same as in striated muscle [112,113].

Using both NADH oxidase and cytochrome oxidase as enzyme markers, we were able to obtain measures of mitochondrial protein content per gram wet weight of muscle. Knowing what the phosphorylation rate for the mitochondria was (see Table 6), we were able to calculate the phosphorylation capacity of the muscle. This really is the phosphorylation rate per gram of muscle and is the parameter of paramount interest in understanding the bioenergetics of muscle contraction. The capacity proved to be 1.40 $\mu$mol of ADP phosphorylation per minute per gram wet weight of muscle. That is almost 10 to 15% of what we obtain for hamster skeletal muscle, and lends support to views that the anaerobic glycolytic pathway provides comparatively more energy in smooth muscle than in striated.

We have also conducted studies of the effect of hypoxia on canine tracheal muscle mitochondrial function and reported that even relatively mild degrees of hypoxia cause uncoupling of their function [114]. This uncoupling is irreversible, then, given severer degrees of damage, it is obvious the muscle will have to depend almost entirely on glycolysis as an energy source. To ensure optimal glycolysis, the muscle cells should be well stocked with glycogen. Whether a regimen of intravenous glucose, insulin, and potassium would achieve the desired effect is not known at this time.

## Anaerobic Glycolysis, Including the Pentose Shunt and the Polyol Pathway

This has not been studied systematically in airway smooth muscle. The Lundholms [105] have studied glycolysis in bovine tracheal smooth muscle and we have investigated some aspects of glycolysis in canine tracheal smooth muscle.

As judged from work on other smooth muscles, it seems that the pathways for carbohydrate metabolism are very similar to those for striated muscles in which a considerable amount of investigation has been carried out. Practically all the enzymes in the glycolytic pathway have been identified and partially characterized by Kirk [78], who has reviewed the field, as has Zemplenyi [115].

In this pathway, glucose or glycogen is metabolized to pyruvate and lactate. Since oxygen is not needed, this is known as the anerobic glycolytic pathway. Pyruvate is fed into the tricarboxyclic acid and is ultimately converted to $CO_2$ and $H_2O$. Reducing equivalents generated in this phase of metabolism are processed by the electron transport chain of mitochondria. Electron energy is coupled to phosphorylation of ADP and results in the production of ATP.

The presence of the *pentose shunt* has not been determined in airway smooth muscle. However, Morrison et al. [116], among others, using [1-$^{14}$C]-glucose, have shown that the pentose shunt exists in aortic smooth muscle, and Mandel and Kempf [117] have suggested that this shunt produces $NADPH_2$ and stimulates lipid synthesis and that this is of significance in the pathogenesis of atherosclerosis. Presumably, a pentose shunt also exists in tracheal smooth muscle. However, it must be admitted that atherosclerosis has not been described in this muscle.

*A polyol pathway* has also been described in rabbit and human aortic smooth muscle [118]. It has also been found in the lens of the eye and has been implicated in the pathogenesis of diabetic cataracts.

In the polyol pathway, glucose is first converted to sorbitol by aldose reduction and then to fructose by sorbitol dehydroglucose. Phosphorylation of glucose is not involved. The pathway requires excess glucose as a starting point and, hence, is probably not operative under normal conditions where intracellular glucose levels are very low either by virtue of being rapidly converted to glycogen or by being processed through the "descending" limb of the Embden-Meyerhof pathway. It is more likely to be active in diabetic states in which intracellular glucose concentrations are higher.

Arnqvist [119] and Bihler et al. [120] have shown in arterial and intestinal smooth muscle, respectively, that *glucose transport* is brought about by facilitated diffusion, which is characterized by substrate stereospecificity, saturation kinetics, and countertransport. No studies of glucose transport have been reported for tracheal smooth muscle, but it is likely to be similar to that of the smooth muscles reported above.

Much more glucose or glycogen is metabolized to lactate in smooth muscle than in skeletal. While this amounts to only 10% in skeletal muscle, in smooth muscle it is about 50 to 80%. This shows the important position of the glycogen-lactate pathway as an energy source in smooth muscle. No data regarding the proportional role of glycolysis in tracheal smooth muscle are available. However, we have shown [25] that oxidative phosphorylation provides only one-seventh the ATP that it does in striated muscle. This indirectly suggests that the glycogen-lactate pathway also plays a predominant role in energy supply for tracheal smooth muscle.

The prominence of the lactate pathway raises questions as to the *status of the Pasteur effect* in smooth muscle. Only a weak Pasteur effect was found in bovine tracheal smooth muscle by Lundholm and Mohme-Lundholm [121]. In other smooth muscle, a stronger Pasteur effect has been reported [116].

**Control of Carbohydrate Metabolism**

This area, just like the other described above, has not yet received enough attention in airway smooth muscle metabolism. Work on other smooth muscles suggests [104] that control is exerted at the same points as in striated muscle. Thus, the key rate-limiting step in smooth muscle carbohydrate metabolism is at the step catalyzed by phosphofructokinase. The factors which stimulate or inhibit this reaction have been well studied in striated muscle; however, nothing is known about them in tracheal smooth muscle. In bovine mesenteric arteries contracted by epinephrine [122], the ratio of fructose-6-phosphate to fructose-1,6-phosphate decreased, which suggests phosphofructokinase activation. A similar response to agonist probably also occurs in tracheal smooth muscle.

With respect to regulation of glycogen breakdown in tracheal smooth muscle, Mohme-Lundholm [123] demonstrated the presence of phosphorylase a and phosphorylase b activities. The presence of the converting enzyme phosphorylase b kinase was also detected in bovine tracheal smooth muscle. Since in vitro cyclic AMP was able to activate phosphorylase b kinase in this muscle, it is probably that the phosphorylase activation and glycogenolysis following stimulation of $\beta$ adrenoceptors in smooth muscle were cyclic AMP mediated.

Currently, there is a controversy about whether elevated levels of cyclic AMP are related to smooth muscle relaxation. The majority of opinion suggests that it is. If that is so, then the biologic significance of the stimulation of carbohydrate metabolism for the cyclic AMP-mediated relaxation is probably that it provides energy for the binding of myoplasmic $Ca^{2+}$ or for its extrusion from the cell.

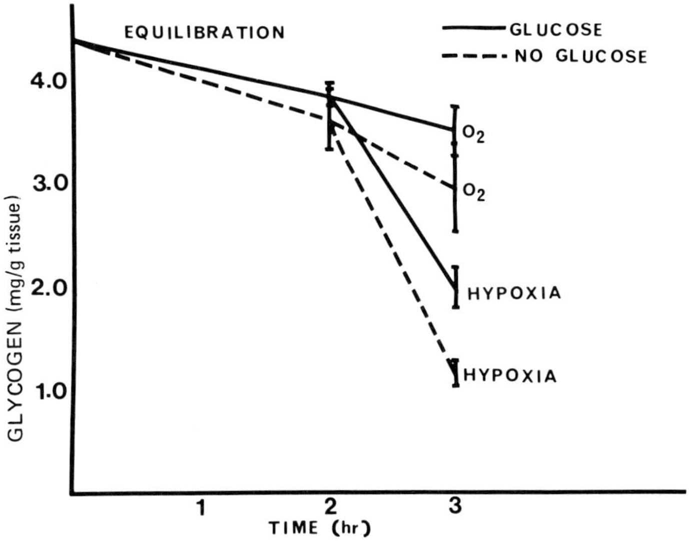


**FIGURE 30** Glycogen concentrations in canine tracheal smooth muscle. Means and standard errors are shown. (From Ref. [31].)

Our own meager data for glycolysis in canine tracheal smooth muscle are given below.

**Glycogen** Glycogen levels were measured in the normal, resting, fully equilibrated muscle held isometrically at its optimal length ($l_o$) at 37°C and bathed in Krebs-Henseleit medium containing 5 mM glucose. They were also measured during hypoxia. The results are shown in Figure 30 [82]. The levels of glycogen seen in the normal muscle are equivalent to values reported for other smooth muscles. On assaying muscle immediately after excision (and using freezing clamps), glycogen content is 4.2 mg/g wet weight of tissue. This falls by a small and statistically significant amount over the first hour. During this hour, the muscle is recovering slowly from the contracture which is always present at the time of dissection. This contracture is said to result from altered permeability to various ions which results in accumulation of increased $Na^+$ inside the cell and efflux of $K^+$. Both of these result in depolarization and development of contracture. With recovery, the ion concentrations are returned to normal levels, the contracture passes, and a mechanically steady state emerges. Presumably, the intense $Na^+$-$K^+$ pump activity is responsible, along with the contracture, for utilization of glycogen. Statistically, there is no significant reduction in tissue glycogen levels for the ensuing 2 hr.

Figure 30 also shows that with hypoxia, instituted at the end of the first hour, there is an increase in glycogenolysis. Omitting glucose from the bath does reduce glycogen levels further, but not by a great deal.

If glycogenolysis is increased by hypoxia, it is reasonable to suppose lactate production will be increased, because oxidative phosphorylation is probably not operative.

In Figure 31, the results of experiments akin to those just described are shown. We have reported these previously [101]. Tissue lactate is expressed per 100 g wet weight of tissue. The medium lactate is expressed as the equivalent amount eliminated into the bathing medium by 100 g of muscle. Note the 10-fold increase in value ordinate units. These data can also be expressed in molar concentrations. When this is done, the lactate gradient is from within the cell to without. From this figure, we conclude that glycolysis, by way of the lactate pathway, is increased considerably.

The next question that arose was whether, in hypoxia, the lactate pathway was able to produce enough ATP for the cells' various functions. To determine this, high-energy phosphate levels were measured [31]. The results are shown in Figure 32. Phosphocreatine (PC), and adenosine triphosphate (ATP) concentrations are similar to those reported for other smooth muscles. With hypoxia, con-

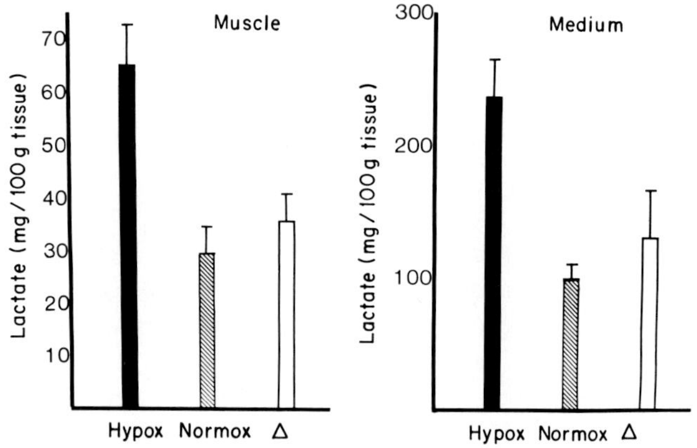


**FIGURE 31** Tissue and medium lactate levels for canine tracheal smooth muscle. Mean and standard errors are shown. (From Ref. [165]; reprinted, by permission, Elsevier/North Holland, Amsterdam.)

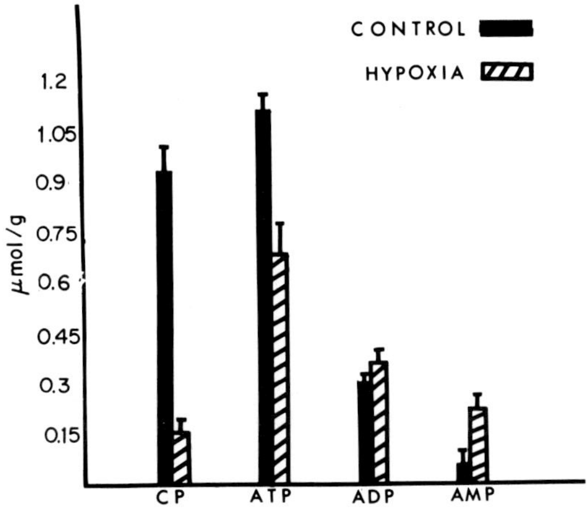


**FIGURE 32** High-energy phosphate levels in canine tracheal smooth muscle. Means and standard errors are shown. (From Ref. [31].)

siderable decreases are seen in both PC and ATP. The reduction in ATP is interesting since changes in it are almost impossible to demonstrate in skeletal muscle. The reason for this is that ATP in skeletal muscle is represented by a small pool turning over at a rapid rate. Levels of adenosine diphosphate (ADP) were unchanged while those for adenosine monophosphate (AMP) were increased. The increase in AMP concentration was less than expected and suggested that its deamination was occurring.

The glycogen, lactate, and high-energy phosphate data indicate that, in hypoxia, energy stores are diminished considerably. Whether this diminution is to levels critical enough to impair contractility is hard to say. It must be remembered, however, that the degree of hypoxia ($P_{O_2}$, 40 mmHg) in the bathing medium was not very severe, and it is conceivable that in clinical hypoxia, which may be more severe, the insult may be greater and result in impairment of mechanical function.

The reduction in ATP and PC levels suggests that the anaerobic glycogenolysis (evidenced by decreasing glycogen and increasing lactate levels) did not compensate adequately for the impairment in energy production, resulting from loss or impairment of mitochondrial function.

*The Role of Intracellular pH* The chief conclusion derived from the above data is that glycolysis is impaired. The obvious step to examine in this regard is that of the activity of phosphofructokinase (PFK), since it is rate limiting for the pathway. It is known, at least in vitro, that PFK works optimally at an alkaline pH [124]. The adicosis resulting from increased lactic acid production would then inhibit PFK. While this is a generally accepted argument it can be

**TABLE 9 $pH_i$ in Tracheal Smooth Muscle**

| | Normoxic resting | Hypoxic resting | Normoxic contracting | Hypoxic contracting | Reversibility normoxic contracting |
|---|---|---|---|---|---|
| Mean | 7.04 | 7.04 | 7.32 | 7.54 | 7.37 |
| ± SE | 0.01 | 0.02 | 0.01 | 0.01 | 0.01 |
| *N* | 10 | 10 | 10 | 10 | 10 |

accepted only after measurements confirm this. To this end, we measured intracellular pH ($pH_i$) employing the dimethyloxazolidine (DMO) method developed by Waddell and Butler [125]. Measurements were made in fully equilibrated, resting, control muscles set at optimal length, at 37°C. Measurements were also made in muscles similarly treated except that they were hypoxic ($P_{O_2}$ 40 mmHg in the bathing medium). In a third group, muscles were under control conditions but were stimulated electrically every 5 min for 2 hr for 15 sec (producing isometric tetani). In a fourth group, in addition to being stimulated, muscles were also hypoxic. The results are given in Table 9.

The pH of the bathing medium was 7.40 in all experiments. The interstitial cell fluid was assumed to be in equilibrium with the bulk of the medium in the bath. Hence, the bath pH was taken to be an accurate index of interstitial fluid pH. This assumption is absolutely crucial to the use of the DMO method in estimating $pH_i$. We have as yet been unable to verify this. If the assumption is incorrect then the validity of our data is questionable. However, the assumption we are making is the one that all workers in the field make.

The $pH_i$ of 7.04 obtained in the resting normoxic muscle is about the same as reported by other workers for striated muscle [126-129]. Hypoxia in the resting muscle does not affect $pH_i$ at all. Either the lactic acid being produced is rapidly extruded from the cell, or it is buffered. Lactate levels are increased threefold when measured in muscles under the same conditions.

Curiously enough, when the normoxic muscle is made to contract periodically, $pH_i$ increases to 7.32. This is in the opposite direction to that expected. Since tracheal smooth muscle is low in mitochondrial protein content, it relies more heavily on the glycogen-lactate pathway for energy production. The resultant increase in lactic acid should have produced, if anything, an acidosis. Even more interesting is the fact that when the hypoxic muscle is made to contract periodically, $pH_i$ increases further to 7.54. We have no data which could provide an explanation. Teleologically, alkalosis would be beneficial because it would ensure the maintenance of optimal pH conditions for PFK activity.

If one is permitted to speculate about this anomalous situation, then one recalls that Embden et al. [130], Meyerhof [131], and Parnas [132], had detected the presence of ammonia in muscle. Since glutamate dehydrogenase did not exist in muscle, glutamate as a source of ammonia was excluded. However, when Schmidt [133] demonstrated the presence of adenylate deaminase in muscle, it was postulated that ammonia was produced by the deamination of AMP.

Adenosine monophosphate breaks down to inosine monophosphate and ammonia. This was substantiated further by our finding that during hypoxia, for example, the amount of AMP detected in the muscle cell was less than expected from the change in levels of ATP and ADP. Obviously, this could be due to the deamination of AMP. Rosado et al. [134] demonstrated that the ammonia liberated could be detected in the cell for several hours and was not driven off from the cell in a few minutes. Hence, the nature of its production could be compatible with the prolonged buffering we find in the hypoxic, contracting muscles.

One other point is that since the reaction is irreversible, synthesis of AMP must be by means of some other reaction. Loewnstein [135] has reviewed this area and adduced evidence to show that the purine nucleotide cycle is involved in this process.

Finally, we would like to indicate once more that the validity of our conclusions is based on the validity of the assumptions inherent in the method. At the present time, we are developing a closed tip, recessed, pH-sensitive microelectrode to obtain $pH_i$ data which will serve as a cross check on the DMO data.

In concluding this section on carbohydrate metabolism, it is fair to say that, with respect to glycolysis, glycogenolysis, and oxidative phosphorylation, smooth and striated muscles are qualitatively similar. Smooth muscle differs in its greater dependance on the lactate pathway as an energy source.

### C. Fatty Acid Metabolism

Hardly any work has been done in smooth muscle with respect to the role of triglycerides and free fatty acids in supplying energy for contractile purposes. The major effort has been directed at studying atherosclerosis of the aorta [136,137]. As far as airway smooth muscle in particular is concerned, almost nothing has been done. The important question of whether airway smooth muscle, like cardiac muscle, uses fatty acid as a substrate in preference to carbohydrate has not been looked at. The only evidence in this regard that we are aware of is with respect to the pregnant uterus, where measurements during surgery revealed the respiratory quotient was 0.70 [111], which suggests that the uterus was preferentially utilizing lipids as an energy source. In arterial tissue in vitro [139], however, it has been shown that oxidation of glucose is not spared by palmitate.

On the other hand, Hashimoto and Dayton [136] suggest from their results that in arterial tissue the brisk oxidation of octanoate had a sparing effect on glucose oxidation. They felt that this may result from the inhibition of glycolysis by the decreased activity of phosphofructokinase [139] activity brought about by the elevation of the intracellular concentration of citrate [140]. The discrepancies in the glucose-sparing effect seem to be related to chain length, octanoate being almost completely oxidized to $CO_2$, whereas palmitate is oxidized to a lesser extent.

For canine tracheal smooth muscle itself, we have no explanatory data dealing with fatty acid metabolism. However, working with isolated mitochondria from this muscle, we have shown [25] that they can use palmityl-L-carnitine and acetyl-L-carnitine as substrates for oxidative phosphorylation. The data are given in Table 9.

### D. Contractile and Regulatory Proteins in Tracheal Smooth Muscle

Considerable research activity has developed in this area with respect to a variety of smooth muscles in the last few years. Much of this has been contributed by investigators of skeletal muscle proteins who are now turning to investigation of smooth muscle. The lure probably is that different mechanisms of contraction and their regulation await discovery, and, furthermore, these may shed some light on mechanisms imperfectly understood in skeletal muscle. Also, contractile proteins are being discovered in almost every type of cell in the body and their properties resemble those of smooth muscle proteins much more closely than those of striated muscle. Hence, study of smooth muscle contractile proteins may develop apace in the near future.

As far as we know, very little work has been done on contractile proteins from airway smooth muscle. We are aware only of work done by Sands and Meyer [141] and by ourselves [142]. Where necessary, reference will be made to data obtained from other smooth muscles.

#### *Contractile Proteins*

These have been isolated from bovine tracheal smooth muscle simply because it is impossible to obtain adequate amounts of this muscle from the dog (the model on which we have conducted all our biophysical and biochemical studies to date) for isolation of these proteins according to methods we are currently employing. Fortunately, Crouch and Kirkpatrick [143] have studied the mechanical properties of the bovine tracheal muscle. These resemble those of the canine and, hence, enable us to carry out studies of bovine tracheal contractile proteins and use these as reasonable models for the canine proteins.

The method we have used is an adaptation of techniques used for obtaining actomyosin from chicken gizzards [144], and platelets [145]. We have previously described this method [142]. It consists of extraction under high ionic strength conditions. Triton X-100 is used to remove membrane ATPases. Lowry's method [146] was used for measuring protein content and Gomori's method [147] for estimating phosphate. In the latter, monomethyl-paraaminophenol sulfate is used as the reducing agent. SDS gel electrophoresis was carried out using 5.6% acrylamide, according to the method of Fairbanks et al. [148]. Coomassie blue was employed for staining of proteins and a Joyce-Leobel densitometer to obtain densitometric patterns of the proteins.

One of the problems that confronted us was the low contractile protein yield. It was only when we used the combination of methods we have described above that we obtained average yields of 2.99 ± 0.3 mg (SE) of contractile proteins per gram of wet weight tissue. Low ionic strength extraction methods, such as those of Sparrow et al. [149], did not improve the yield. The RNA content of our preparations was 0.72 ± 0.04 $\mu$g (SE) per milligram of actomyosin. With respect to protein yield, published values usually range between 5 and 10 mg/g wet weight of muscle [150]. However, Sobieszek and Bremel [151] have developed a new technique for obtaining a myofibril-like preparation from vertebrate smooth muscle. Using this method, their actomyosin yields are 80 to 100 mg/g of wet gizzard muscle. Their striking success is probably due to better extraction of actin. Actin is notoriously more difficult to extract, perhaps because of attachment of the filaments to other proteins in the superstructure of the muscle cell. At any rate, we propose to employ their technique to see if we can improve our yields in the future.

### *Actomyosin Mg-ATPase Activity*

At low ionic strength, at 37°C, with a pH of 7.0 (using imidazole buffer) and a concentration of 2.5 mM ATP-Na, the highest values we obtained for Mg-ATPase activity were 50 nmol $mg^{-1}$ $min^{-1}$. Comparable values for intestinal smooth muscle are 20 nmol $mg^{-1}$ $min^{-1}$. Reported values for arterial actomyosin [152], and chicken gizzard actomyosin [144], are higher. The values we obtained for tracheal smooth muscle actomyosin ATPase activity are between 5 and 10% of the values for skeletal muscle. It must be pointed out that Sands (personal communication, 1978), while succeeding in obtaining an actomyosin preparation (from bovine tracheal muscle) which demonstrated ATPase activity, superprecipitation upon addition of ATP, and the solubility and the extraction characteristics of actomyosin, was unable to demonstrate any calcium sensitivity for his preparation.

Perhaps the lack of use of Triton X-100, which Driska and Hartshorne [144] recommend to ensure isolation of a preparation with calcium sensitivity, may account for Sand's results.

*Densitometry*

Figure 33 shows a densitometric trace. Peaks are seen which correspond to those of the myosin heavy chain, four bands in the 17 to 20 × $10^4$ molecular weight

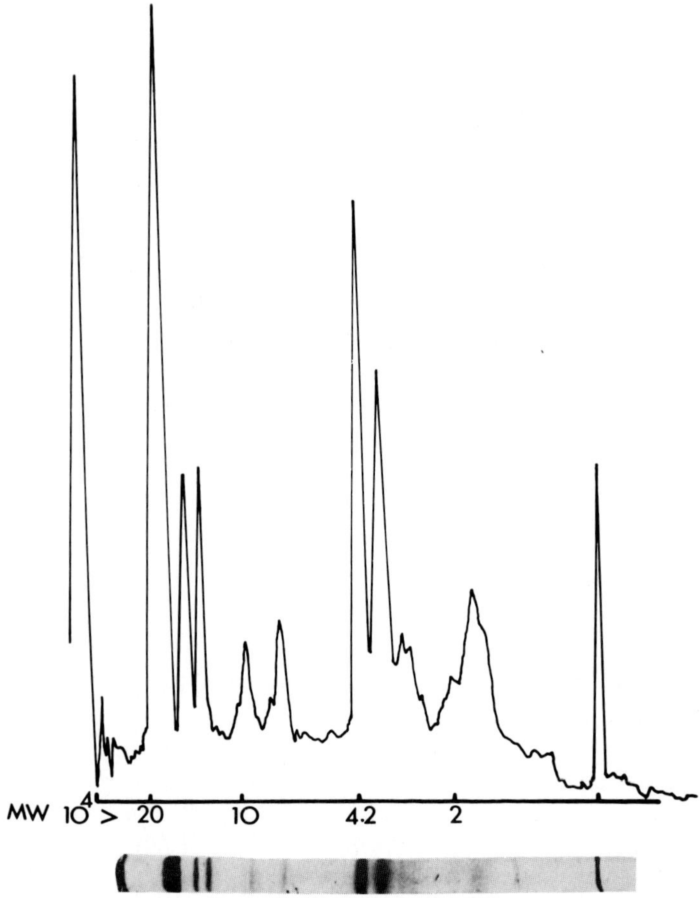


**FIGURE 33** Densitometric trace of SDS gel electrophoresis of a Ca-sensitive preparation from bovine tracheal smooth muscle: 5.6% acrylamide; pH 7.4; 28 μg of a Ca-sensitive preparation. (From Ref. [165]; reprinted, by permission, Elsevier/North Holland, Amsterdam.)

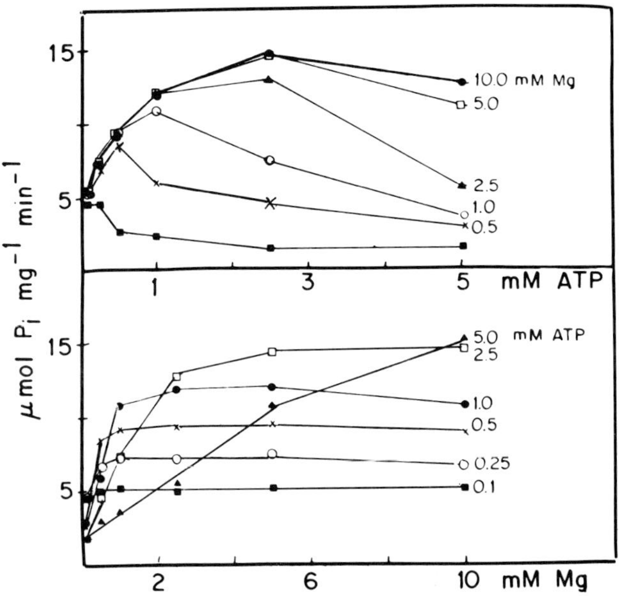


**FIGURE 34** Mg-ATPase assay of tracheal muscle actomyosin. Assay mixture contained imidazole buffer (pH 7.6), 20 mM; $CaCl_2$, $10^{-5}$ M; protein, 460 μg/ml; at 37°C. ATP and Mg were varied as shown. (From Ref. [142].)

range, actin, tropomyosin (so far we have only been able to find one chain in place of the two which are usually present in skeletal muscle), and two light chains. One is clearly seen here with a molecular weight close to 20,000. Another of even lower molecular weight has been found in other gels. Standard molecular weight markers were used in determining molecular weights of the muscle proteins.

Protein 34 reveals that the $Mg^{2+}$ and ATP requirements for ATPase activity differ from those of skeletal muscle actomyosin. The top panel shows that when ATP is present in excess of $Mg^{2+}$, activity is inhibited. However, the reverse is not true, as shown in the bottom panel. The apparent $K_m$ for ATP when $Mg^{2+}$ was present in equimolar amounts was 0.238 mM. This is similar to the values reported for arterial [152] and esophageal [153] smooth muscle actomyosin. The value for skeletal muscle myosin, which is $1.2 \times 10^{-6}$ M, is much lower. It is possible that structural differences between striated and smooth muscle actomyosins account for the differing affinities seen.

Figure 35 demonstrates that Mg-ATPase activity of tracheal smooth muscle actomyosin has only one pH optimum at 5.5. At this point, activity in the pres-

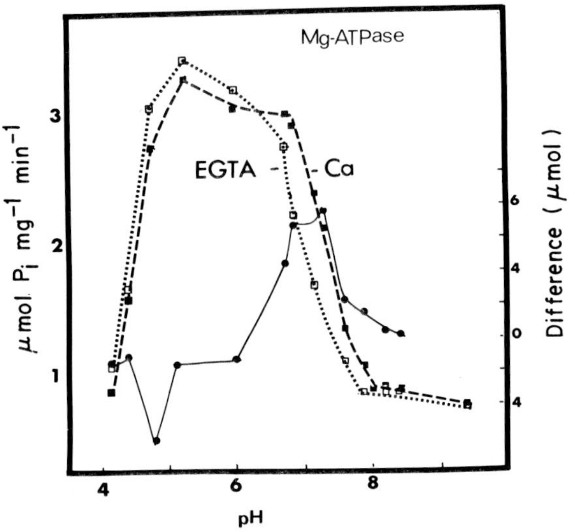


**FIGURE 35** Effect of pH on Mg-ATPase activity. Assay mixture contained 50 mM buffer; 10 mM $MgCl_2$ ; 2.5 mM ATP; actomyosin, 320 $\mu g/ml$; 2.5 mM Ca-EGTA; at 37°C. Acetate, imidazole, TRIS, and glycly-glycine buffers were used for the required pH. (From Ref. [142].)

ence of EGTA was greater than in the presence of $Ca^{2+}$. Calcium ion sensitivity, as determined from the increase in activation, was greatest at pH 7.0. This can be assessed by the difference between the EGTA and $Ca^{2+}$ curves. The difference is depicted by the solid line, which peaks at a pH of about 7.0. The pCa for half-maximal activation was decreased by 0.4 units for every half unit on the alkaline side and increased by the same amount on the acid side.

In the presence of 1 mM $Ca^{2+}$ and 0.2 M KCl, two pH optima were seen. This is akin to what is seen in skeletal muscle. The alkaline peak is the more prominent ot the two.

At low ionic strength the calcium requirement for actomyosin Mg-ATPase activity is depicted in Figure 36. The pCa for half-maximal activation in the presence of 10 mM $Mg^{2+}$ was found to be 6.5. Under these experimental conditions minimal ATPase activity was seen at a pCa of about $5 \times 10^{-8}$ M and maximal at $10^{-6}$ M.

### *Superprecipitation Studies*

These were carried out by monitoring turbidity changes at 600 nm in a Unicam SP 1800 spectrophotometer equipped with a temperature regulator. In Figure 37 the EGTA curve shows clearing, which results from the absence of $Ca^{2+}$. The +Ca curve demonstrates the requirement of this ion for superprecipitation in tracheal smooth muscle contractile proteins. These findings qualitatively confirm those for the Mg-ATPase studies.

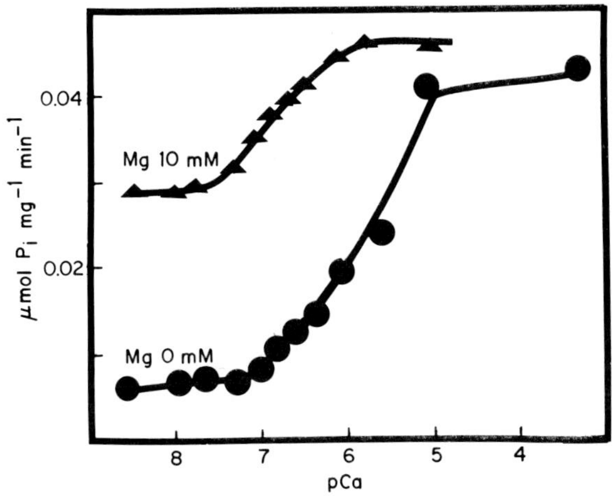


**FIGURE 36** Effect of Ca on Mg-ATPase activity. Assay mixture contained 20 mM imidazole buffer, pH 7.0, 2.5 mM ATP, 10 or 0 mM Mg, 2.5 mM Ca-EGTA buffer, and 350 μg/ml of actomyosin; at 37°C. (From Ref. [142].)

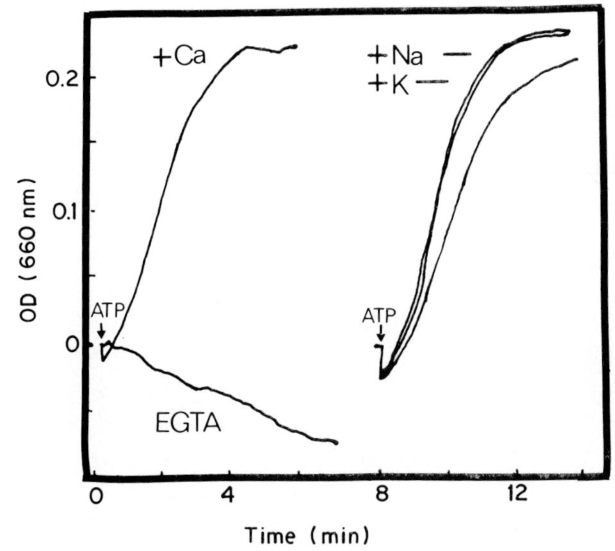


**FIGURE 37** Superprecipitation measured at 26°C. Assay mixture contained 20 mM imidazole buffer, pH 7.0; 10 mM $MgCl_2$; 2.5 mM ATP, to mg of protein per ml; and 2.5 mM Ca-EGTA buffer; 30 mM $K^+$ or 30 mM $Na^+$ were added as needed. The last curve on the right is a control.

The +Na and the +K curves in the figure reveal that these produce almost identical superprecipitation. In this regard, tracheal smooth muscle differs from arterial smooth muscles, in which Shibata and Hollander [152] have shown greater superprecipitation to $Na^+$ than to $K^+$.

### Effect of Hypoxia

We have shown in the past that hypoxia impairs contractility (leftward shift of the force-velocity curves with respect to control) in tracheal smooth muscle [79]. This is associated with a partial defect in oxidative energy production [114]. We have also studied the effect of hypoxia on energy utilization processes. In these studies, we determined the changes induced in Mg-ATPase activity of actomyosin isolated from hypoxic bovine tracheal smooth muscle. The contractile protein yields were the same in the control and hypoxic muscles. Mg-ATPase and Ca-ATPase activities were significantly lower in the actomyosin from hypoxic muscle.

### Regulatory Proteins

Again, as far as we are aware, only Sands and Mayer [141] have studied regulatory proteins in airway smooth muscle. They have noted the absence of a troponin regulatory system in bovine tracheal smooth muscle. Murphy et al. [154], Driska et al. [144], and Sobieszek and Bremel [151] have also reported similar findings in chicken gizzard proteins. Ebashi [155] and Carsten [27] were the only investigators to report that a troponin-like system constituted the regulatory proteins in smooth muscle. The consensus at this time seems to be that in smooth muscle the regulatory proteins do not belong to the troponin system and that calcium sensitivity of actomyosin ATPase activity is a property of the myosin molecule. In this, smooth muscle differs from skeletal and cardiac muscles and resembles molluscan muscles [156]. Driska and Hartshorne [144] suggest that the activity of gizzard actomyosin is regulated by a protein on the thin filaments with a subunit weight of about 130,000. However, they point out the possibility that myosin light chains may also function as part of the regulatory mechanism.

Interest has developed recently in recognizing tissue-specific substrates for a cyclic AMP-dependent protein kinase in different muscles. It is speculated that phosphorylation of the substrate (in all likelihood a regulatory protein) is related in some way to activation of regulation of actomyosin ATPase activity. The substrate has been termed the "P light chain" (molecular weight 18,000-20,000) by Frearson et al. [157] in both skeletal and smooth muscle myosins. For tracheal smooth muscle, similar findings have been reported by Sands and Mayer [141].

In recent unpublished studies of isolated tracheal smooth muscle from ovalbumen-sensitized pups, we have found that while $P_o$ (maximum isometric tetanic tension development) is unchanged when compared to controls, $V_{max}$, or the maximum velocity of shortening, is significantly increased. The only interpretation of this finding is that the properties of the actomyosin ATPase have changed. Since actomyosin ATPase activity basically resides in one light chain in the globular head of heavy meromyosin, further research in the area should be directed at isolating and characterizing this light chain and comparing it with the corresponding chain from the control muscle.

In summing up this section, we would like to point out that no work has been done regarding structural protein in airway smooth muscle. It is very likely that all the structural proteins already described for other smooth muscles (which are similar to those in striated muscle) are also present in airway smooth muscle.

In concluding this chapter on the airway smooth muscle, it is evident that much work remains to be done before one can say that the fundamental biophysics and biochemistry of this muscle have been elucidated to the same extent as in striated muscle. Hopefully, it is then that basic investigations into disorders of airway smooth muscle, such as one sees in human disease, can be meaningfully conducted.

## References

1. Bouhuys, A., *Lung Cells in Disease.* New York, North-Holland, 1977.
2. Lenfant, C., Nonrespiratory aspects of lung physiology, *Fed. Proc.,* **36**(13): 2651-2652 (1977).
3. Permutt, S., Physiological changes in the acute asthmatic attack. In *Asthma.* Edited by K. Frank Austen and L. M. Lichtenstein. New York, Academic, 1973, pp. 15-27.
4. Nadel, J. A., Neurophysiological aspects of asthma. In *Asthma.* Edited by K. Frank Austen and L. M. Lichenstein. New York, Academic, 1973, pp. 29-38.
5. Luschka, H., *Anatomie des Menschen, Bd. 1, Abt. 2.* Tubingen, 1963.
6. Suzuki, H., K. Morita, and H. Kuriyama, Innervation and properties of the smooth muscle of the dog trachea, *Jpn. J. Physiol.,* **26**:303-320 (1976).
7. Silva, D. G., and G. Ross, Ultrastructural and fluorescence histochemical studies on the innervation of the tracheobronchial muscle of normal cats and cats treated with 6-hydroxyodopamine, *J. Ultrastruct. Res.,* **47**:310-328 (1974).
8. Fay, F. S., P. H. Cooke, and P. G. Canaday, Contractile properties of isolated smooth muscle cells. In *Physiology of Smooth Muscle.* Edited by E. Bulbring and M. F. Shuba. New York, Raven, 1976, pp. 249-264.
9. Somlyo, A. P., and A. V. Somlyo, Ultrastructure of smooth muscle. In *Methods in Pharmacology.* Edited by E. E. Daniel and D. M. Paton. New York, Plenum, 1975, pp. 3-45.

10. Langer, G. A., and J. S. Frank, Calcium exchange in cultured cardiac cells. In *Developmental and Physiological Correlates of Cardiac Muscle.* Edited by M. Lieberman and T. Sano. New York, Raven, 1975, pp. 117-126.
11. Hajdu, S., and E. J. Leonard, Minireview: A calcium transport system for mammalian cells, *Life Sci.,* **17**:1527-1534 (1976).
12. Burnstock, G., Structure of smooth muscle and its innervation. In *Smooth Muscle.* Edited by E. Bulbring, A. F. Brading, A. N. Jones, and T. Tomita. London, Edward Arnold, 1970, pp. 1-69.
13. Oosaki, T., and S. Ishii, Junctional structure of smooth muscle cells. The ultrastructure of the regions of junction between smooth muscle cells in the rat intestine, *J. Ultrastruct. Res.,* **10**:567-577 (1964).
14. Nagasawa, J., and T. Suzuki, Electron microscopic study of the cellular interrelationships in the smooth muscle, *Tohoku J. Exp. Med.,* **91**:299-313 (1967).
15. Sjostrand, F. S., and L. G. Elfvin, The layered asymmetric structure of the plasma membrane in the exocrine pancreas cells of the cat, *J. Ultrastruct. Res.,* 7:504-536 (1962).
16. Farquhar, M. G., and G. E. Palade, Junctional complexes in various epithelia, *J. Cell Biol.,* **17**:375-412 (1963).
17. Gabella, G., Fine structure of smooth muscle, *Philos. Trans. R. Soc. Lond. [Biol.],* **265**:7-16 (1973).
18. Pease, D. C., and S. Molinari, Electron microscopy of muscular arteries; pial vessels of the cat and monkey, *J. Ultrastruct. Res.,* **3**:447-468 (1960).
19. Devine, C. E., and A. P. Somlyo, Thick filaments in vascular smooth muscle, *J. Cell. Biol.,* **49**:636-649 (1971).
20. Somlyo, A. P., J. Vallieres, R. E. Garfield, H. Shuman, A. Scarpa, and A. V. Somlyo, Calcium compartmentatization in vascular smooth muscle: Electron probe analysis and studies on isolated mitochondria. In *The Biochemistry of Smooth Muscle.* Edited by N. L. Stephens. Baltimore, University Park Press, 1977, pp. 563-584.
21. Cooke, P. H., and F. S. Fay, Thick filaments in contracted and relaxed mammalian smooth muscle cells, *Exp. Cell. Res.,* **71**:265-272 (1972).
22. Nonomura, Y., and S. Ebashi, Isolation and identification of smooth muscle contractile proteins. In *Methods in Pharmacology.* Edited by E. E. Daniel and D. M. Paton. New York, Plenum, 1975, pp. 141-162.
23. Lazarides, E., and B. D. Hubbard, Immunological characterization of the subunit of the 100 Å filaments from the muscle cells, *Proc. Natl. Acad. Sci. USA,* **73**:4344-4347 (1976).
24. Schollmayer, J. S., D. E. Boll, R. M. Robson, and M. H. Stormer, Localization of actinin and tropomyosin in different muscles, *J. Cell Biol.,* **59**:306a (1973).
25. Stephens, N. L., and K. Wrogemann, Oxidative phosphorylation in smooth muscle, *Am. J. Physiol.,* **219**:1796-1801 (1970).
26. Hackenbrock, C. R., Ultrastructurally linked basis for metabolically linked mechanical activity in mitochondria. I. Reversible ultrastructural changes

with change in metabolic steady state in isolated liver mitochondria, *J. Cell Biol.,* **30**:269-297 (1966).

27. Carsten, M. E., Uterine smooth muscle: Troponin, *Arch. Biochem.,* **147**: 353-357 (1971).
28. Hurwitz, L., D. F. Fitzpatrick, G. Debbas, and E. S. Landon, Localization of calcium pump activity in smooth muscle, *Science,* **179**:384-386 (1973).
29. De Duve, C., The participation of lysosomes in the transformation of smooth muscle cells to foamy cells in the aorta of cholesterol fed rabbits, *Acta Cardiol.,* Suppl., **20**:9 (1974).
30. Paul, R. J., J. W. Peterson, and S. R. Caplan, Oxygen consumption rate in vascular smooth muscle: Relation to isometric tension, *Biochim. Biophys. Acta,* **305**:476-480 (1973).
31. Kroeger, E. A., and N. L. Stephens, Effect of hypoxia on energy and calcium metabolism in airway smooth muscle, *Am. J. Physiol.,* **220**(5):1199-1204 (1971).
32. Stephens, N. L., and E. A. Kroeger, Effect of hypoxia in airway smooth muscle mechanics and electrophysiology, *J. Appl. Physiol.,* **28**:630-638 (1970).
33. Yamauchi, A., Electronmicroscopic studies on the autonomic neuromuscular junction in the taenia coli of the guinea-pig, *Acta Anat. Nippon,* **39**: 22-38 (1964).
34. Rogers, D. C., Comparative electronmicroscopy of smooth muscle and its innervation. Ph.D. Thesis, Zoology Department, University of Melbourne, 1964.
35. Somlyo, A. P., C. E. Devine, A. V. Somlyo, and R. V. Rice, Filament organization in vertebrate smooth muscle, *Philos. Trans. R. Soc. [Biol.],* **265**:233-229 (1973).
36. Yamauchi, A., and G. Burnstock, Post-natal development of smooth muscle cells in the mouse vas deferens. A fine structural study, *J. Anat.,* **104**:1-5 (1969).
37. Gansler, H., Phasenkontrast und electronenmikros-kopische. Untersuchungen zum morphologie und funktion der glatten muskulatur, *Zellforsch Mikrosk. Anat.,* **52**:60-92 (1960).
38. Conti, G., B. Haenni, L. Laszt, and C. H. Rouiller, Structure et ultrastructure de la cellule musculaire lisse de paroi carotidienne a l'état de repos et a l'état de contraction, *Angiologica,* **1**:119-140 (1964).
39. Choi, J. K., Fine structure of the smooth muscle of the chicken's gizzard. In *Electron Microscopy.* Proceedings of the Fifth International Congress for Electron Microscopy, Vol. 2. Edited by S. S. Breese. New York, Academic, 1962, pp. M-9.
40. Needham, D. M., and C. F. Shoenberg, Proteins of the contractile mechanism of mammalian smooth muscle and their possible location in the cell, *Proc. R. Soc. B,* **160**:517-522 (1964).
41. Small, J. V., The contractile apparatus of the smooth muscle cells: Structure and composition. In *The Biochemistry of Smooth Muscle.* Edited by N. L. Stephens. Baltimore, University Park Press, 1977, pp. 379-441.

42. Sobieszek, A., Vertebrate smooth muscle myosin. Enzymatic and structural properties. In *The Biochemistry of Smooth Muscle.* Edited by N. L. Stephens. Baltimore, University Park Press, 1977, pp. 413-433.
43. Rice, R. V., G. M. McManus, C. E. Devine, and A. P. Somlyo, A regular organization of thick filaments in mammalian smooth muscle, *Nature New Biol.,* **231**:242-243 (1971).
44. Lowy, J., F. R. Poulsen, and P. J. Vibert, Myosin filaments in vertebrate smooth muscle, *Nature,* **225**:1053-1054 (1970).
45. Lowy, J., P. J. Vibert, J. C. Haselgrove, and F. R. Poulsen, The structure of the myosin elements in vertebrate smooth muscle, *Proc. R. Soc. Lond. B,* **265**:191-196 (1973).
46. Somlyo, A. V., C. E. Devine, A. V. Somlyo, and R. V. Rice, Filament organization in vertebrate smooth muscle, *Philos. Trans. R. Soc. [Biol.],* **265**:223-229 (1973).
47. Kapanci, Y., P. M. Costabella, and G. Gabbiani, Location and function of contractile interstitial cells of the lungs. In *Lung Cells in Disease.* Edited by A. Bouhuys. Amsterdam, Elsevier/North Holland, 1977, pp. 69-84.
48. von Hayek, H., *The Human Lung.* New York, Hafner, 1960, pp. 127-226.
49. Baltisberger, W., Uber die glatte muskulatur der menschliehen lunge, *Anatomy,* **61**:249-282 (1921).
50. Widdicombe, J. G., and J. A. Nadel, Airway volume, airway resistance and work force of breathing: Theory, *J. Appl. Physiol.,* **18**:863-868 (1963).
51. Olsen, C. R., H. J. H. Colebatch, P. E. Mebel, J. A. Nadel, and N. C. Staub, Motor control of pulmonary airways studied by nerve stimulation, *J. Appl. Physiol.,* **20**:202-208 (1965).
52. Macklem, P., and L. A. Engel, The physiological role of airways smooth muscle constriction, *Postgrad. Med. J.* (Suppl. 1), **51**:45-50 (1975).
53. Hakansson, C. H., and N. G. Toremalm, Studies on the physiology of the trachea. V. Histology and mechanical activity of the smooth muscles, *Ann. Otol. Rhinol. Laryngol.,* **77**(2):255-263 (1968).
54. Krahl, V. E., Anatomy of the mammalian lung. In *Handbook of Physiology, Sec. 3, Respiration, Vol. I.* Edited by W. O. Fenn and H. Rahn. Washington, D.C., American Physiological Soc., 1964, pp. 213-284.
55. Larsell, O., and R. S. Dow, Innervation of the human lung, *Am. J. Anat.,* **52**:125-146 (1933).
56. Hebb, C., Motor innervation of the pulmonary blood vessels of mammals. In *The Pulmonary Circulation and Interstitial Spaces.* Edited by A. P. Fishman and H. H. Heent. Chicago, University of Chicago Press, 1969, pp. 1-52.
57. Widdicombe, J. G., The regulation of bronchial calibre. In *Advances in Respiratory Physiology.* Edited by C. G. Caro. London, Edward Arnold, 1966, pp. 48-82.
58. Karczewski, N., and J. G. Widdicombe, The role of the vagus nerve in the respiratory and circulatory reactions to anaphylaxis in rabbits, *J. Physiol. (Lond.),* **201**:293-304 (1969).
59. Coburn, R. F., and T. Tomita, Evidence for nonadrenergic inhibitory

nerves in the guinea pig trachealis muscle, *Am. J. Physiol.*, **224**:1072-1080 (1973).

60. Cameron, A. R., and C. T. Kirkpatrick, The distribution of autonomic nerves within the smooth muscle layer of the bovine trachea, *J. Physiol. (Lond.)*, **259**:48P (1976).

61. Mann, S. P., Innervation of mammalian bronchial smooth muscle: Localization of catecholamines and cholinesterases, *Histochem. J.*, **3**:319-331 (1971).

62. Golla, F. L., and W. L. Symes, The reversible action of adrenaline and some kindred drugs in the bronchioles, *J. Pharmacol.*, **5**:87-103 (1913).

63. Daly, I. de B., and C. Hebb, *Pulmonary and Bronchial Vascular Systems.* London, Edward Arnold, 1966.

64. Richardson, J. B., and J. Beland, Nonadrenergic inhibitory system in human airways, *J. Appl. Physiol.*, **41**:764-771 (1976).

65. Akasaka, K., K. Konno, Y. Ono, S. Mue, C. Abe, M. Kumagai, and T. Tse, A new electrode for electromyographic study of bronchial smooth muscle, *Tokoku J. Exp. Med.*, **117**:49-54 (1975).

66. Akasaka, K., K. Konno, Y. Ono, S. Mue, C. Abe, M. Kumagai, and T. Tse, Electromyographic study of bronchial smooth muscle in bronchial asthma, *Tokoku J. Exp. Med.*, **117**:55-59 (1975).

67. Bose, R., D. Bose, and I. R. Innes, Induction of rhythmicity in multiunit smooth muscle in glucose free media, *Fed. Proc.*, **35**:77 (1976).

68. Kirkpatrick, C. H., Excitation and contraction in bovine tracheal smooth muscle, *J. Physiol. (Lond.)*, **244**:263-281 (1975).

69. Bahler, A. S., Series elastic components of mammalian skeletal muscle, *Am. J. Physiol.*, **213**:1560-1564 (1967).

70. Burnstock, G., and C. L. Prosser, Responses of smooth muscles to quick stretch: Relation of stretch to conduction, *Am. J. Physiol.*, **198**:921-925 (1960).

71. Burnstock, G., and C. L. Prosser, Conduction in smooth muscle comparative electrical properties, *Am. J. Physiol.*, **199**:533-559 (1960).

72. Prosser, C. L., G. Burnstock, and J. Kahn, Conduction in smooth muscle: Comparative structural properties, *Am. J. Physiol.*, **199**:545-552 (1960).

73. Barr, L., W. Bergen, and M. M. Dewey, Electrical transmission at the nexus between smooth muscle cells, *J. Gen. Physiol.*, **51**:347-368 (1968).

74. Daniel, E. E., V. L. Daniel, G. Duchon, R. E. Garfield, M. Nicholas, S. K. Malhotra, and M. Oki, Is the nexus necessary for cell-to-cell coupling of smooth muscle? *J. Membr. Biol.*, **28**:207-239 (1976).

75. Kroeger, E. A., and N. L. Stephens, Effect of tetraethylammonium on tonic airway smooth muscle: Initiation of phasic electrical activity, *Am. J. Physiol.*, **228**:633-663 (1975).

76. Stephens, N. L., E. A. Kroeger, and U. Kromer, Induction of myogenic response in tonic airway smooth muscle by tetraethylammonium, *Am. J. Physiol.*, **228**:628-632 (1975).

77. Tomita, T., Electrical properties of mammalian smooth muscle. In *Smooth*

*Muscle.* Edited by E. Bulbring, A. F. Brading, A. W. Jones, and T. Tomita. London, Edward Arnold, 1970, pp. 197-243.
78. Kirk, J. E., *Enzymes of the Arterial Wall.* New York, Academic, 1969, pp. 1-494.
79. Stephens, N. L., Effect of hypoxia on contractile and series elastic components of smooth muscle, *Am. J. Physiol.,* **224**(2):318-321 (1973).
80. Stephens, N. L., Physical properties of contractile systems. In *Methods in Pharmacology,* Vol. 3, *Smooth Muscle.* Edited by E. E. Daniel and D. M. Paton. New York, Plenum, 1975, pp. 265-296.
81. Sonnenblick, E. H., Force-velocity relations in mammalian heart muscle, *Am. J. Physiol.,* **202**:931-939 (1962).
82. Huxley, A. F., and A. M. Gordon, Striation patterns in active and passive shortening of muscle, *Nature (Lond.),* **193**:280-281 (1962).
83. Huxley, A. F., Muscle structure and theories of contraction, *Prog. Biophys. Chem.,* **7**:255-318 (1957).
84. Taylor, S. R., Decreased activation in skeletal muscle fibers at short lengths. In *The Physiological Basis of Starling's Law of the Heart,* Ciba Symposium 24 (New Series). Edited by R. Porter and D. W. Fitzsimons. London, Elsevier/Excerpta Medica-North Holland, 1974, pp. 93-116.
85. Zebe, E., W. Meinrenken, and J. C. Ruegg, Superkontraktion glycerinextramerter asynchroner insektenmuskeln in gegenwart von ITP, *Z. Zellforsch.,* **87**:603-621 (1968).
86. Matsumoto, Y., and B. C. Abbott, Folding muscle fibers of the *Goldfingia gouldii, Biochem. Physiol.,* **26**:927-936 (1968).
87. Buchtal, F., and E. Kaiser, Factors determining the tension development in skeletal muscle, *Acta Physiol. Scand.,* **8**:38-74 (1944).
88. Burton, A. C., Physical principles of circulation phenomena: The physical equilibrium of the heart and wood vessels. In *Handbook of Physiology Circulation,* Set 2, Vol. 1. Washington, D.C., American Physiology Soc., 1962, pp. 85-106.
89. Abbott, B. C., and D. R. Wilke, The relation between velocity of shortening and the length tension curve of skeletal muscle, *J. Physiol. (Lond.),* **120**: 214-223 (1953).
90. Rosenblueth, A., J. Alanis, and R. Rubio, A comparative study of the isometric and isotonic contractions of striated muscles, *Arch. Int. Physiol. Biochem.,* **66**:330-353 (1958).
91. Huxley, A. F., and Simmons, R. N., Proposed mechanism of force generation in striated muscle, *Nature (Lond.),* **233**:533-538 (1971).
92. Ford, L. E., and R. Forman, Tetanized cardiac muscle. In *The Physiological Basis of Starling's Law of the Heart,* Ciba Foundation Symposium 24 (New Series). Edited by R. Porter and D. N. Fitzsomons. London, Elsevier/Excerpta Medica/North-Holland, 1974, pp. 137-154.
93. Stephens, N. L., E. A. Kroeger, and J. A. Mehta, Force-velocity characteristics of respiratory airway smooth muscle, *J. Appl. Physiol.,* **26**:685-692 (1969).

94. Hill, A. V., The heat of shortening and the dynamic constants of muscle, *Proc. R. Soc. Lond. B,* **126**:136-195 (1938-39).
95. Hill, A. V., The effect of load on the heats of shortening of muscle, *Proc. R. Soc. Lond. B,* **159**:297-318 (1964).
96. Woledge, R. C., The energetics of tortoise muscle, *J. Physiol. (Lond.),* **1973**:685-707 (1968).
97. Barany, M., ATPase activity of myosin correlated with speed of muscle shortening, *J. Gen. Physiol.,* **50**:197 (1967).
98. Stephens, N. L., R. W. Mitchell, U. Kromer, and L. A. Antonissen, A study of asthma. Alterations in airway smooth muscle contractility, Part 2, *Am. Rev. Respir. Dis.,* **115**(4):75 (1977).
99. Hill, A. V., The series elastic component of muscle, *Proc. R. Soc. Lond. B,* **137**:272-280 (1956).
100. Stephens, N. L., and U. Kromer, Series elastic component of tracheal smooth muscle, *Am. J. Physiol.,* **220**:1890-1895 (1971).
101. Stephens, N. L., E. A. Kroeger, and W. Loh, Intracellular pH in hypoxia smooth muscle, *Am. J. Physiol.,* **232**:E330-E335 (1977).
102. Gasser, H. S., and A. V. Hill, The dynamics of muscular contraction, *Proc. R. Soc. B,* **96**:398-437 (1924).
103. Paul, R. J., J. W. Peterson, and S. R. Caplan, A nonequilibrium thermodynamic description of vascular smooth muscle mechanochemistry. I. The rate of oxygen consumption: A measure of the driving chemical reaction, *J. Mechanochem. Cell. Motil.,* **3**(1):19-32 (1974).
104. Lundholm, L., and E. Mohme-Lundholm, Energetics of isometric and isotonic contraction in isolated vascular smooth muscle under anaerobic conditions, *Acta Physiol. Scand.,* **64**:274-282 (1965).
105. Mohme-Lundholm, E., Effect of adrenaline, nor-adrenaline, isopropylnoradrenaline and ephedriae on tone and lactic acid formation in bovine tracheal muscle, *Acta Physiol. Scand.,* **37**:1-4 (1956).
106. Stephens, N. L., and C. M. Skoog, Tracheal smooth muscle and rate of oxygen uptake, *Am. J. Physiol.,* **226**:1462-1467 (1974).
107. Woledge, R. C., The thermoelastic effect of change of tension in active muscle, *J. Physiol. (Lond.),* **155**:187-208 (1968).
108. Clinch, N. F., On the increase in rate of heat production caused by stretch in frog's skeletal muscle, *J. Physiol. (Lond.),* **196**:397-414 (1968).
109. Pantesco, V., E. Kempf, P. Mendel, and R. Fontaine, Studies metaboliques comparees des parois arterielles et veineuse chez les bevides. Leurs variations au cours du vieillissement, *Pathol. Biol. Sem. Hop.,* **10**:1301-1306 (1962).
110. Chance, B., and B. Hagihara, Direct spectroscopic measurements of interaction of compounds of the respiratory chain with ATP, ADP, phosphate and uncoupling agents, *Proceedings of the Fifth International Congress on Biochemistry* held in Moscow, Vol. 5, 1973, pp. 3-37.
111. Beatty, C. H., G. M. Barsinger, and R. M. Bocek, Carbohydrate metabo-

lism of myometrium from the pregnant rhesus monkey, *J. Reprod. Fert.*, **19**:443-454 (1969).
112. Ernster, L., and K. Nordenbrand, Skeletal muscle mitochondria, *Methods Enzymol.*, **10**:86-94 (1967).
113. Lehninger, A., The transfer of energy in oxidative phosphorylation, *Bull. Soc. Chim. Biol. (Paris)*, **46**:1555-1575 (1964).
114. Stephens, N. L., and J. Vogel, Oxidative phosphorylation in hypoxic airway smooth muscle, *Can. J. Physiol. Pharmacol.*, **52**:84-89 (1974).
115. Zemplenyi, T., J. Hladovec, and O. Mrhova, Vascular changes accompanying the induction of experimental atherosclerosis. I. Rats fed Hartroft's diet, *J. Atheroscler. Res.*, **5**:540-547 (1965).
116. Morrison, A. D., R. S. Clements, Jr., and A. I. Winegrad, Effects of elevated glucose concentrations on the metabolism of the aortic wall, *J. Clin. Invest.*, **51**:3114-3123 (1972).
117. Mandel, P., and E. Kempf, The pentose phosphate pathway in the degradation of glucose by aortic tissue, *J. Atheroscler. Res.*, **3**:233-236 (1963).
118. Clements, R. S., A. D. Morrison, and A. I. Winegrad, Polyol pathway in aorta: Regulation by hormones, *Science*, **166**:1007-1008 (1969).
119. Arnqvist, H. J., Glucose transport and metabolism in smooth muscle: Action of insulin and diabetes. In *The Biochemistry of Smooth Muscle.* Edited by N. L. Stephens. Baltimore, University Park Press, 1977, pp. 127-158.
120. Bihler, I., P. C. Sawh, and J. Elbrink, Membrane transport of sugars in smooth muscle: Its relationship to carbohydrate metabolism and its regulation by physiological and pharmacological factors. In *The Biochemistry of Smooth Muscle.* Edited by N. L. Stephens. Baltimore, University Park Press, 1977, pp. 113-126.
121. Lundholm, L., and E. Mohme-Lundholm, The carbohydrate metabolism and tone of smooth muscle, *Acta Pharmacol. Toxicol.*, **16**:374-388 (1960).
122. Beviz, A., L. Lundholm, E. Mohme-Lundholm, and N. Vamos, Hydrolysis of ATP and CP in isometric contraction of vascular smooth muscle, *Acta Physiol. Scand.*, **65**:268-272 (1965).
123. Mohme-Lundholm, E., Smooth muscle phosphorylase and enzymes affecting its activity, *Acta Physiol. Scand.*, **59**:74-84 (1963).
124. Michio, U., A role of phosphofructokinase in pH-dependent regulation of glycolysis, *Biochim. Biophys. Acta*, **124**:310-322 (1966).
125. Waddell, W. J., and T. C. Butler, Calculation of intracellular pH from the distribution of 5,5-dimethyl-2,4-oxazolidine-dion (DMO). Application to skeletal muscle of the dog, *J. Clin. Invest.*, **38**:720-729 (1959).
126. Adler, S., A. Roy, and A. S. Relman, Intracellular acid-base regulation. I. The response of muscle cell to changes in $CO_2$ tension and extracellular bicarbonate concentration, *J. Clin. Invest.*, **44**:8-20 (1965).
127. Heisler, N., and J. Piiper, Determination of intracellular buffering properties in rat diaphragm muscle, *Am. J. Physiol.*, **222**:747-753 (1972).

128. Izutsu, K. I., Intracellular pH, H-ion flux and H-ion permeability coefficient in bull frog toe muscle, *J. Physiol. (Lond.)*, **221**:15-27 (1972).
129. Lavallee, M., Intracellular pH of rat atrial muscle fibers measured by glass micropipette electrodes, *Circ. Res.*, **15**:185-193 (1969).
130. Embden, G., M. Carsten, and H. Schumacher, Über die bedeutung der adenylsaure für die Muskelfunktion. 4. Sparling und wideraufbau der ammonia K-bildenden substanz bei der muskettätigkeir, *A. Physiol. Chem.*, **179**:186-225 (1928).
131. Meyerhof, O., Die chemischen vorgange in muskel und ihr zusammenhand mit arbeitsleistung und wasmebildung. In *Physiologie der Pflanzen und der Tiere.* Berlin, Springer, 1930.
132. Parnas, J. K., Ammonia formation in muscle and its source, *Am. J. Physiol.*, **90**:467 (1929).
133. Schmidt, G., Uber gementative desaminierung im muskel, *Z. Physiol. Chem.*, **179**:243-282 (1928).
134. Rosado, A., G. Flores, J. Mora, and G. Sobirn, Distribution of an ammonia load in the normal rat, *Am. J. Physiol.*, **203**:37-42 (1962).
135. Loewenstein, J. M., Ammonia production in muscle and other tissues. The purine nucleotide cycle, *Physiol. Rev.*, **52**(2):382-412 (1972).
136. Hashimoto, S., and S. Dayton, Fatty acid metabolism of normal aortic tissue and its alteration induced by atherosclerosis. In *The Biochemistry of Smooth Muscle.* Edited by N. L. Stephens. Baltimore, University Park Press, 1977, pp. 219-240.
137. Stein, Y., and O. Stein, Incorporation of fatty acids into lipids by aortic slices of rabbits, dogs, rats, baboons, *J. Atheroscler.*, **2**:400-412 (1962).
138. Winegrad, A. I., S. Yalein, and P. D. Mulcahy, Alterations in aortic metabolism in diabetes. In *On the Nature and Treatment of Diabetes.* Edited by B. S. Leibel and G. A. Wrenshall. Amsterdam, Excerpta Medica Foundation, 1965, pp. 452-462.
139. Newsholme, E. A., P. J. Randle, and K. L. Manchester, Inhibition of the phosphofructokinase reaction in perfused rat heart by respiration of ketone bodies, fatty acid and pyruvate, *Nature (Lond.)*, **193**:270-271 (1962).
140. Parmeggiani, A., and R. H. Bowman, Regulation of phosphofructokinase activity by citrate in normal and diabetic muscle, *Biochem. Biophys. Res. Commun.*, **12**:268-273 (1963).
141. Sands, H., and T. A. Meyer, Phosphorylation of muscle proteins by cyclic adenosine 3,5′-monophosphate-dependent protein kinase from muscle, *Biochim. Biophys. Acta*, **321**:489-495 (1973).
142. Bose, R., and N. L. Stephens, Mechanism of action of hypoxia in smooth muscle: Role of contractile proteins. In *The Biochemistry of Smooth Muscle.* Edited by N. L. Stephens. Baltimore, University Park Press, 1977, pp. 499-512.
143. Crouch, C. M., and C. H. Kirkpatrick, Smooth muscle from respiratory tract: Effects of altered gas tensions, *Irish J. Med. Sci.*, **144**:157-165 (1975).

144. Driska, S., and D. J. Hartshorne, The contractile proteins of smooth muscle. Properties and components of a Ca-sensitive actomyosin from chicken gizzard, *Arch. Biochem. Biophys.*, **167**:203-212 (1975).
145. Hanson, J. P., D. I. Repke, A. M. Katz, and L. M. Aledort, Calcium in control of platelet thrombosthenin ATPase activity, *Biochim. Piophys. Acta,* **344**:382-389 (1973).
146. Lowry, O. H., N. J. Rosebrough, A. L. Farr, and R. J. Randall, Protein measurement with the Folin reagents, *J. Biol. Chem.*, **193**:265-275 (1951).
147. Gomori, C. J., A modification of the colorimetric phosphorus determination for use with the photoelectric colorimeter, *J. Lab. Clin. Med.*, **27**: 955-960 (1941).
148. Fairbanks, G., T. L. Steck, and D. F. H. Wallach, Electrophoretic analysis of the major polypeptide of the human erythrocyte membrane, *Biochemistry,* **10**:2606-2617 (1971).
149. Sparrow, M. P., L. C. Maxwell, J. C. Ruegg, and D. F. Bohr, Preparation and properties of a calcium sensitive actinomyosin from arteries, *Am. J. Physiol.,* **219**:1366-1372 (1970).
150. Needham, D. M., *Machina Carnis.* Cambridge, England, The University Press, 1971, p. 62.
151. Sobieszek, A., and R. D. Bremel, Preparation and properties of vertebrate smooth muscle myofibrils and actomyosin, *Eur. J. Biochem.*, **55**:49-60 (1975).
152. Shibata, N., and W. Hollander, Biochemical and Morphological characteristics of arterial actomyosin, *Exp. Mol. Pathol.,* **20**:313-328 (1974).
153. Tonomura, T., and A. T. Saske, Some observations on contractile proteins from smooth muscle of oesphagus, *Enzymolgia,* **18**:111-119 (1957).
154. Murphy, R. A., and J. Megerman, Protein interactions in the contractile system of vertebrate smooth muscle. In *The Biochemistry of Smooth Muscle.* Edited by N. L. Stephens. Baltimore, University Park Press, 1977, pp. 398-473.
155. Ebashi, S., T. Toy-oka, and Y. Nonomura, Gizzard troponin. In *The Biochemistry of Smooth Muscle.* Edited by N. L. Stephens. Baltimore, University Park Press, 1977, pp. 551-556.
156. Kendrick-Jones, J., W. Lehman, and A. G. Szent-Gyorgyi, Regulation in molluscan muscle, *J. Mol. Biol.,* **54**:313-326 (1970).
157. Frearson, N., B. W. W. Focant, and S. V. Perry, Phosphorylation of a light chain component of myosin from smooth muscle, *FEBS Lett.,* **63**: 17-32 (1976).
158. Sonnenblick, E. H., Series elastic and contractile elements in heart muscle: Changes in muscle length, *Am. J. Physiol.,* **207**:1330-1338 (1964).
159. Meiss, R. A., Some mechanical properties of cat intestinal muscle, *Am. J. Physiol.,* **220**:2000-2007 (1971).
160. Aberg, A. K. G., The series elasticity of active taenia coli in vitro, *Acta Physiol. Scand.,* **69**:348-364 (1967).

161. Herlihy, J. T., and R. A. Murphy, Force-velocity and series elastic characteristics of smooth muscle from the hog carotid artery, *Circ. Res.,* **34**: 461-466 (1974).
162. Johansson, B., Active state in the smooth muscle of the rat portal vein in relation to electrical activity and isometric force, *Circ. Res.,* **32**:246-258 (1973).
163. Stephens, N. L., R. Cardinal, and B. Simmons, Mechanical properties of tracheal smooth muscle: Effects of temperature, *Am. J. Physiol.,* **233**(3): C92-C98 (1977).
164. Stephens, N. L., and W. Van Niekerk. Isometric and isotonic contractions in airway smooth muscle, *Can. J. Physiol. and Pharmacol.,* **55**:833-838 (1977).
165. Stephens, N. L., Airway smooth muscle. In *Lung Cells in Disease.* Edited by A. Bouhuys. Elsevier/North Holland, Amsterdam, 1976, pp. 113-138.

# 3

# Role of Cyclic Nucleotides in Airway Smooth Muscle

*WARREN M. GOLD*

University of California, San Francisco
School of Medicine
San Francisco, California

*The work performed in the author's laboratory was the collaborative effort of D. B. Barnett, S. E. Chesrown, S. C. Lazarus, T. Mjörndal, B. Reed, M. Frey, H. R. Bourne, and K. L. Melmon and was supported in part by grants from the U.S. Public Health Service: Pulmonary SCOR Grants HL-19156 and HL-14201 and Program Project Grant HL-06285.*

Dr. Barnett had a Merck International Traveling Fellowship in Clinical Pharmacology (present address: University of Leicester School of Medicine, Department of Clinical Pharmacology, Leicester LE1 7RH, England). Dr. Chesrown was a Trainee supported by Training Grant HL-05251 (present address: Pediatric Pulmonary Center, University of Florida College of Medicine, Gainesville, Florida, 32610). Dr. Lazarus had a Young Investigator Pulmonary Research Award, Division of Lung Diseases, Grant IR23 HL-19604. Dr. Mjörndal had a Merck International Traveling Fellowship in Clinical Pharmacology (present address: Department of Pharmacology, University of Umeå, S-90187 Umeå, Sweden). B. Reed (present address: Gladstone Foundation Laboratories, P.O. Box 40608, San Francisco, California, 94140). M. Frey (present address: 1427 Corcoran Street, N.W., Washington, D.C., 20009). K. Melmon (present address: Department of Medicine, Stanford University Medical Center, Stanford, California, 94305).

## I. General Considerations

There is increasing evidence that the regulation of cellular metabolism involves several intracellular chemical mediators, including calcium ion, cyclic 3′,5′-adenosine monophosphate (cyclic AMP) and cyclic 3′,5′-guanosine monophosphate (cyclic GMP). (See Figure 1.) These intracellular mediators are involved in a variety of functions within a specific tissue. The final biochemical control of the activity of a particular type of cell within a tissue requires critical regulation of these chemicals at specific intracellular effector sites. In certain processes, such as IgE-mediated secretion of histamine from pulmonary mast cells, diverse evidence supports the concept that mast cell secretion is modulated by cyclic nucleotides [1]. Although cyclic AMP may facilitate antigen-induced mediator release under certain conditions, increased cyclic AMP inhibits the intensity of inflammation and release reactions in basophils, mast cells, neutrophils, lymphocytes, and platelets [1]. Other data suggest that activation of muscarinic cholinergic receptors by acetylcholine induces transient increases in cyclic GMP and enhanced release of histamine and other mediators from passively sensitized human lung in vitro [1,2].

It has also been suggested that cyclic nucleotides are involved in the regulation of contraction and relaxation of smooth muscle. Unlike the mast cell, however, the role of the nucleotides in regulating smooth muscle is highly controversial. Early workers [3] proposed that increased cyclic AMP mediated relaxation of smooth muscle induced by β-adrenergic agonists (Fig. 2). Later, Robison et al. [4] proposed that decreased cyclic AMP mediated contraction of smooth muscle induced by α-adrenergic agonists. Then, Amer [5] suggested that the contractile state of smooth muscle may be a general function of the concentration of cyclic AMP. At the same time, Lee et al. [6] proposed that increased concentrations of cyclic GMP may mediate contraction of smooth muscle induced by cholinergic agonists, some α-adrenergic agonists, and other contractile stimuli (Fig. 2). De-

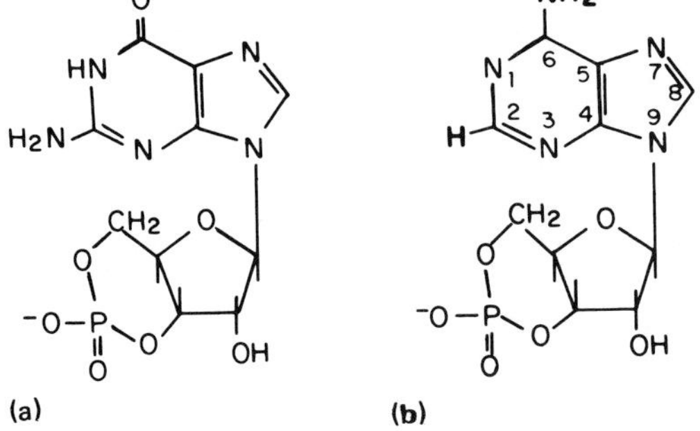


**FIGURE 1** Chemical structure of cyclic GMP (a) and cyclic AMP (b).

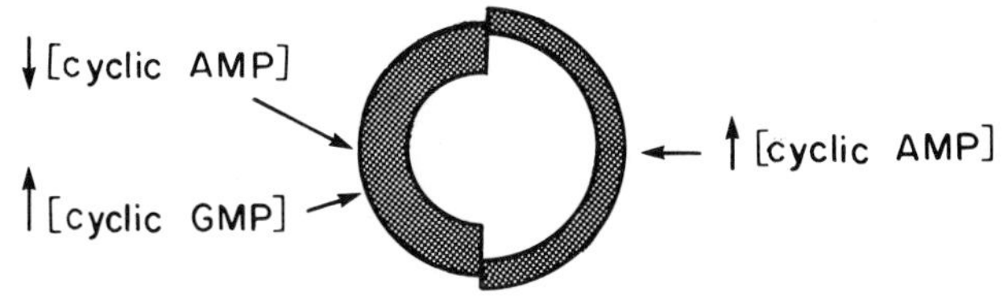


**FIGURE 2** Postulated relationship between changes in cyclic nucleotide concentrations and airway smooth muscle tone (see text for details).

spite notable exceptions, in which relaxing and contracting mechanisms do not involve cyclic AMP [7,8], there appears to be sufficient evidence to justify the hypothesis that contractility of at least some smooth muscles can be modulated by cyclic nucleotides.

The mechanisms by which calcium regulates the interactions of the contractile components of smooth muscle, the numbers and nature of these contractile components, the structures and systems involved in the delivery of calcium to and removal of calcium from the contractile apparatus of smooth muscle are matters of debate and uncertainty. Similar controversy and uncertainty exist concerning the roles of calcium and cyclic nucleotides in the metabolism of carbohydrates during contraction and relaxation of smooth muscle. Investigations of the role played by cyclic nucleotides in the physiology of smooth muscle may provide answers to fundamental questions concerning the regulation of basic contractile elements found in a variety of cells.

## II. Problems in Evaluating Data

In order to resolve the increasing numbers of apparently conflicting reports in this field, it is important to remember that different workers have used a variety of tissues from diverse species, different experimental conditions, and different methods of assay. Furthermore, in preparations of isolated tissues, normal anatomical relationships may be disrupted, receptors may be exposed that are not accessible in the living organism, and neurohumoral control mechanisms that influence the tissues in the intact organism usually cannot be evaluated.

All smooth muscles need not be expected to share similar mechanisms of regulation. Smooth muscle in different organs, even within the same species, may behave differently in response to the same agonist; smooth muscle in large airways (e.g., trachea) may behave differently than smooth muscle in other airways (e.g., small bronchi)—a reflection of the specificity of pharmacologic receptors associated with cellular differentiation (see Chapter 4).

Specimens of muscle used in vitro contain many different cells. For example, preparations from the gastrointestinal tract contain smooth muscle, but also contain excitatory parasympathetic and inhibitory sympathetic nerve endings. Moreover, the intestine contains an intrinsic neural plexus [9]. Thus, catecholamines may stimulate intestine by way of at least four receptors: (1) inhibitory β-adrenergic receptors on the plasma membrane of smooth muscle cells; (2) inhibitory α-adrenergic receptors on the plasma membrane of smooth muscle cells; (3) inhibitory α-adrenergic receptors in the myenteric plexus; and (4) excitatory α-adrenergic receptors in the sphincters and terminal ileum [10-13].

$K^+$ ions have mixed effects on intestinal smooth muscle which also reflect the heterogeneous nature of the tissue: Paton and Aboo Zar [14] used preparations of both innervated and denervated intestinal smooth muscle and demonstrated an effect of $K^+$ on the smooth muscle itself and on the nerve plexus. Andersson [15] showed that the effects of $K^+$ on intestinal smooth muscle were partially inhibited by adrenergic and cholinergic antagonists, but increased concentrations of cyclic AMP still occurred.

The airways are also a heterogeneous tissue containing endothelial cells, epithelial cells, fibroblasts, mast cells, smooth muscle cells, and so on. Anatomical and physiological evidence indicates the presence of excitatory parasympathetic nerve endings in all species, but adrenergic innervation is variable and the subject of controversy [16]. In contrast to the intestine, there appears to be no evidence for intrinsic tone in airway smooth muscle of many species, little evidence for significant excitatory α-adrenergic endings on smooth muscle (in human, cat, or dog), little evidence for significant α- or β-adrenergic inhibitory endings on the parasympathetic ganglia, and only preliminary evidence concerning the presence of a nonadrenergic inhibitory nervous system (in guinea pig and human, but not in dog; see Chapter 1).

Differences in the behavior of different preparations of smooth muscle may be related to the local release of mediators. For example, the local release of prostaglandins may modify the response of both the contractile apparatus and the cyclic nucleotides in smooth muscle. In guinea pigs, airways appear to have high myogenic tone attributable to prostaglandin production. Furthermore, Bouhuys showed that inhibitors of prostaglandin synthesis (indomethacin and aspirin) enhance the contractile responses to large concentrations of agonists (e.g., acetylcholine and $K^+$) [17]. Andersson showed that inhibitors of prostaglandin synthesis also blocked the increase in cyclic AMP induced by cholinergic agonists without altering the increase in tension in rabbit colon [8].

Thus, humoral and neurotransmitter activation of the contractile mechanisms in smooth muscle may initiate a sequence of reactions, including feedback mechanisms, that may override the primary stimulus. This complexity may lead to misinterpretation of the effects of various agonists on cyclic nucleotide metabolism in smooth muscle, particularly when observers ignore the possible contribution of other cells (mast cells, endothelial cells, fibroblasts, and so on) to changes in total concentrations of cyclic nucleotides measured chemically. Yet some workers assume that if increased concentrations of cyclic AMP do not always accompany agonist-induced relaxation, or increased concentrations of cyclic GMP do not always accompany agonist-induced contraction, these nucleotides must not participate in agonist-induced responses of the contractile system. There is also a tendency to assume that the increased concentration of cyclic AMP (or cyclic GMP) in tissues, coincident with altered smooth muscle tension, means that the particular cyclic nucleotide must be mediating the effect of the agonist on the contractile state. Both assumptions may be misleading. The ability of a mediator (e.g., cyclic nucleotide) to regulate a certain cellular function in a given tissue does not necessarily imply that the mediator *must* regulate that function in that tissue, or even that it can regulate that function in other tissues. Smooth muscle, like other biologic systems, has multiple regulatory mechanisms, and these may vary in relative importance in different types of smooth muscle cells.

Therefore, in evaluating the role of cyclic nucleotides in smooth muscle function, it is important to control the number of mechanisms activated at one time. It is also important to relate changes in chemical concentrations of cyclic nucleotides to specific cells within the tissue. In heterogeneous tissues, even when smooth muscle predominates (e.g., rat ductus deferens is estimated to be 70% smooth muscle), the evidence for the role of cyclic nucleotides in regulatory function, when based on measurements of their total chemical content, is probably circumstantial at best.

There are several experimental approaches to this problem: (1) studying individual smooth muscle cells in tissue culture, Goldberg et al. [18] found markedly different effects of methacholine on cyclic GMP in isolated myometrial cells compared to the effects reported in the intact uterus [19,20] ; (2) to identify individual cells contributing to total chemical changes by immunocytochemical staining for cyclic AMP and cyclic GMP [21] and their substrates [22] ; and (3) to dissociate the change in cyclic nucleotide concentration from airway smooth muscle function by appropriate pharmacological interventions.

In this chapter, I shall review (1) the enzymes related to cyclic nucleotide metabolism and function in the lung; (2) cyclic nucleotide content of the lung and factors that affect it; (3) cyclic nucleotide metabolism in mast cells in which evidence for the biologic role of cyclic nucleotides is reasonably well developed; and (4) current concepts of the relationship of cyclic nucleotides to airway smooth muscle function, including their possible roles in the metabolism of calcium and carbohydrates.

## III. Enzymes Related to Cyclic Nucleotide Metabolism

### A. Adenylate Cyclase

There are several extensive reviews which summarize recent advances in this field resulting from newer techniques [23-25] and classic modes of study [22,26-28]. Hormone-induced activation of adenylate cyclase involves binding of the hormone to a tissue-specific receptor in the cell membrane. The complex formed by the hormone and receptor then functionally couples to adenylate cyclase. The coupled complex interacts with guanine nucleotides which activate adenylate cyclase. In many cells, this activation diminishes the capacity of the cell to respond to further stimuli. Studies of radiolabeled hormones and neurotransmitters have demonstrated that most agonists bind to specific high-affinity sites on the plasma membrane. These sites contain a heterogeneous population of molecules composed of several different components of plasma membrane, including proteins, carbohydrates, and lipids [28]. When the hormone binds to these molecules, the interaction alters the receptor number and affinity: In some instances, receptors increase and in other instances, receptors decrease in number subsequent to binding the agonist [29] (see below). Binding studies with radiolabeled agonists and antagonists show that binding of the agonist, but not antagonist, involves formation of a high-affinity hormone-receptor intermediate which is stabilized by divalent cations ($Mg^{2+}$, $Mn^{2+}$, and $Ca^{2+}$; Fig. 3).

Certain cells (e.g., mast cell, airway smooth muscle cell) respond to several different hormones with increased synthesis of cyclic AMP. This has led to the "mobile receptor hypothesis" [27] to explain coupling under these circumstances. A set of adenylate cyclase molecules exists which is capable of activation by a number of different hormone-receptor complexes; these complexes can diffuse laterally in the plasma membrane until they couple with the enzyme. Cell hybridization techniques have provided critical support for this hypothesis. One cell line was prepared containing β-adrenoceptors without adenylate cyclase; another line was prepared containing adenylate cyclase but *without* β-adrenoceptors. Cell fusion produced hybrid cells with both functions intact [24]. That cyclase and receptor are separable chemical entities has gained further support from workers who have chemically isolated the β receptor from the adenylate cyclase [30,31].

In more recent studies [32], Dufau and coworkers separated lipid vesicles containing luteinizing hormone (LG) receptors devoid of adenylate cyclase activity from ovarian homogenates. Subsequently, they incubated these receptors with isolated rat adrenal fasiculata cells and obtained a time-dependent uptake of 40 to 125 receptors per cell by 4 hr. When the cells were then incubated with $10^{-9}$ M human chorionic gonadotropin (HCG), increased intracellular and extra-

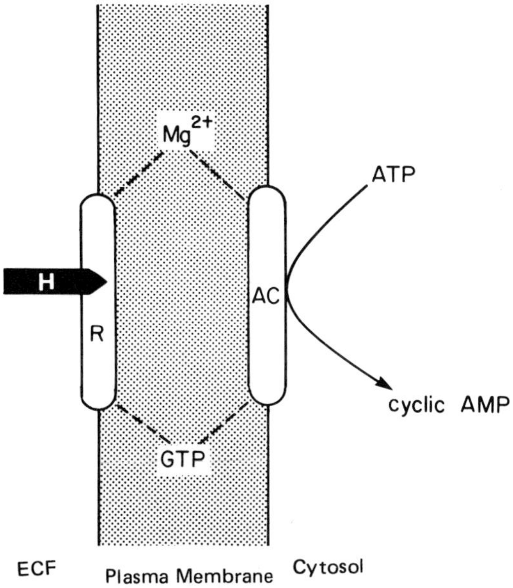


**FIGURE 3** Schematic relationship between hormone (H) and receptor (R) on plasma membrane. Binding of the agonist but not antagonist involves formation of a high-affinity hormone-receptor intermediate stabilized by divalent cations (e.g., $Mg^{2+}$). Activation of adenylate cyclase (AC) involves an allosteric guanine nucleotide (GTP) regulatory site on adenylate cyclase. This nucleotide can activate the enzyme, enhance hormone stimulation, and alter binding affinity of hormone for the receptor. Activated adenylate cyclase synthesizes cyclic AMP from ATP.

cellular cyclic AMP associated with production of corticosterone was observed. These changes were similar to those produced by $5 \times 10^{-10}$ M ACTH in normal adrenal cells. These experiments also demonstrate that hormone receptors exist as separate entities from adenylate cyclase in the gonadal cell membrane and can be functionally coupled to the adenylate cyclase of the host cell [32].

Other studies have demonstrated that in the sequence of hormone-receptor coupling and activation of adenylate cyclase, an allosteric guanine nucleotide regulatory [33] site exists on adenylate cyclase. These nucleotides can activate the enzyme, enhance hormone stimulation [33,34], and, in some systems, alter the binding affinity of the hormone [35] for the receptor.

Among the complex interrelationships between intracellular regulatory mechanisms, the effect of $Ca^{2+}$ on cyclic AMP is of critical importance. $Ca^{2+}$ seems necessary in the coupling process to transmit the hormone signal into the intact cell. $Ca^{2+}$ binds to a specific protein which activates adenylate cyclase in vitro [36,37]. This same protein ($Ca^{2+}$-dependent regulator protein) can also activate phosphodiesterase when bound to $Ca^{2+}$, providing two mechanisms to regulate cyclic nucleotide metabolism. The cyclic nucleotides function effectively as so-called second messengers because they are synthesized and hydrolyzed rapidly. This enables them to act as efficient, transient signals to regulate biochemical events.

In addition, regulation of hormone responsiveness of adenylate cyclase provides another level of control to prevent continual stimulation of these systems. Several mechanisms provide this type of autoregulation. When hormones such as catecholamines occupy receptor sites, a decrease in number of surface receptors occurs [38]. In other cells, stimulation by catecholamines or prostaglandins decreases adenylate cyclase responsiveness to both agonists, apparently by inhibiting coupling of receptor and cyclase [39]. Two different low molecular weight inhibitors have been isolated (one from adipocytes and the other from liver) which block activation of adenylate cyclase by several agonists. Conceivably, one or several of these mechanisms operate to effect compartmentalization of cyclic AMP within a single cell so that adenylate cyclase can be activated in selective loci only. Conversely, the diverse controls of adenylate cyclase in different tissues contribute to the tissue specificity of the response to hormones.

### B. Guanylate Cyclase

Most current evidence suggests that guanylate cyclase is not regulated by direct interaction with hormones or neurotransmitters. The indirect regulation of this enzyme by hormone is probably related to its subcellular distribution. Guanylate cyclase can be found in particulate (membrane-bound) or soluble form, and the partitioning varies from 90% particulate in rat small intestine [40] to 80% soluble in rat lung and liver [41-43]; cell-specific differences in soluble to particulate fraction vary within each tissue.

There are calcium-dependent mechanisms which regulate guanylate cyclase activity. A classic example of the indirect regulation of the enzyme by acetylcholine was reported by Schultz et al. [44]. When rat vas deferens was stimulated by acetylcholine in a medium containing $Ca^{2+}$, cyclic GMP was synthesized rapidly. In a $Ca^{2+}$-free medium, acetylcholine did not increase cyclic GMP. These workers concluded that acetylcholine caused $Ca^{2+}$ influx into the cell, resulting in activation of guanylate cyclase and synthesis of cyclic GMP.

There are also calcium-independent mechanisms which regulate guanylate cyclase activity [45]. $Ca^{2+}$ appears to be able to alter the activity of both particulate and soluble enzyme; thus, hormonal regulation of localized $Ca^{2+}$ pools might alter cyclic GMP production directly. A metal-adenine nucleotide site on guanylate cyclase appears to regulate its activity [46]. This is similar to the regulation of adenylate cyclase by guanine nucleotides. Moreover, cyclic AMP itself appears to stimulate nuclear guanylate cyclase in vitro [47], but whether this effect is direct or a result of cyclic AMP-dependent protein kinase is uncertain. In any event, modulation of nucleotide pools and cyclic AMP may also affect guanylate cyclase activity.

Oxidation-reduction reactions appear critically important in regulating guanylate cyclase. Kimura et al. [48] suggest that catalase [49,50] converts $NaN_3$ to a nitric oxide-containing compound which increases guanylate cyclase activity 30-fold. Other similar compounds including nitric oxide isolated from cigarette smoke [51], nitroprusside [52], and certain carcinogens such as nitrosoguanidine [53] activate the enzyme. Autoactivation of soluble guanylate cyclase occurs with $O_2$ and with $H_2O_2$ under certain conditions [54], and by direct effects of fatty acids [55] (which may also depend on the oxidation-reduction state of the system). Stimulation of membrane-bound enzyme by fatty acids may be a direct effect, or a result of solubilization of latent enzyme activity [56,57].

Another example of the complex and perplexing interactions involving these intracellular mediators is the report by Murad et al. [58] that soluble guanylate cyclase from lung and other tissues activated by sodium nitroprusside, sodium nitrite, N-methyl-N′-nitro-N-nitrosoguanidine, and nitric oxide gas causes synthesis of cyclic GMP from GTP and cyclic AMP from ATP. The significance of this new pathway for cyclic AMP synthesis remains to be determined, but suggests that effects of some agonists on cyclic AMP may result from alteration of guanylate cyclase activity.

In addition to acute regulation of existing guanylate cyclase activity, there are also mechanisms which appear to regulate the total concentration of the two forms independently [59].

Thus, guanylate cyclase exists in several different forms localized to certain specific sites within the cell. Mechanisms exist which modify the subcellular distribution and total concentration of the enzyme. Acute regulation appears to depend on local interactions of ions, nucleotides, oxides, and fatty acids with guanylate cyclase. The synthesis of cyclic GMP is probably localized to specific pools within the cell and responds indirectly to hormones, neurotransmitters, and mediators of inflammation.

### C. Cyclic Nucleotide Phosphodiesterases

Cyclic nucleotide phosphodiesterase activity is found in multiple forms which differ in their affinity for substrates, specificity for hydrolysis, and distribution in membrane-bound or soluble form within tissues. The most common classification of these enzymes is based on three fractions extracted from rat liver [60]. Fraction I hydrolized cyclic GMP, but not AMP, and was not inhibited by cyclic AMP. It was soluble and, as mentioned previously, was activated by calcium-dependent regulator [61]. Fraction II hydrolyzed both nucleotides with low substrate affinities. This fraction predominated in rat liver and hydrolyzed cyclic AMP when activated by small concentrations of cyclic GMP at pH 7.4 [60, 62]. Fraction III was a high-affinity enzyme that hydrolyzed cyclic AMP, not cyclic GMP, was associated with membranes, and was inhibited by cyclic GMP.

Recent studies suggest that each form of cyclic AMP phosphodiesterase can be generated from the others and represents different states of aggregation of the enzyme [63]. Furthermore, cyclic GMP phosphodiesterase appears to be chemically distinct from cyclic AMP phosphodiesterase.

Phosphodiesterase activity is also critically modulated by calcium-dependent regulator protein [61] which selectively increases soluble, but not membrane-bound phosphodiesterase, and does not alter the equilibrium between the interconvertible forms of the enzyme [63]. This same protein increases adenylate cyclase activity [37] and is very similar to the calcium-binding subunit of muscle troponin. Earp and Steiner have suggested that $Ca^{2+}$ may not only modulate synthesis and degradation of cyclic nucleotides, but may also regulate contractile events in cells, including stimulus-secretion coupling [22]. According to these authors, calcium-dependent regulator protein may provide a potent mechanism for compartmentalization of control of cyclic AMP. When a hormone stimulates cyclic AMP, the calcium-dependent regulator may accelerate cyclic AMP synthesis initially and then cause rapid hydrolysis of cyclic GMP at a specific intracellular locus. When critical levels of cyclic AMP are synthesized, the calcium-dependent regulator may next accelerate cyclic AMP hydrolysis until levels return to control. Some experiments suggest that the calcium activator complex may move from one site to another in the cell [64], thus providing another means to control both cyclic nucleotides at different intracellular sites [22].

Certain hormones, including insulin and norepinephrine, can activate phosphodiesterase in vivo but not in vitro, and do not depend on calcium-dependent regulator protein [65,66]. These observations suggest that still another possible intracellular messenger may be involved. Leichter and Anderson [67] confirmed this hypothesis in studies of insulin and acetylcholine on glucagon-stimulated cyclic AMP accumulation and gluconeogenesis in liver. Insulin, acetylcholine, and cyclic GMP all decreased glucagon-stimulated gluconeogenesis and cyclic AMP increases. Insulin, acetylcholine, and exogenous cyclic GMP all stimulated low $K_m$, cyclic AMP phosphodiesterase in liver slices. Cyclic GMP had similar effects in liver homogenates, but insulin and acetylcholine were ineffective, suggesting their action on phosphodiesterase requires the intact cell. Neither hormone altered adenylate cyclase activity. These results suggest cyclic GMP may mediate certain effects of insulin and acetylcholine on hepatic gluconeogenesis by stimulation of phosphodiesterase which decreases the effect of glucogen on cyclic AMP.

### D. Cyclic Nucleotide-Dependent Protein Kinase

*Cyclic AMP-Dependent Protein Kinases*

There are at least two types of soluble cyclic AMP-dependent protein kinases [68]. Each is composed of two regulatory and two catalytic units. The isoenzymes differ in their receptor units, but appear to have a common catalytic unit [68]. When cyclic AMP binds to the regulatory subunit, the catalytic unit is dissociated, freed from inhibition, and phosphorylates specific serine residues in protein substrates (Fig. 4) [69]. Phosphorylation can be inhibited by a protein kinase inhibitor protein [69].

A small protein that inhibits cyclic AMP-dependent protein kinase is found in many tissues. It is thermostable, and binds to the catalytic unit, but not to the intact enzyme [68]. Although its physiologic significance is unknown, Earp and Steiner [22] speculate that it may inhibit phosphorylation directly and require generation of larger amounts of cyclic AMP to sustain a cyclic AMP-mediated response. If the protein were present in selected sites within the cell, it could block the effect of cyclic AMP there while permitting small amounts of cyclic AMP to induce effects elsewhere in the same cell.

Many studies have shown a marked dissociation between cyclic AMP and steroid production during stimulation of steroidogenic target cells by the appropriate trophic hormone. Recently, Sala et al. [70] showed that in testis, adrenal fasciculata, and ovarian luteal cells, this discrepancy can be resolved by measuring cyclic AMP bound to regulatory subunits of protein kinase; this component of cyclic AMP increases in a dose-related manner with trophic hormone stimulation of steroid production. Increments of two- to threefold in the quantity of cyclic AMP bound to protein kinase consistently accompany the stimulation of steroidogenesis by trophic hormone and substantiate the fact that peptide hormones mediate steroid secretion by very small changes in cyclic AMP, indeed without increased extracellular or total levels. This finding provides further substantiation for the physiological significance of evaluating cyclic AMP metabolism by immunocytochemistry which detects bound nucleotides only.

A second, smaller inhibitor protein has also been identified [71] which inhibits phosphorylation by both protein kinases which are dependent on cyclic nucleotides and others which are independent of the nucleotides. This inhibitor and its ratio to the original inhibitor varies from tissue to tissue.

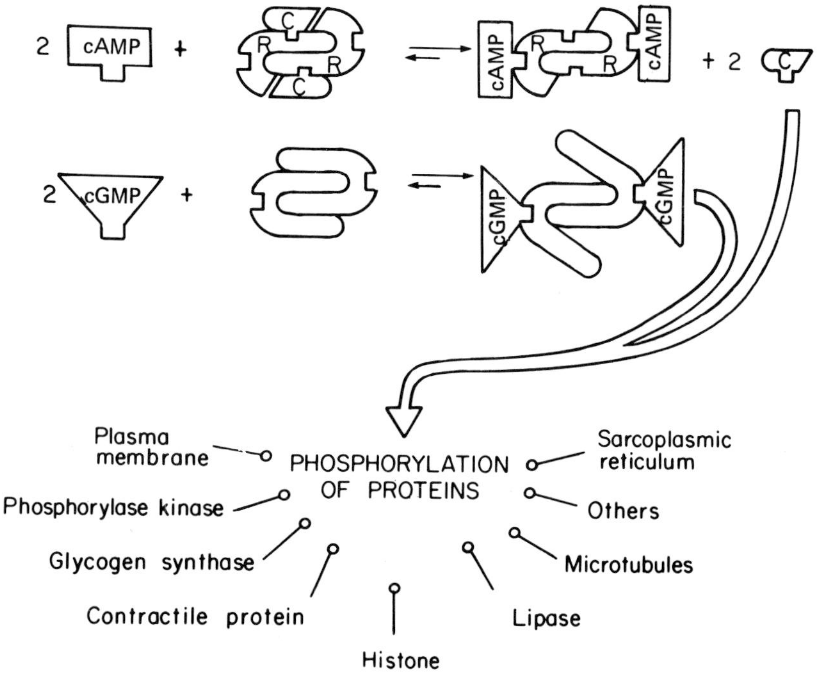


**FIGURE 4** Cyclic AMP-dependent protein kinase (top) and cyclic GMP-dependent protein kinase (bottom). Cyclic GMP-dependent protein kinases differ from cyclic AMP-dependent protein kinases in that the receptor and catalytic units do not dissociate when activated by cyclic GMP in most tissues.

Translocation of catalytic subunits or protein kinase from cytoplasm to nucleus has been described in liver [72], adrenal medulla [73], and ovary [74]. Other studies suggest that the cyclic AMP receptor unit may also be translocated to the nucleus of rat liver cells. This suggests that the cyclic AMP-receptor complex may also play a physiologic role in addition to that played by the catalytic unit. Confirmation of these translocations by immunofluorescence has been obtained by Steiner et al. [75].

*Cyclic GMP-Dependent Protein Kinases*

Cyclic GMP-dependent protein kinases have been reviewed recently [76]. These enzymes differ from cyclic AMP-dependent protein kinases, in that receptor and catalytic units do not dissociate when activated by cyclic GMP in most tissues (Fig. 4) [77]. Present evidence does not indicate whether the biologic function of cyclic GMP depends entirely on this kinase. Immunocytochemical studies utilizing antibodies to cyclic GMP-dependent protein kinase might provide clues as to the biologic role of cyclic GMP by locating substrates of its kinase within the cell.

### E. Compartmentalization of Cyclic Nucleotides

Current evidence suggests that the different components of the so-called second messengers are compartmentalized within the cell, thus promoting localization of cyclic nucleotides and diverse interrelationships with other factors involved in mediating the response to hormones, neurotransmitters, and mediators of inflammation. Whereas adenylate cyclase is bound to membranes, guanylate cyclase is bound and free in the cytosol. There are bound and soluble cyclic nucleotide phosphodiesterases and bound and soluble cyclic AMP-dependent protein kinases. Translocation of subunits of cyclic AMP-dependent protein kinase and further regulation by protein kinase inhibitors enhance intracellular specificity. Finally, there is increasing evidence of intracellular compartmentalization of divalent cations which provides further modulation of cyclic nucleotide levels and actions [78].

Previous concepts that a stimulus to a cell turned it off or on as reflected by tissue levels of second messengers are oversimplified. A stimulus may initiate a small change in cyclic nucleotide level with a resultant response in a confined region of the cell (e.g., at the microtubule); a different or more intense stimulus may provoke a more global response of the entire cell or even tissue. This concept has been confirmed qualitatively by immunocytochemical studies of hormone stimulation of specific intracellular sites [21], by localized binding of antisera to surface immunoglobulins on lymphocyte membranes [21], by studies of steroidogenesis [70], and by studies of liver regeneration in which changes in cyclic GMP staining were detected without associated changes in chemical levels [21].

In summary, cyclic AMP acts as a biochemical messenger in response to perturbation of cell membranes. Its biologic effect results from binding either to a local receptor unit (usually a protein kinase) or by penetration into the interior of the cell. Translation of the catalytic unit of cyclic AMP-dependent protein kinase provides another mobile effector of cyclic AMP. The magnitude of response of cyclic AMP to a given stimulus may determine the intracellular location of the biologic response; that is, large amounts of free cyclic AMP generated in some circumstances may be required to stimulate receptors located at a distance from the cell membranes.

Guanylate cyclase is found in almost all compartments of the cell. Synthesis of cyclic GMP seems regulated by local biochemical conditions under hor-

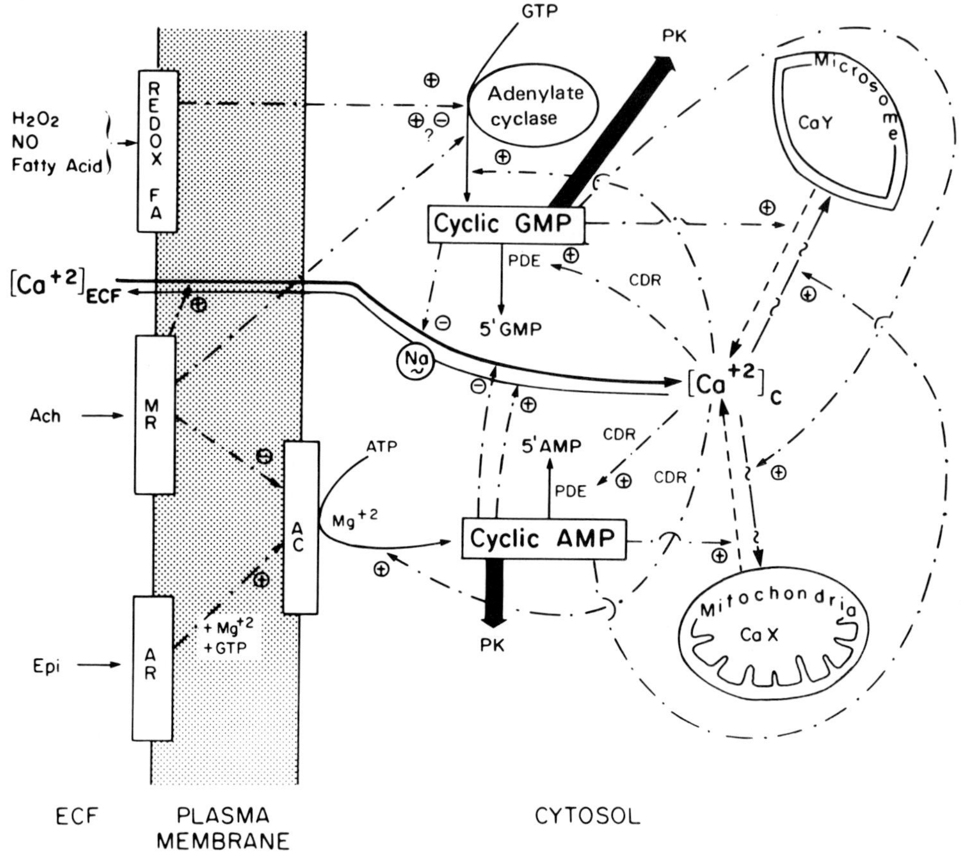


**FIGURE 5** Generalized model indicating possible relationships between calcium and the cyclic nucleotides. Active transport of calcium is indicated by (–Na–) or (–∼–). The former symbol implies that energy for active transport of calcium out of the cell across the plasma membrane is the $Na^+$ gradient across the membrane. Passive movements of calcium are indicated by dashed arrows. CaX and CaY represent nonionic calcium pools in the mitochondria and microsomes, respectively. A broken arrow with dots indicates a control signal; ⊕ and ⊖ indicate that the control chemical enhances or inhibits the process. $[Ca^{2+}]_C$ indicates cytosol calcium concentration. Adrenergic agonists and other hormones that relax smooth muscle stimulate adenylate cyclase and increase cyclic AMP. Cyclic AMP promotes removal of calcium from $[Ca^{2+}]_C$ to $Ca_{ECF}$ (extracellular pool) or to inactive intracellular pools (e.g., to microsomes or mitochondria). CDR indicates calcium-dependent regulator protein which stimulates adenylate cyclase and phosphodiesterase. Cholinergic agonists, and other hormones that cause contraction, increase influx of calcium from extracellular pools or inactive intracellu-

monal influences. Since synthesis of cyclic GMP is so flexible, there is no need to translocate this molecule long distances. Small changes in local levels of cyclic GMP within the cell may be sufficient to alter cell function. The localized nature of both control and action of cyclic GMP may explain why the concentration of this nucleotide is always much less than cyclic AMP. Some of these interrelationships are illustrated in Figure 5.

### F. Negative Interactions between Cyclic Nucleotides and Calcium

As reviewed above, an increasing body of data suggests that cyclic AMP, calcium, and cyclic GMP interact in various ways. In some cells, agonists that increase calcium in the cytoplasm decrease cyclic AMP. Calcium appears to stimulate at least one form of cyclic nucleotide phosphodiesterase and to inhibit adenylate cyclase in many cells. Cyclic AMP stimulates calcium removal from the cytoplasm of myocardium and from some smooth muscle cells. Cyclic GMP can stimulate hydrolysis of cyclic AMP by some phosphodiesterases, and vice versa. Thus, frequent negative interactions seem to occur between cyclic AMP, calcium, and cyclic GMP. Van Cauter et al. [79] have developed a model in which one agonist stimulates the formation of two mediators which interact via cross inhibitions (Fig. 6). Agonist $H_1$, synthesized and degraded outside the target cell, binds to the receptors, $R_1$ and $R_2$, and stimulates the synthesis or release of mediator X from precursor pool A and mediator Y from precursor pool C. X and Y are degraded within the cell. X inhibits accumulation of Y, and vice versa. Mediator X could be cyclic AMP, A the ATP pool, Y could be cyclic GMP or free cytoplasmic calcium, and C could be the GTP pool or the sequestered or extracellular calcium pool. This single model can account for complex experimental results without the need to postulate elaborate molecular models of agonist-receptor interaction. The computer-simulated results offer a possible explanation for some apparent contradictory effects of hormones and neurotransmitters on intracellular concentrations of cyclic AMP, cyclic GMP, and

---

**FIGURE 5** (continued)
lar pools (e.g., from microsomes) to cytoplasm. Reduction of cyclic AMP by these agents may involve inhibition of adenylate cyclase or activation of phosphodiesterase by calcium. Elevation of cyclic GMP by these agents appears to be secondary to increased $[Ca^{2+}]_C$ and probably not to direct effects on guanylate cyclase. Increased cyclic GMP also causes uptake of $Ca^{2+}$ by mitochondria, providing a positive feed-forward loop in cellular control. Certain smooth muscle relaxants (e.g., nitroglycerin) and fatty acids also stimulate cyclic GMP but do not require extracellular $Ca^{2+}$. Cyclic GMP may decrease tissue excitation by reducing $Ca^{2+}$ influx from inactive sties or by affecting an earlier step in the excitation process.

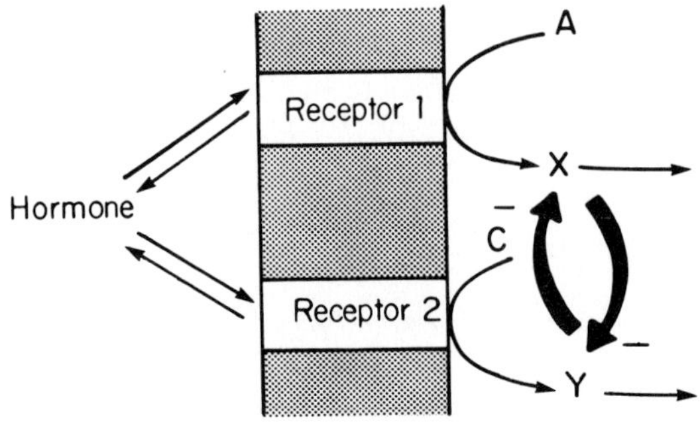


**FIGURE 6** Model of negative interactions between cyclic nucleotide and calcium. One agonist stimulates the formation of two mediators which interact by means of cross inhibitions. [From E. Van Cauter, J. G. Hardman, and J. E. Dumont [79], Implications of cross inhibitory interactions of potential mediators of hormone and neurotransmitter action, *Proc. Natl. Acad. Sci. USA,* **73**: 2982-2986 (1976).]

$Ca^{2+}$ in different tissues and experimental preparations. Apparent contradictions in some data may simply result from investigation of different ranges of agonist concentration by different investigators. These results show that studies of an agonist on each of its possible intracellular mediators must be conducted over a wide range of concentrations.

## IV. Cyclic Nucleotide Content of the Lung

### A. Basal Values

The concentration of cyclic nucleotides, particularly cyclic GMP, in mammalian lung tissues is relatively large compared to that of most other tissues [80,81]. Murine lung contains relatively large concentrations of the inhibitor of cyclic AMP reported by Murad et al. [82].

In part, the variability of cyclic nucleotide concentrations reported by different workers appears to be due to the procedures used for removing and fixing the tissue. Kimura et al. [83] reported that when rats were killed by immersion in liquid nitrogen, lung tissue contained 1 pmol cyclic GMP and 10 pmol cyclic AMP per milligram of protein. When lungs were removed and fixed in liquid nitrogen 30 to 45 sec after decapitation of the rats, the lungs contained approximately twice as much cyclic GMP and cyclic AMP. Barrett-Bee and Green [84] studied cyclic nucleotide metabolism in lungs of guinea pigs by stunning the animals 90 sec after an experimental intervention, then irradiating the animals for 20 sec in a microwave oven, prior to removing their lungs for assay. The interval of 90 sec was used to avoid increases in cyclic AMP postmortem. Polson et al. [85] decapitated rats, removed their lungs "rapidly," and froze the lungs in liquid nitrogen. In my own laboratory, cyclic nucleotide metabolism in canine lung tissue is studied in vivo by freezing samples of lung tissue in situ with clamps cooled in liquid nitrogen prior to resecting the tissue for assay [86].

A variety of methods have been used to sedate, anesthetize, or kill experimental animals, which may have altered the content of cyclic nucleotides. For example, when Kimura anesthetized rats with ether and surgically resected lung tissue instead of killing the animals by immersion in liquid nitrogen, cyclic GMP increased from 1 to 17 pmol/mg protein, but the concentration of cyclic AMP was unaltered. Kimura found that atropine prevented the increased cyclic GMP induced by ether and surgical removal of lung tissue in rats, suggesting a cholinergic mechanism was involved [83].

Other causes of variable "basal levels" of cyclic nucleotide concentrations in lungs include:

1. Sympathetic activity. Anesthesia and surgical trauma may increase sympathetic discharge and cause changes in either cyclic nucleotide, depending on the species of animal and the type of catecholamine released (see below).
2. Pattern of respiration. Failure to fix the pattern of respiration prior to obtaining samples of lung may lead to variable effects on cyclic nucleotide content. Inflation of the lung causes release of prostaglandins [87]; other workers report that synthesis of prostaglandins after a given stimulus may not reach maximal levels for 10 to 60 min [88]. Therefore, depending on the pattern of breathing and the time when samples of lung tissue are taken after inflating the lung, the concentration of cyclic nucleotides in lung tissue may vary markedly. Few workers have tried to control this possible influence [86].
3. Oxygen. Clyman et al. showed that cyclic GMP in human arteries and the response of this tissue to hormones and calcium depend on oxygen [45]. Similarly, DeRubertis has reported that adenylate cyclase activity in renal medulla of the rat is enhanced by increased $O_2$ pressure resulting in increased concentrations of cyclic AMP. This effect is probably mediated, at least in part, by local metabolism of prostaglandins.
4. Acid-base disturbances. Variations in cyclic nucleotides may be due to lack of control of acid-base balance, since Goodman et al. [89]

reported that chronic metabolic alkalosis increased cyclic GMP and chronic acidosis decreased cyclic GMP content of the lungs in rats.

Additional variability in the reported values for cyclic GMP and cyclic AMP in lung tissues may be related to variations in the methods of preparing and assaying the tissues. Many workers add phosphodiesterase inhibitors to their assay mixtures. This step is usually taken to augment the sensitivity of the assay to detect small quantities of the nucleotide. Most authors rationalize the possible effect of the phosphodiesterase inhibitor on the observed "basal" nucleotide content, or the change in content caused by the experimental intervention, by asserting that the addition of the phosphodiesterase inhibitor does not change the "basal" content of the nucleotides. Since the agonist acts by changing the kinetics of hydrolysis of the nucleotides, it is difficult to assume that the kinetics of the response to an agonist or to another experimental intervention are unaltered.

These possible causes of variability in the concentration of cyclic nucleotides have not been studied systematically by most investigators. However, Barnett et al. have reported recently on the content of cyclic GMP and cyclic AMP in peripheral canine lung in vivo by methods in which many of these influences were controlled systematically [86]. In dogs anesthetized with either barbiturate or chloralose-urethane, paralyzed with gallamine triethiodide, and mechanically ventilated with pure $O_2$ to maintain an end-tidal $CO_2$ of 4.5 ± 0.5%, samples of lung were obtained in situ from within 3 cm of the edge of a lobe through the open chest with clamps cooled in liquid nitrogen. All samples were obtained at end-inspiration and at least 10 min after inflating the lung three times to a transpulmonary pressure of 30 $cmH_2O$.

Control levels of cyclic GMP were 1.87 ± 0.32 pmol/100 mg wet weight (0.18 ± 0.02 pmol/mg protein) and of cyclic AMP were 88.3 ± 7.9 pmol/100 mg wet weight (9.8 ± 0.87 pmol/mg protein). Under these conditions, propranolol decreased cyclic AMP to 62.4 ± 3.2 pmol/100 mg wet weight; a similar change in concentration of cyclic AMP was not caused by cutting the sympathetic nerves to the lungs, suggesting that the control levels were not due to sympathetic nerve stimulation. Infusion of phentolamine during administration of propranolol did not reverse the effect of propranolol, suggesting that the decreased cyclic AMP was *not* due to an unopposed α-adrenergic effect. Rather, these results suggest that circulating catecholamines, probably released from the adrenal medulla, stimulate the β receptor in peripheral canine lung causing increased synthesis of cyclic AMP. In this preparation, neither cholinergic blockade (by cervical vagotomy or atropine sulfate), nor blockade of histamine receptors by $H_1$ or $H_2$ antagonists, nor blockade of prostaglandin synthesis altered the control levels of cyclic GMP or cyclic AMP. Table 1 summarizes basal levels in respiratory tissue of cyclic AMP and cyclic GMP reported in a variety of mammalian species.

**TABLE 1 Cyclic Nucleotide Concentrations in Respiratory Tissue of Different Species**

| Species | Respiratory tissue | Method of sacrifice | Cyclic AMP (pmol/mg protein ± SE) | Cyclic GMP (pmol/mg protein ± SE) | References |
|---|---|---|---|---|---|
| Guinea pig | Chopped parenchyma | Cervical dislocation | 8 ± 2 | — | 84 |
| Guinea pig | Homogenized parenchyma | Stunned, exsanguinated, perfused | 2.21 ± 0.16 | 0.69 ± 0.088 | 115 |
| Guinea pig | Sliced parenchyma | — | 9 ± 1<br>16 ± 0 | 1.4 ± 0.1<br>3.0 ± 0.6 | 95, 96 |
| Guinea pig | Tracheal ring | Cervical dislocation | 17.3 ± 1.7 | 0.74 ± 0.13 | 99 |
| Rat | Sliced parenchyma | Decapitation | 6.4 ± 0.3 | 4.8 ± 0.4 | 94 |
| Rat | Homogenized parenchyma | Liquid $N_2$ | 11.34 ± 1.35 | 1.02 ± 0.23 | 83 |
| | Homogenized parenchyma | Decapitation | 19.21 ± 2.96 | 2.43 ± 0.43 | 83 |
| | Homogenized parenchyma | Ether | 14.37 ± 1.69 | 17.14 ± 2.51 | 83 |
| | Homogenized parenchyma | Pentobarbital | 9.78 ± 2.42 | 3.39 ± 1.27 | 83 |
| Human | Chopped parenchyma | General anesthesia, resected at surgery | 4.3 ± 1.7 | 0.24 ± 0.11 | 2 |
| Dog | Parenchyma | Pentobarbital or chloralose-urethane, frozen in situ | 9.8 ± 0.87 | 0.18 ± 0.02 | 86 |
| Dog | Trachea | Frozen in situ | 2.31 ± 0.14 | — | †[a] |
| Dog | Bronchus | Pentobarbital | 29.4 ± 2.4 | — | 149 |

[a]†, W. M. Gold and A. Leff, unpublished data.

## B. Effect of Pharmacologic Agonists

*β-Adrenergic Agonists*

Many laboratories have reported that β-adrenergic agonists increase cyclic AMP by activating adenylate cyclase in rat, guinea pig, and rabbit without concomitant changes in cyclic GMP [90-96]. Kaliner incubated human lung fragments with [$^{14}$C] adenine and found that β-adrenergic agonists increased [$^{14}$C] cyclic AMP and that the response was potentiated by blocking phosphodiesterase-induced catabolism with methylxanthine [97]. Similar effects have been reported in perfused rat lung, after administration of isoproterenol intraperitoneally, in mouse lung [98]. We found that isoproterenol increased cyclic AMP from 80 ± 10 pmol/100 mg wet weight to 550 ± 25 pmol in peripheral canine lung in vivo (unpublished observation).

*α-Adrenergic Agonists*

The effect of α-adrenergic agonists on cyclic nucleotides in lung tissue is more controversial. Some workers report no effect in guinea pig trachea [99], while others demonstrate a consistently decreased cyclic AMP in human (peripheral) lung fragments [100-102]. There are also several reports that α-adrenergic agonists inhibit increases in the concentrations of cyclic AMP caused by other agonists in diverse types of target cells [103-106]. It has been suggested that α agonists decrease accumulation of cyclic AMP, thus causing the metabolic responses attributed to them [103]. Schultz et al. [107,108] and Butcher et al [106] report that α-adrenergic agonists increase levels of cyclic GMP in widely different rat tissues (ductus deferens and parotid gland, respectively). α Agonists increase cyclic GMP in mouse and rabbit parotid gland [109].

Cyclic GMP may be involved in a variety of secretory processes. Some examples include the effect of acetylcholine on cyclic GMP and function in isolated pancreatic islets; the effect of cholinergic stimulation on release of insulin [110]; the capacity of 8-bromo-GMP to mimic the action of carbamylcholine and phenylephrine on release of histamine from lung [102]; and the capacity of 8-bromo-cyclic GMP to mimic the action of acetylcholine on the release of lysosomal enzyme from human neutrophils [111].

Goldberg et al. [18] suggest there is a reciprocal relationship between concentrations of cyclic AMP and cyclic GMP in the same tissue. Cholinergic agonist-induced increased cyclic GMP is inhibited by β-adrenergic agonists [92,111]. Conversely, cholinergic agonists antagonize isoproterenol-induced increases in cyclic AMP [6,94]. Butcher et al. [106] observed that isoproterenol (β) inhibited the increased cyclic GMP caused by phenylephrine (α). Norepinephrine (with α and β effects) equalled the effect of phenylephrine on cyclic GMP. Moreover, propranolol (which blocked the effect of norepinephrine on cyclic AMP) did not enhance its effect of cyclic GMP [106]. Schultz [107], with Hardman [108], also reports that a reciprocal relationship does not always exist between cyclic AMP and cyclic GMP.

### *Prostaglandins*

Butcher and Baird [90] first demonstrated that prostaglandin $E_1$ ($PGE_1$) increased the concentration of cyclic AMP in rat lung tissues as it does in many other tissues. $PGE_1$ increases the concentration of cyclic AMP but not cyclic GMP in guinea pig lung tissue [95,96]; $PGA_2$ and $PGF_{2a}$ have no effect on cyclic GMP in this preparation [95,99].

More recent studies suggest that the effects of prostaglandins are more complex. In certain species, $PGF_{2a}$ appears to increase concentrations of cyclic GMP [2]; other workers suggest that prostaglandins modulate effects of autonomic neurotransmitters [113,114]. Dilute concentrations of $PGE_1$ and $PGF_{2a}$ decrease cyclic AMP and augment antigen-induced mediator release, whereas high concentrations of the prostaglandins increase cyclic AMP and inhibit release of mediators [101].

### *Histamine*

Histamine increases the concentration of cyclic GMP in slices of guinea pig lung. This effect is inhibited completely by promethazine in a concentration that only partly prevents the increase in concentration of cyclic AMP [96]. Histamine also increases the concentration of cyclic AMP in lung slices from rat, guinea pig, and rabbit [92,93,96]. Stoner showed that indomethacin prevented the increase in cyclic AMP, but not the increase in cyclic GMP induced by histamine in slices of guinea pig lung. These results suggest that enhancement of local prostaglandin synthesis may be one of the consequences of stimulating cyclic GMP metabolism. This hypothesis requires that there are cells in the tissue that can accumulate cyclic GMP, cells that can produce prostaglandins, and cells that can accumulate detectable amounts of cyclic AMP in response to the production of prostaglandins. Thus, the composition of this tissue in terms of numbers and capacities of different types of cells will determine whether all these steps can occur, or be detected [96].

Mathé has reported that in perfused guinea pig lungs, histamine causes increased cyclic GMP prevented by pyrilamine (an $H_1$ antagonist) and increased cyclic AMP prevented by burimamide (an $H_2$ antagonist) [115]. The explanation for the differences between results obtained in studies using slices of guinea pig lung and studies using perfused guinea pig lung is uncertain. The former studies were performed in the presence of theophylline, while the latter were not. Conceivably, anatomical relationships may have been more altered (and certain receptors exposed) in the slices of lung than in whole perfused lungs.

In preparations using central airways, Murad showed that histamine increased concentrations of both cyclic GMP and cyclic AMP in tracheal rings from guinea pigs [99]. The effects of histamine on the cyclic nucleotides were inhibited by both atropine and diphenhydramine, suggesting that acetylcholine was released locally and mediated the action of histamine. On the other hand, Andersson et al. [8] found that histamine increased both cyclic AMP and cyclic GMP associated with increased tension in bovine tracheal smooth muscle. Whereas spontaneously contracting tracheal smooth muscles and those contracted by histamine were relaxed completely by isoproterenol ($5 \times 10^{-7}$ g/ml), trachea contracted by carbamylcholine was not relaxed at all by isoproterenol, nor did the $\beta$-adrenergic agonist increase cyclic AMP at this concentration [116].

In vivo, Polson et al. [117] reported that histamine increased cyclic GMP in lung tissues from pertussis-treated and propranolol-treated mice, but not in lung tissues from normal mice. Histamine increased cyclic AMP in lung tissues from normal as well as pertussis-treated mice [117].

Barnett et al. [86] demonstrated that in the anesthetized dog in vivo, histamine increased both cyclic GMP and cyclic AMP associated with alveolar duct and central airway constriction. This effect was blocked completely by chloraphenirimine maleate, indicating that histamine acted on $H_1$ receptors. Indomethacin prevented the increase in cyclic AMP but did not block the increase in cyclic GMP or the physiologic reaction. This result is consistent with the hypothesis of Stoner et al., namely, that local synthesis of prostaglandins due to histamine, smooth muscle contraction, or increased cyclic GMP caused a secondary increase in cyclic AMP.

### *Bradykinin*

Bradykinin, lyslbradykinin, or kallidin increase the concentrations of both cyclic GMP and cyclic AMP in slices of guinea pig lung [96]. This effect is not inhibited by atropine and therefore appears to be independent of local cholinergic mechanisms. The increased cyclic AMP is not affected by propranolol but is blocked completely by indomethacin or aspirin, while the increased cyclic GMP is unaffected. The latter drugs inhibit synthesis of prostaglandins in homogenates of lung tissue [118] and prevent the release of $PGE_2$, $PGF_{2a}$, and "rabbit aorta contracting substance" stimulated by bradykinin in perfused rabbit lung [118]. On the basis of these studies, Stoner suggested that bradykinin, acetylcholine, and other stimuli may enhance local synthesis and release of prostaglandins from lung as a consequence of their effects on cyclic GMP metabolism.

### *Cholinergic Agonists*

Cholinergic agonists acting on muscarinic receptors increase the concentration of cyclic GMP in a variety of tissues, including lung [94-96,116]. Kuo and Kuo reported that acetylcholine not only increased the concentration of cyclic GMP in rat lung, without affecting the basal level of cyclic AMP, but inhibited the response of cyclic AMP to isoproterenol. In slices of guinea pig lung, acetylcholine increased the concentration of both cyclic nucleotides. Atropine blocked the cholinergic effect on both nucleotides; indomethacin blocked the increase in cyclic AMP only, suggesting that it was a secondary effect due to changes in local metabolism of prostaglandins stimulated by acetylcholine or increased cyclic GMP, or both.

In isolated tracheal rings from guinea pigs, Murad found that acetylcholine and carbamylcholine increased cyclic GMP (prevented by atropine) and increased cyclic AMP (prevented by atropine or propranolol), suggesting that the cholinergic agonist caused the local release of catecholamines, which then stimulated a β-adrenergic receptor [99]. Andersson found that carbamylcholine caused a short-lasting decrease in the concentration of the cyclic AMP in bovine tracheal smooth muscle preceding the onset of tension; this was followed by an increase in both cyclic nucleotides, paralleling the increased muscle tension. Both the actions on tension and cyclic nucleotides were blocked by atropine. If the muscle was incubated first with indomethacin, then the basal concentration of cyclic GMP decreased, and carbamylcholine caused a decrease in cyclic AMP and a later increase in cyclic GMP without inhibiting the increased tension. Finally, Andersson found that in contrast to histamine-contracted muscle, carbamylcholine-contracted trachea was much less sensitive to β-adrenergic stimulation and was not relaxed by a concentration of isoproterenol that relaxed the histamine-treated muscle completely [8] (see below).

Chesrown and Gold (unpublished data) studied the effect of acetylcholine on cyclic nucleotide metabolism in lungs in vivo. They infused acetylcholine (3 mg/min) into the pulmonary circulation of dogs anesthetized with chloralose-urethane, paralyzed with gallium triethiodide, and mechanically ventilated with pure oxygen. The animals had bilateral cervical vagotomy to block reflex, vagally mediated mechanisms and propranolol infusion to block homeostatic β-adrenergic mechanisms. Cholinergic stimulation caused cyclic GMP to increase from $1.7 \pm 0.2$ to $3.2 \pm 0.9$ pmol/100 mg wet weight, associated with alveolar duct constriction.

## C. Effect of Antigen

The effect of specific antigen or anti-IgE on concentrations of cyclic nucleotides in sensitized respiratory tissues is controversial.

*In Vitro*

Schmutzler and Derwall used chopped lungs from sensitized guinea pigs and observed a 20% increase in concentration of cyclic AMP following challenge with specific antigen [119]. Barrett-Bee and Green [84] found a fourfold increase in cyclic AMP in chopped lungs from sensitized guinea pigs after challenge with antigen in vitro. These same workers challenged sensitized guinea pigs in vivo and found an increase in concentration of cyclic AMP in lung tissue similar to that found in studies in vitro [84].

Since mepyramine ($H_1$), and burimamide ($H_2$), and ICI 74,917 (prevents release of histamine from guinea pig lung and rat mast cells) did not affect the increase in concentration of cyclic AMP induced by antigen in vivo or in vitro, these results suggest that histamine release is not a critical factor in the effect of antigen on cyclic AMP. Propranolol did not alter the effect of antigen on cyclic AMP; therefore, the increase was not due to $\beta$-adrenergic stimulation. $PGE_2$ and $PGF_{2\alpha}$ are released when sensitized guinea pig lung is challenged with antigen in vitro [120]. Barrett-Bee and Green found that indomethacin prevented the increased cyclic AMP induced by antigen in vitro and in vivo and prevented prostaglandin release, but did not prevent release of histamine [84]. They concluded that antigen-induced increased cyclic AMP in guinea pig lung was due to $PGE_2$.

Mathé et al. studied effects of histamine and antigen in perfused guinea pig lungs [115]. Antigen (and histamine) increased both cyclic nucleotides and increased the cyclic AMP:cyclic GMP ratio fourfold. Burimamide (an $H_2$ antagonist) diminished the antigen-induced increase in cyclic AMP, but did not alter the increase in cyclic GMP. Pyrilamine (an $H_1$ antagonist) prevented the histamine-induced increase in cyclic GMP, but had no effect on cyclic GMP changes in anaphylactic lungs [115].

More recently, Kaliner studied these effects of antigen in passively sensitized human lung in vitro. He found that aspirin inhibited IgE-mediated release of PGE and $PGF_{2\alpha}$, but had no effect on release of histamine on SRS-A. Furthermore, in his experiments, the increased cyclic GMP was blocked by an $H_1$ antagonist, whereas the increased cyclic AMP was blocked by an $H_2$ antagonist [88, 120]. The basis for the differences in these observations is unclear, but may be related to differences in species, respiratory tissues sampled, or the assays themselves.

Most of our current concepts concerning regulation of IgE-mediated release of chemical mediators rely heavily on the extensive studies of Austen and Orange [1] (Fig. 7). Using passively sensitized human lung fragments in vitro, they found that stimulation of adenylate cyclase by $\beta$-adrenergic agonists [100] and prostaglandins [100] increased cyclic AMP and inhibited mediator generation and release. Phosphodiesterase inhibitors also blocked mediator release and

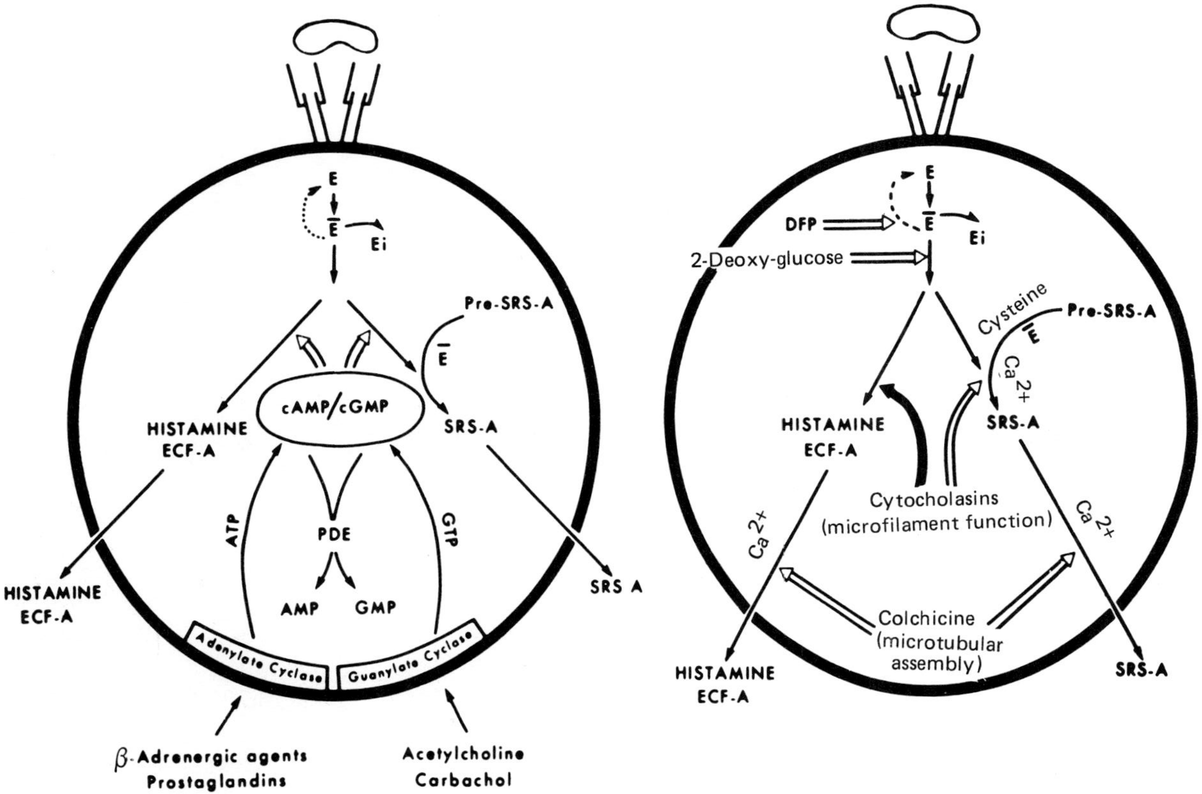


**FIGURE 7** Theoretical sites of pharmacologic modulation of the immunologic release of chemical mediators. See text for details and explanations of abbreviations. (From K. F. Austen and R. P. Orange [1], Bronchial asthma: The possible role of the chemical mediators of immediate hypersensitivity in the pathogenesis of subacute chronic disease, *Am. Rev. Respir. Dis.*, **112**:423-436 (1975).)

acted synergistically with β-adrenergic agonists. Imidazole stimulated phosphodiesterase, decreased tissue concentrations of cyclic AMP, and augmented mediator release [1]. α-Adrenergic agonists and small concentrations of prostaglandin, especially $PGF_{2a}$, decreased tissue concentrations of cyclic AMP and enhanced release of mediators [1]. While increased intracellular levels of cyclic AMP are almost always associated with decreased release of histamine in lung fragments (and leukocytes), in situations where antigen concentration is suboptimal or calcium concentration is limited, dibutyryl cyclic AMP potentiates the rate and extent of release of histamine [121].

Kaliner has examined the relationship between cyclic GMP and cholinergic augmentation of mast cell secretion in detail [2]. Acetylcholine, $10^{-7}$ to $10^{-11}$ M, caused parallel increases in both cyclic GMP and immunologic release of mediators from passively sensitized human lung fragments. Blockade of the muscarinic receptor by atropine blocked both effects. The capacity of acetylcholine to augment IgE-mediated secretion of mediators (Table 2) and to increase cyclic GMP (Fig. 8) followed the same time course: onset within 30 sec, peak by 120 sec, followed by an abrupt return to control levels. $PGF_{2a}$ also augmented mediator release and increased cyclic GMP in lung fragments.

In passively sensitized human lung, the intracellular events modulated by cyclic GMP and cyclic AMP are evanescent and reversible. These results suggest that the portion of the secretory process susceptible to augmentation by cyclic GMP and inhibition by cyclic AMP is only modulated if the cyclic nucleotide is increased during the activation period. The identical kinetics for augmentation of histamine and SRS-A suggest that the events modulated by cyclic GMP occur coincidentally for both mediators, the same event controls augmentation of both mediators, or increase in SRS-A release is secondary to increased histamine release.

Certain chemicals cause striking dissociation of the release of histamine and SRS-A. In the presence of the fungal metabolites cytochalasin A and B, the release of histamine is enhanced and SRS-A formation is inhibited. These agents appear to act before the calcium-dependent release phase [122] and may be analogous to a variety of secretory processes which are all dependent on a subcortical web of microfilaments which may act as a cytochalasin-sensitive barrier to exocytosis of granules (Fig. 7) [123,124].

Cysteine treatment of sensitized lung fragments also dissociates histamine and SRS-A secretion (Fig. 7). Cysteine selectively and markedly augments formation of SRS-A [125], whether by contributing a reactive sulfide required for synthesis of SRS-A, or by stabilizing or activating an enzyme is not clear. Cysteine and other thiols increase the total amount of SRS-A formed, but do not alter the percentage released. The amount of SRS-A synthesized is augmented by 8-bromocyclic GMP and diminished by dibutyryl cyclic AMP, suggesting that endogeneous nucleotides may influence other steps in the antigen-induced reaction besides secretion of mediators.

**TABLE 2 Kinetic Relationship between the Addition of Acetylcholine, the Time of Antigen Challenge, and Mediator Release[a]**

| Acetylcholine ($10^{-8}$ M) added: | | | |
|---|---|---|---|
| Before antigen (sec) | After antigen (sec) | Histamine (% release) | SRS-A release (U/g) |
| – | – | 20.6 | 750 |
| 180 | | 20.5 | 630 |
| 150 | | 21.0 | 750 |
| 120 | | 19.0 | 750 |
| 90 | | 25.0 | 1250 |
| 60 | | 24.5 | 1030 |
| 30 | | 32.0 | 2205 |
| 5 | | 41.0 | 1800 |
| | 30 | 34.5 | 2500 |
| | 60 | 24.0 | 2125 |
| | 90 | 21.5 | 1000 |
| | 120 | 23.0 | 830 |

[a]The antigen-induced release of mediators was determined simultaneously with the cyclic GMP levels demonstrated in Figure 8.

*Source:* From M. Kaliner [2], Human lung tissue and anaphylaxis. I. The role of cyclic GMP as a modulator of the immunologically induced secretory process, *J. Allergy Clin. Immunol.*, **60**:204-211 (1977).

Microtubules are also involved in the release of mediator. Colchicine binds the microtubular subunit protein to prevent assembly and function [126] and appears to act in the calcium-dependent phase of release. Agents that chelate calcium ions, alter cyclic nucleotide concentrations, or inhibit assembly of microtubules all act in later phases of the release reaction.

Kaliner has also used passively sensitized human lung fragments to study the effect of cyclic nucleotides on microtubules during IgE-mediated reactions [127]. His approach was indirect and based on the fact that colchicine appears to inhibit mast cell secretion by binding to the disassambled 6S form of microtubules (Fig. 7). Thus, inhibition of mast cell secretion by colchicine was used as an index that microtubules were disassembled; conversely, failure of colchicine to inhibit mast cells was used as an index that microtubules were polymerized. Exogenous cyclic GMP prevented colchicine inhibition, suggesting that this nucleotide stabilizes polymerized microtubules. Increased cyclic AMP (exogenous 8-bromo-cyclic AMP or isoproterenol-stimulated endogenous cyclic AMP) enhanced colchicine

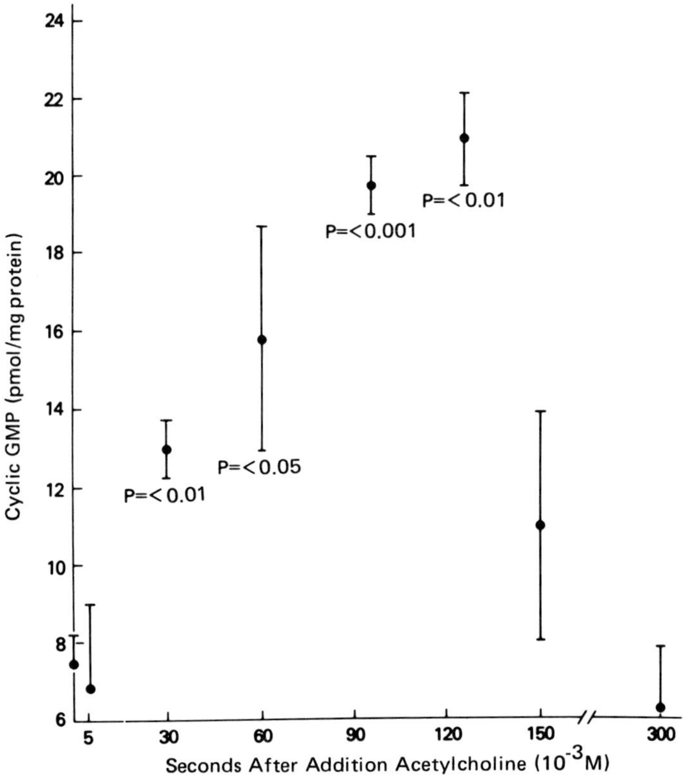


**FIGURE 8** The time curve of the effects of acetylcholine upon the cyclic GMP content of human lung tissue. Acetylcholine ($10^{-8}$ M) was added to lung fragments for 5 to 300 sec before determination of cyclic GMP levels. Data represent mean ± SEM. (From M. Kaliner [2], Human lung tissue and anaphylaxis. I. The role of cyclic GMP as a modulator of the immunologically induced secretory process, *J. Allergy Clin. Immunol.*, **60**:204-211 (1977).)

inhibition of mediator release. This suggested that this nucleotide promoted disassembly of microtubules. Anatomical correlates of these findings have not been obtained in lung fragments. However, in neutrophils, increased cyclic GMP is associated with increased numbers of microtubules, whereas increased cyclic AMP is associated with decreased numbers of microtubules [127].

This suggests an integral relationship between calcium ion flux, relative concentrations of cyclic nucleotides, and assembly and function of microtubules. As suggested earlier, a calcium-binding regulator protein may control adenylate cyclase, guanylate cyclase, and phosphodiesterase activators. The concentrations of cyclic nucleotides may affect the degree of phosphorylation or dephosphorylation of the protein associated with assembled microtubules that control movement of intracellular granules [128-132] (see above).

### *In Vivo*

Lazarus et al. [133] studied the effect of antigen in natively allergic dogs in vivo and reported findings similar to those of Kaliner in human lung in vitro. Antigen increased cyclic GMP from 2.1 ± 3.5 to 5.1 ± 1.4 pmol, increased cyclic AMP from 73 ± 6 to 388 ± 1.5 pmol/100 mg wet weight and decreased histamine content (20.4 ± 3.7%) in peripheral canine lung. This was associated with elution of histamine from the lung and increased arterial plasma histamine (709 ± 274 ng/ml), increased airflow resistance, decreased pulmonary compliance, and decreased arterial blood pressure. These results do not define the effect of the changes in tissue concentrations of cyclic AMP and cyclic GMP on the initiation of IgE-mediated secretion of chemical mediators, but the increased nucleotides may modulate the effects of antigen and mediators on subsequent function of primary and secondary target cells [133].

Although clear dose-response relationships have been demonstrated between cyclic nucleotide concentrations and inhibition of mediator release following treatment of tissues with different agonists, and the kinetics of the changes of cyclic nucleotide concentrations parallel the kinetics of the effects on IgE-mediated release of mediators, the causal relationships between cyclic nucleotides and IgE-induced release of mediators remain circumstantial. Relatively few experiments with pure basophils or mast cells isolated from primate lungs have been carried out. Moreover, chemical and immunocytochemical studies with partially purified cells suggest inconsistencies in the conclusions drawn from passively sensitized human lung fragments (see below).

## V. Cyclic Nucleotide Metabolism in Mast Cells

I have reviewed the literature concerning the metabolism of the cyclic nucleotides in the whole lung. Most of these data concern heterogeneous tissues, so that only rarely is it possible to postulate the significance of changes in the metabolism of these chemicals with respect to regulation of cellular or tissue function. Since most preparations of smooth muscle, except for those in tissue culture, contain numerous other cells, including mast cells, endothelial cells, and fibroblasts, I shall review studies of cyclic nucleotides in two specific types of cells found in the lung: (1) mast cells (since the role of cyclic nucleotides in regulating their function is relatively well defined, and (2) smooth muscle cells.

**TABLE 3 Effect of Optimal Concentrations of Agents Which Affect Cell Cyclic AMP Content on 48/80-Induced Histamine Release[a]**

| Agent | Concentration | % of Control 48/80 histamine release | P | *N* |
|---|---|---|---|---|
| Theophylline | 20 mM | 11 ± 2 | 0.001 | 6 |
| DBcAMP | 1 mM | 55 ± 7 | 0.001 | 4 |
| $PGE_1$ | 27 μM | 58 ± 5 | 0.001 | 5 |
| Isoproterenol | 1 mM | 107 ± 8 | NS[b] | 6 |
| Epinephrine | 1 mM | 114 ± 5 | NS | 6 |
| Diazoxide | 10 μM | 120 ± 6 | 0.025 | 4 |
| Adenine | 1 μM | 135 ± 9 | 0.003 | 4 |
| Carbamylcholine | 1 nM | 135 ± 10 | 0.001 | 5 |

[a]After a 15-min preincubation of $1.5 \times 10^5$ mast cells at 37°C with the indicated agents, 48/80 at a final concentration of 1 μg/ml in medium or medium alone was then added and the incubation was continued for another 5 min. Data are presented as the mean ± SEM.
[b]NS, not significant.

*Source:* From T. J. Sullivan et al. [136], Modulation of cyclic AMP in purified rat mast cells. II. Studies on the relationship between intracellular cyclic AMP concentrations and histamine release, *J. Immunol.*, **114**:1480-1485 (1975); © The Williams & Wilkins Co., Baltimore.

and cyclic AMP localized immunocytochemically. At 2 min, no cyclic AMP could be localized by the anti-cyclic AMP antibody, but by 30 min staining returned to control levels of intensity. These experiments indicate that changes in concentration of cyclic AMP measured chemically are reflected in immunofluorescent staining patterns [21].

### C. Human Mast Cells

Ts'ao, Patterson, and co-workers have carefully studied morphology and function of histamine-containing cells isolated from bronchial lumens of humans, monkeys, and dogs [139]. Their electron microscope comparisons with mast cells from airways, lung parenchyma, bone marrow, and blood basophils indicate that these cells are mast cells. Their physiological studies show that bronchial lumen mast cells release histamine following stimulation by 48/80, anti-IgE, and specific antigen. Thus, viable immunoreactive mast cells in the lumen of the airways provide the first line of response to immunologic and other stimuli which activate these cells. Boucher and coworkers [140] have demonstrated that IgE-mediated reactions increase the permeability of the airway epithelium, permitting large molecules of antigen access to the mast cells deep to the basement membrane.

**TABLE 4 Effects of Epinephrine and Theophylline on 48/80-Induced Histamine Release and Changes in Cyclic AMP Content[a]**

| Preincubation | Addition | Histamine release (%) | Cyclic AMP (pmol/1.5 × $10^5$ cells) |
|---|---|---|---|
| Experiment 1 | | | |
| Medium | Medium | 1 ± 0.1 | 9.9 ± 1.4 |
| Medium | 1 μg/ml 48/80 | 60 ± 7 | 1.1 ± 0.1 |
| 1 mM epinephrine | Medium | 2 ± 0.1 | 38 ± 0.8 |
| 1 mM epinephrine | 1 μg/ml 48/80 | 61 ± 7 | 2.6 ± 0.2 |
| Experiment 2 | | | |
| Medium | Medium | 2 ± 0.4 | 3.0 ± 0.2 |
| Medium | 1 μg/ml 48/80 | 44 ± 3.1 | 0.5 ± 0.1 |
| 20 mM theophylline | Medium | 1 ± 0.1 | 5.8 ± 0.4 |
| 20 mM theophylline | 1 μg/ml 48/80 | 7 ± 0.6 | 6.0 ± 0.2 |

[a]After a 15-min preincubation at 37°C with the drugs in medium, 1.5 × $10^5$ mast cells were challenged with medium or 1 μg/ml 48/80 in medium and the incubation continued for another 10 min. Data are presented as mean and standard error of values from representative experiments.

*Source:* From T. J. Sullivan et al. [136], Modulation of cyclic AMP in purified rat mast cells. II. Studies on the relationship between intracellular cyclic AMP concentrations and histamine release, *J. Immunol.*, **114**:1480-1485 (1975); © The Williams & Wilkins Co., Baltimore.

This provides an anatomical mechanism to amplify the IgE-medicated response to antigen.

Paterson et al. [141] have concentrated human mast cells to greater than 50% purity from enzymatically digested lung fragments by sedimentation in isopyknic and velocity gradients. Ultrastructural studies of these cells showed features characteristic of mast cells, including granules with scroll or reticular structures surrounded by perigranular membranes. Histamine and preformed eosinophilic chemotactic activity sedimented with the mast cells. Histamine content of the cells ranged from 1.0 to 5.5 pg/cell and was released by anti-IgE or specific antigen. SRS-A generation by anti-IgE or specific antigen was limited, but confined to fractions rich in mast cells and was associated with release of histamine and eosinophilic chemotactic activity. Although dispersed human lung cells sensitized with IgE and stimulated with specific antigen maintain a ratio of SRS-A generation to histamine release comparable to the starting lung fragments, this ratio decreases markedly as the mast cells are progressively separated from other cells. SRS-A has been generated from rat peritoneal macrophages [142] and from dispersed human lung cells depleted of mast cells by calcium ionophore [141]. These observations suggest that such cells or other secondary target cells may respond to the primary mediators released from mast cells and contribute significantly to the total SRS-A generated [143]. The role of cyclic nucleotides and other regulators in modulating the antigen-induced reaction of these cells remains to be determined.

## VI. Cyclic Nucleotide Metabolism in Smooth Muscle

### A. Cyclic AMP

*Increased Cyclic AMP*

**Increased Synthesis**

A relatively small number of hormones and neurotransmitters stimulate synthesis of cyclic AMP in smooth muscle. β-Adrenergic agonists increase concentrations of cyclic AMP in cells and decrease tone in most tissues containing smooth muscle [144]. Prostaglandins of the E series cause similar effects in some blood vessels, including canine and bovine veins [145], canine pulmonary arteries and veins, human umbilical arteries [146], and in tracheal rings from guinea pigs [99]. The C-terminal octapeptide of cholecystokinin causes a similar increase in cyclic AMP content and decreased tone in the sphincter of Oddi [147]. Although many investigators have not compared carefully the time course of the change in concentrations of cyclic AMP and muscle tone, or the dose-response curves of a given agonist for cyclic AMP and relaxation of smooth muscle, Andersson and others [8,116] have shown temporal and quantitative correlations in diverse smooth muscles between increased cyclic AMP and decreased muscle tone. Moreover, the relative potency in causing relaxation of bronchial smooth muscles obtained from rat, guinea pig, and dog correlated well with the relative potency in stimulating cyclic AMP synthesis: isoproterenol > epinephrine > norepinephrine [148]. The actions of the catecholamines are blocked by propranolol and enhanced by phentolamine, indicating that their effects are produced by a β-adrenergic receptor.

Vulliemoz et al. [149] showed that the increased cyclic AMP content of canine bronchial tissue induced by isoproterenol, epinephrine, and norepinephrine (Fig. 11) results from their stimulation of adenylate cyclase in bronchial tissue homogenates. Epinephrine and norepinephrine, when compared to isoproterenol, behave like partial agonists for cyclic AMP. In contrast to their effect on synthesis of cyclic AMP, all three β-adrenergic agonists have the same maximal relaxing effect, and their order of potency to relax bronchial smooth muscle is the same as that to stimulate adenylate cyclase. The maximal relaxing effect is obtained at concentrations which induce a submaximal increase in cyclic

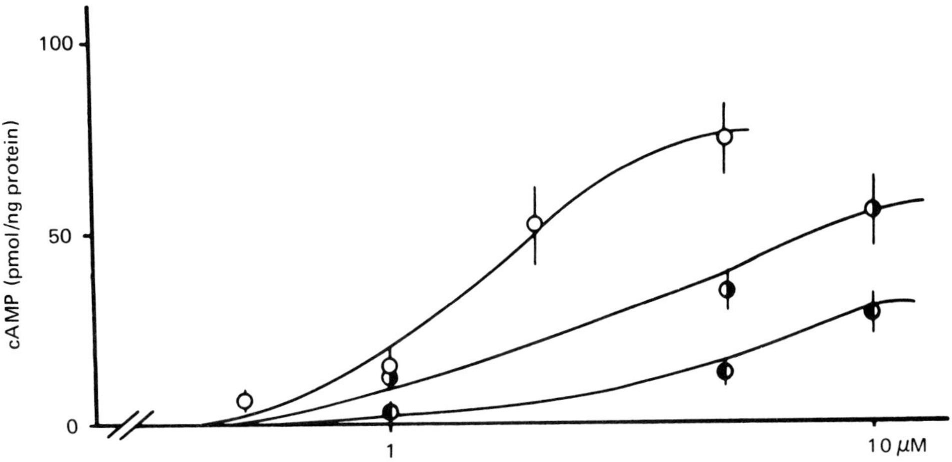


**FIGURE 11** Catecholamine-induced increase in cAMP in dog bronchial tissue after a 5-min incubation in Krebs-Ringer bicarbonate medium in the presence of 10 mM theophylline. Values represent the mean net increase over control (20.05 ± 1.4 pmol/mg of protein) in 10 to 11 experiments ± SE. ○ isoproterenol; ◑ epinephrine; ◐ norepinephrine. (From Y. Vulliemoz et al. [149], The cyclic adenosine 3′:5′-monophosphate system in bronchial tissue. In *The Biochemistry of Smooth Muscle.* Edited by N. L. Stephens. Baltimore, University Park Press, 1977, pp. 293-314; © University Park Press, Baltimore.)

AMP concentration; the agonist concentrations which cause maximal relaxation (0.5-5 μM) cause similar increases in cyclic AMP content (Fig. 12).

The fact that only a submaximal response of cyclic AMP to β-adrenergic agonists is associated with a maximal relaxing effect is in agreement with results in other tissues (isolated fat cells, myocardium) [148]. This suggests that the maximal increase in cyclic AMP content is far in excess of that required for a normal functional effect.

Vulliemoz et al. [149] showed that both the cyclic AMP and relaxation dose-response curves for epinephrine and norepinephrine were shifted to the right of isoproterenol. This may have reflected a decreased affinity for the β receptor, but also an interaction between the synthesis of cyclic GMP and cyclic AMP proportional to the α-adrenergic action of each agonist. Conceivably, the increased intracellular $Ca^{2+}$ secondary to α-adrenergic agonist activity is related to the decreased cyclic AMP. Increased calcium ion modifies activities of adenylate cyclase and phosphodiesterases and may be related to synthesis of cyclic GMP (see below) [108,150-153].

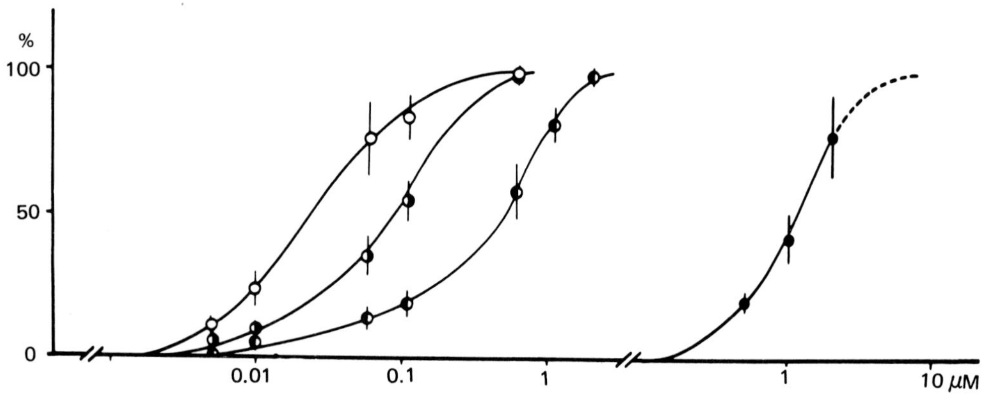


**FIGURE 12** Relaxing effect of isoproterenol (○——○), epinephrine (◑——◑), norepinephrine (◐——◐), and dibutyryl cyclic AMP (●——●) on a carbachol-induced contraction in dog bronchial strip. Catecholamines dose-response curves: mean values of seven experiments; dibutyryl cyclic AMP dose-response curve: mean values of four experiments. (From Y. Vulliemoz et al. [149], The cyclic adenosine 3′:5′-monophosphate system in bronchial tissue. In *The Biochemistry of Smooth Muscle.* Edited by N. L. Stephens. Baltimore, University Park Press, 1977, pp. 293-314; © University Park Press, Baltimore.)

Changes in adenylate cyclase activity in bronchial tissue homogenates can result not only from hormones or neurotransmitters, but also from changes in hydrogen ion concentration. This effect then modifies agonists acting on the enzyme: the basal activity of adenylate cyclase and the synthesis of cyclic AMP induced by isoproterenol and sodium fluoride are significantly decreased at pH 7.0 compared to pH 7.4 [149].

**Adenylate Cyclase** An important criterion for involvement of cyclic AMP in mediation of a cellular response is that an agonist causing a change in cell function can also activate adenylate cyclase in cell-free preparations. However, adenylate cyclase isolated from smooth muscle has not been studied carefully in cell-free systems. Agonists that increase concentrations of cyclic AMP in cells have been shown to stimulate adenylate cyclase in cell-free preparations obtained from some tissues [104]; other workers have been unsuccessful in demonstrating that β-adrenergic agonists stimulate the enzyme [154].

Hardman et al. [155] isolated adenylate cyclase from porcine coronary arteries. They found that the enzyme was extremely labile, with a half-life of 7 to 10 min at 37°C and 90 min at 0°C, when incubated in the absence of components of the reaction mixture (including $MgCl_2$, ATP, dithiotreitol, cyclic AMP, isobutylmethylxanthine, bovine serum albumin, and TES buffer. Alternative methods of homogenization and individual components of the reaction mixture failed to stabilize the enzyme. This lability of the enzyme has prohibited extensive study of its kinetics.

Thus, difficulties encountered in demonstrating stimulation of adenylate cyclase may be due in part to lability of the enzyme under assay conditions. Preliminary studies by Hardman et al. [155] of adenylate cyclase isolated from vascular smooth muscle suggest that the status of the smooth muscle prior to homogenization is also important. For example, if vessels are homogenized immediately after dissection, isoproterenol increases cell-free adenylate cyclase 15 to 20%; if vessels are incubated in oxygenated, glucose-containing, balanced salt solution for several hours after dissection, but before homogenization, isoproterenol increases adenylate cyclase activity more than twofold. These results suggest that some of the problems encountered in studying adenylate cyclase activity may be dependent on the state of oxygenation, nutrition, and perhaps integrity of the tissue membranes.

**Decreased Hydrolysis**

Diverse inhibitors of cyclic nucleotide phosphodiesterases cause relaxation of smooth muscle [144]. Pöch and Kukovetz [156] correlated inhibition of phosphodiesterase and decreased tone in vascular smooth muscle. These workers and Andersson and Mohme-Lundholm [10] showed that phosphodiesterase inhibitors potentiated relaxation induced by β-adrenergic agonists, while Takagi et al. [13] showed that activation of phosphodiesterases by imidazole, inhibited relaxation induced by β-adrenergic agonists. The relative importance of the increased concentration of cyclic AMP compared to the parallel increased concentration of cyclic GMP caused by phosphodiesterase inhibitors and the associated decreased tone in smooth muscle is uncertain (see below) [44].

Vulliemoz et al. [149] studied homogenates of canine bronchus and showed that cyclic AMP and cyclic GMP phosphodiesterases have kinetic behavior suggesting two forms of activity, one with a high affinity and the other with a lower affinity for the substrate. At low concentrations of substrate, the hydrolysis of cyclic AMP and cyclic GMP is inhibited by theophylline and papaverine. Papaverine is a 20-fold stronger inhibitor of phosphodiesterase than theophylline; their $K_i$ values for cyclic AMP and cyclic GMP phosphodiesterase are in the same range. Cyclic GMP is a competitive inhibitor of cyclic AMP phosphodiesterase at low concentrations of substrate (0.1 μM cyclic AMP), while at higher concentrations (10 μM cyclic AMP), cyclic GMP stimulates hydrolysis of cyclic AMP markedly at concentrations of cyclic GMP of 0.1 to 10 nM; at higher concentrations of cyclic GMP, its effect is to inhibit cyclic AMP hydrolysis.

Similar observations have been made in preparations from liver, brain, uterus, and vascular smooth muscle. The $K_i$ for cyclic GMP differs from its $K_m$

value, suggesting that cyclic GMP is probably not an alternate substrate for the enzyme hydrolyzing cyclic AMP. However, alteration of cyclic AMP hydrolysis may be a mechanism by which cyclic GMP affects intracellular concentrations of cyclic AMP in airways. Moreover, the activity of cyclic AMP phosphodiesterase decreases with pH, while the effect of theophylline, a phosphodiesterase inhibitor, is relatively unaltered. The effects of acidosis and theophylline on phosphodiesterase are thus additive, resulting in more marked inhibition of the enzyme at low pH compared to normal pH [149].

**Cell-Free Phosphodiesterases** Hardmann et al. [155] have studied two cyclic nucleotide phosphodiesterases from the soluble fraction of the media-intima layer of pig coronary arteries. One peak (I) has a greater affinity for cyclic GMP than for cyclic AMP, shows classic kinetic behavior, and is activated three- to eightfold by a heat-stable, nondialyzable factor that requires $Ca^{2+}$ ions. The other peak (II) has a greater affinity for cyclic AMP than for cyclic GMP and is not affected by the activator of peak I. Preliminary studies with this system show that substituted xanthines are capable of inhibiting one form of phosphodiesterase activity in a relatively selective manner [157]. These studies, as well as those of others [158-160], suggest that it may be possible to use certain agonists to selectively inhibit the hydrolysis of cyclic AMP and cyclic GMP and induce the increase in concentration of one cyclic nucleotide only. This approach would permit analysis of which, if either, cyclic nucleotide is participating in relaxation caused by the phosphodiesterase inhibitor. This would be especially useful in studying cyclic GMP which is often increased by agonists that cause both contraction and presumably increased $Ca^{2+}$ ion in the cytoplasm. In these situations, the increased cyclic GMP often appears to be secondary to the increased $Ca^{2+}$ [108]. It would be useful to study the contractile response to an agonist that increased cyclic GMP without increased cyclic AMP or $Ca^{2+}$. Although substituted xanthines show some selectivity in other, nonvascular systems, more studies are needed because particular xanthines are not equally selective in their actions on phosphodiesterases isolated from all types of cells.

### *Decreased Cyclic AMP*

The relevance of drug-induced decreases in cyclic AMP to the tone of smooth muscle is uncertain [144]. The pharmacologic basis for this drug effect may be related to changes in $Ca^{2+}$ concentration and inhibition of adenylate cyclase, or stimulation of phosphodiesterase (see above).

### *Exogenous and Synthetic Cyclic AMP*

Cyclic AMP and synthetic cyclic AMP derivatives applied to isolated smooth muscle reproduce many effects of hormones or other agonists that are associated with increased concentrations of endogenous cyclic AMP and decreased smooth muscle tone. Dibutyryl cyclic AMP causes relaxation in all smooth muscle preparations [144]. This agonist also induces hyperpolarization of vascular smooth muscle caused by β-adrenergic agonists [161]. Cyclic AMP itself causes relaxation in some smooth muscles, but causes contraction or augments contraction caused by other agonists in diverse smooth muscles [144]. This is analogous to the cyclic AMP-induced augmentation of mediator release from leukocytes under conditions of antigen excess (see above). The fact that controls were not established for a variety of chemicals which may contract or relax smooth muscle undoubtedly has contributed to the present confusion in this field [162,163].

Alternatively, the confusion may be a result of the fact that cyclic AMP and cyclic GMP and their synthetic derivatives are competitive inhibitors of the hydrolysis of each other by phosphodiesterase [161]. Apparent $K_i$ values (2 μM for cyclic GMP and 60 μM for cyclic AMP) are the same as $K_m$ values for the nucleotides as substrates for peak I; the hydrolysis of 1 μM of cyclic AMP is inhibited 50% by about 10 μM cyclic GMP for peak II.

To produce 50% inhibition of 1 μM of cyclic AMP or cyclic GMP by peak I (in presence of activator), 30 to 40 μM dibutyryl cyclic GMP, 20 to 30 μM 8-bromo-cyclic GMP, and 1 μM dibutyryl cyclic AMP are required; concentrations 10-fold larger for cyclic GMP derivatives and 10-fold smaller for dibutyryl cyclic AMP produce 50% inhibition of hydrolysis of 1 μM cyclic AMP by peak II.

In view of the ability of both cyclic nucleotides and their derivatives to inhibit both cyclic AMP and cyclic GMP phosphodiesterases, results obtained with these chemicals applied to intact cell systems must be interpreted cautiously (e.g., see Sec. V.B).

### *Smooth Muscle Relaxation Independent of Cyclic AMP*

Several preparations of isolated smooth muscle undergo relaxation without a change in the concentration of cyclic AMP. Even when increased concentrations of cyclic AMP occur, some agonists appear to relax smooth muscle by cyclic AMP-independent mechanisms. Most examples of this type involve smooth muscle isolated from uterus or colon. Andersson [164], with Mohme-Lundholm [10], showed that epinephrine, norepinephrine, isoproterenol, and phenylephrine in sufficient concentration stimulate α and β receptors, which both relax colon smooth muscle. Stimulation of α-adrenergic receptors in rabbit colon caused decreased cyclic AMP content and relaxation associated with inhibition of cholinergic neurons in the intestine [165] and *not* direct effects on the smooth muscle. There are a few drugs that relax smooth muscle under all conditions by one mechanism.

### *Cyclic AMP and Cellular Function*

Hormones and drugs that increase cellular cyclic AMP levels also cause increased phosphorylation of proteins by cyclic AMP-dependent protein kinases. This phosphorylation step is thought to be essential in producing the hormone or drug effect on the target cells. Cyclic AMP-dependent protein kinases have been demonstrated in some smooth muscles, but the critical substrates of these enzymes are unknown. Similarly, the physiological significance of the demonstration of phosphorylation of some smooth muscle plasma membrane proteins is unknown. The relationship to cell function of the fact that β-adrenergic agonists can hyperpolarize vascular smooth muscle or that cyclic AMP can stimulate uptake of $Ca^{2+}$ by microsomes from intestinal and vascular smooth muscle remains to be determined.

### *Biologic Role of Cyclic AMP*

It is not certain which metabolic functions in smooth muscle cells are regulated by the concentration of cyclic AMP. In many tissues, hormones and drugs which cause increased concentrations of cyclic AMP in cells cause increased phosphorylation of proteins by cyclic AMP-dependent protein kinases [166,167]. Cyclic AMP-dependent protein kinases have been demonstrated in some smooth muscles [168], but the physiologic substrates of these enzymes have not been identified. Cyclic AMP phosphorylates some proteins in membranes of certain smooth muscles [169], but the implication of this finding for physiologic function is uncertain; it may be related to the fact that β-adrenergic agonists cause hyperpolarization of vascular smooth muscle.

Cyclic AMP (high concentration) can stimulate binding of calcium by microscomal fractions of smooth muscle isolated from blood vessels and from colon, but these results need confirmation. Studies of mechanisms of inhibition of smooth muscle tone by Kroeger et al. [170] in rat uterus show the following. (1) Inhibition by relaxants (e.g., isoproterenol) affecting cyclic AMP can be qualitatively differentiated from that produced by relaxants (e.g., D-600) that have no direct effect on metabolism of cyclic AMP [171]. (2) There is good temporal correlation of mechanical, electrical, and metabolic respones to isoproterenol [172]. (3) The two different types of relaxants act at different sites on the control of cellular calcium ion: isoproterenol stimulates outwardly directed $Ca^{2+}$ pumping, and D-600 inhibits $Ca^{2+}$ influx activated by depolarization [173]. (4) Various contractile agonists inhibit the increase in cyclic AMP produced by isoproterenol and decrease the period of inhibition following exposure to isoproterenol, although they are not effective in broken cells.

In summary, possible mechanisms of cyclic AMP on relaxation of smooth muscle include increased removal of $Ca^{2+}$ from the cytoplasm, increased membrane potential, decreased influx of calcium ion into the muscle cell, and decreased effect of calcium at the contractile apparatus.

Although relaxation of many smooth muscles is often associated with increased concentration of cyclic AMP, contraction of smooth muscle is *not* generally associated with decreased concentration of cyclic AMP. In rabbit colon contracted by carbamylcholine [174], or in bovine mesenteric artery contracted by phenylephrine or histamine [175], or in bovine tracheal smooth muscle contracted by carbamylcholine [116], there is an initial decrease in cyclic AMP lasting 10 sec which precedes the increase in smooth muscle tension. The decrease is followed by an increase in concentration of cyclic AMP in proportion to the increased tension (Fig. 13) [8].

The mechanism causing the increased cyclic AMP during contraction does not involve β-adrenergic stimulation or phosphodiesterase inhibition. In preparations of smooth muscle incubated in calcium-free media, β-adrenergic agonists or phosphodiesterase inhibitors still increase cyclic AMP, whereas the increase following contraction is absent during this condition. In preparations of smooth muscle (rabbit colon, bovine tracheal smooth muscle) incubated with indomethacin, carbamylcholine-induced contraction is not followed by increased cyclic AMP and the increase in tension is potentiated (Fig. 14) [8]. Indomethacin blocks synthesis of prostaglandins in smooth muscles [176]. Prostaglandins are released from smooth muscle when distortion of the cell membrane occurs; the effect is inhibited in $Ca^{2+}$-free muscle which cannot contract. Since indomethacin inhibits the secondary increase in cyclic AMP, and this increase is absent in $Ca^{2+}$-free muscle and in muscle contracted submaximally, the effect is probably caused by the release of prostaglandins. Since the contractile effect is potentiated by indomethacin, it seems likely that the increased cyclic AMP counteracts the contractile action. This large, secondary increase in cyclic AMP during contraction makes the small transient decrease caused by some contractile agonists of questionable significance.

Furthermore, the enzymatic basis for an agonist-induced decrease in concentration of cyclic AMP is uncertain. Contraction involves increased free calcium in the cytoplasm; this change in calcium concentration may change the metabolism of cyclic AMP. For example, calcium inhibits adenylate cyclase activity [177-179] and stimulates phosphodiesterase activity in various cell-free enzyme systems [180]. α-Adrenergic agonists inhibit adenylate cyclase activity directly without involving calcium ion in lysates of human platelets. If the hypothesis is to be accepted, there must be separate pools of cyclic AMP to influence the contractile system differently. Contraction may be mediated by mechanisms not involving cyclic AMP.

When bovine mesenteric arteries are contracted by $K^+$ ions, a secondary increase in cyclic AMP occurs if α-adrenergic receptors are blocked. $K^+$, in the

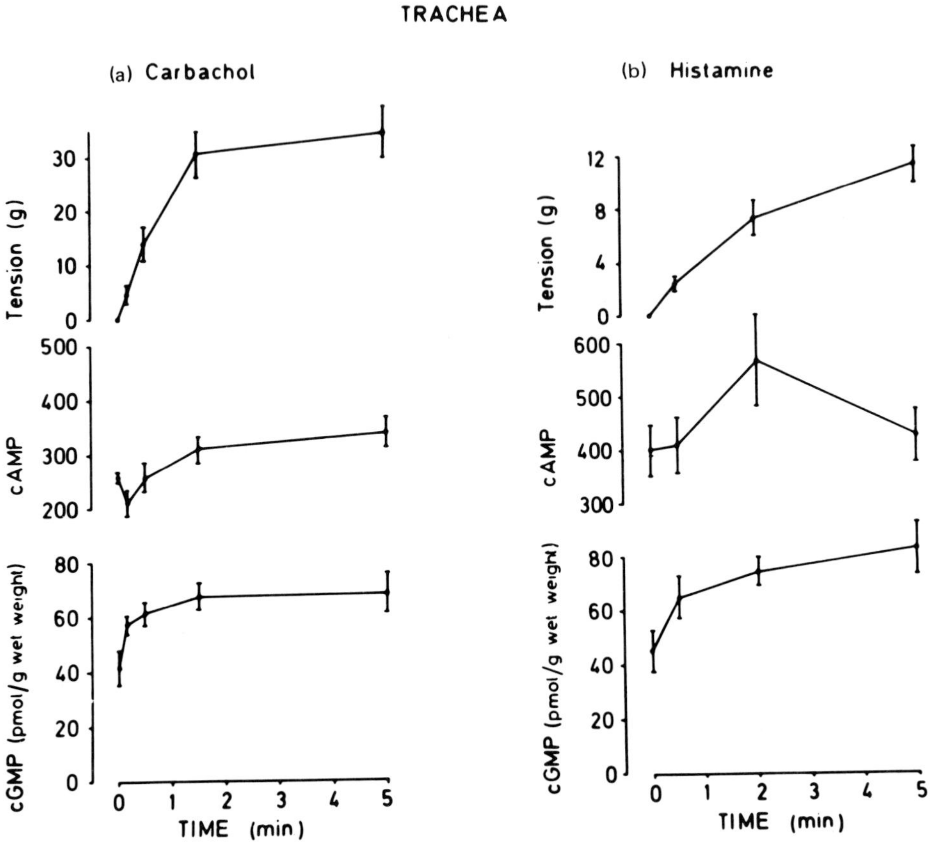


**FIGURE 13** Effects of carbachol, $8 \times 10^{-7}$ g/ml (a), and histamine, $3 \times 10^{-6}$ g/ml (b), on tension and cyclic nucleotide levels in bovine tracheal muscle. Mean ± SEM ($N = 6$–8). (From R. Andersson et al. [8], Cyclic nucleotides and the contraction of smooth muscle. In *Advances in Cyclic Nucleotide Research,* Vol. 5. Edited by G. I. Drummond, P. Greengard, and G. A. Robinson. New York, Raven Press, 1975, pp. 491–518. Reprinted, by permission, Raven Press.)

absence of α-adrenergic antagonists, causes release of norepinephrine from sympathetic nerve endings and an initial decreased cyclic AMP [15].

When rat uterus is contracted by epinephrine, acetylcholine, oxytocin, $BaCl_2$, or prostaglandin $F_{2\alpha}$, no change occurs in basal concentrations of cyclic AMP. If basal cyclic AMP is increased by isoproterenol, contracting agents then decrease the concentration of cyclic AMP [172,181,182]. Conversely, stimulating agonists such as $PGE_2$ [182] and $K^+$ increase cyclic AMP in rat uterus after a delay [116].

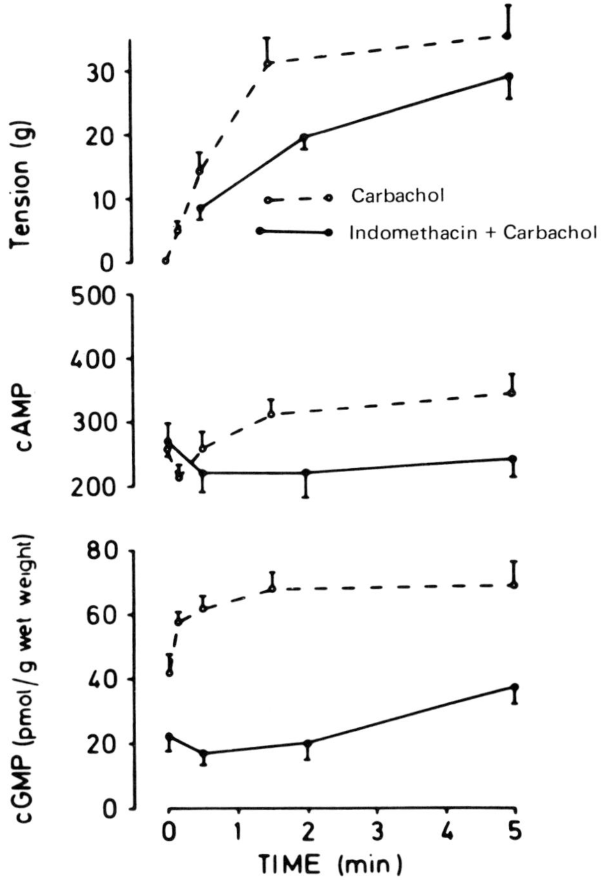


**FIGURE 14** Effect of indomethacin ($3 \times 10^{-6}$ g/ml) on carbachol-induced changes of tension and cyclic nucleotides in bovine trachea. Indomethacin treatment was started 15 min prior to the carbachol addition. Mean ± SEM ($N = 6$). (From R. Andersson et al. [8], Cyclic nucleotides and the contraction of smooth muscle. In *Advances in Cyclic Nucleotide Research,* Vol. 5. Edited by G. I. Drummond, P. Greengard, and G. A. Robinson. New York, Raven Press, 1975, pp. 491-518. Reprinted, by permission, Raven Press.)

In summary, cyclic AMP probably activates carbohydrate metabolism to provide energy necessary to bind $Ca^{2+}$ within the cell, pump $Ca^{2+}$ out of the cell, decrease $Ca^{2+}$ influx into the cell, or inhibit $Ca^{2+}$ effects on the contractile elements. Many more data are required to define these speculations.

## B. Cyclic GMP

Previous reports which suggested that agonists causing contraction of smooth muscle also caused increased concentration of cyclic GMP and decreased cyclic AMP led to the hypothesis that cyclic GMP plays a causal role in contraction and that cyclic GMP and cyclic AMP play opposing roles in regulation of tone in smooth muscle [8,112,116].

### *Increased Cyclic GMP*

**Effects of Hormones and Neurotransmitters**

Diverse hormones and neurotransmitters that cause contraction of smooth muscle (including acetylcholine, α-adrenergic agonists, histamine, serotonin, oxytocin, bradykinin, and prostaglandin $F_{2a}$, and large depolarizing concentrations of $K^+$) also increase the intracellular concentration of cyclic GMP three- to five-fold [183].

The cellular responses, increased intracellular cyclic GMP, and increased smooth muscle tone induced by hormones [150,184] appear to be due to an increase in the concentration of calcium ion in the cytoplasm. Furthermore, there is a temporal discrepancy between the increase in concentration of cyclic GMP and increased smooth muscle tone in different tissues. In the ductus deferens of the rat, the increased cyclic GMP induced by acetylcholine and potassium was detected as early as the onset of tension, whereas the increased cyclic GMP induced by α-adrenergic agonists occurred only after the increased tension was maximal [44]. In longitudinal smooth muscle from guinea pig small intestine, acetylcholine and histamine caused increased smooth muscle tone of similar magnitude, whereas histamine increased the concentration of cyclic GMP much more than acetylcholine [108].

Diamond has reported similar discrepancies between the effect of agonists on cyclic GMP and smooth muscle tone. Carbamylcholine caused contraction of guinea pig ileum without any change in cyclic GMP; carbamylcholine and potassium contracted rat myometrium without changing cyclic GMP [185,186]. During spontaneous contraction of rat uterus, no detectable change in concentration of cyclic GMP occurred (Fig. 15) [187]. In guinea pig myometrium and tenia coli, contraction induced by carbamylcholine preceded increased concentrations of cyclic GMP (Fig. 16) [185]. In dog femoral arteries, carbamylcholine increased cyclic GMP without changing smooth muscle tone [188]. In human umbilical arteries, prostaglandins induced contraction of smooth muscle without change in concentration of cyclic GMP [146].

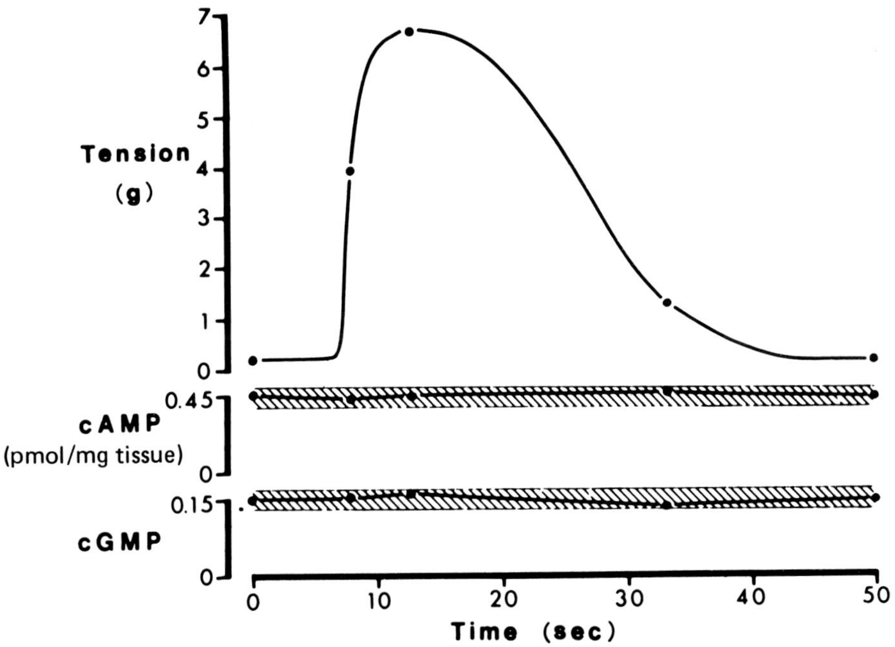


**FIGURE 15** Temporal relationships between cyclic nucleotide levels and isometric tension during spontaneous contractions of isolated rat uterus. Shaded areas represent mean values ± SE for cyclic AMP and cyclic GMP levels in relaxed muscles. Each point represents an average of 7 to 13 determinations. (From J. Diamond and D. K. Hartle [187], Cyclic nucleotide levels during spontaneous uterine contractions, *Can. J. Physiol. Pharmacol.*, **52**:763-767 (1974). Reproduced by permission of the National Research Council of Canada.)

### Effects of Divalent Cations

**Calcium** $Ca^{2+}$ appears critical in mediating the increased concentrations of cyclic GMP induced by hormones [44,107]. If $Ca^{2+}$ is omitted from the extracellular medium, hormones have little or no effect on cyclic GMP. In rat ductus deferens and other tissues, $Ca^{2+}$ also appears important in regulating the basal concentration of cyclic GMP [44,107]. However, the original concept that hormones or neurotransmitters increased cyclic GMP by their effect on increasing cytoplasmic $Ca^{2+}$ concentration no longer seems feasible. Increased smooth muscle tone and increased cyclic GMP are apparently $Ca^{2+}$-dependent phenomena, but they correlate poorly; therefore, other $Ca^{2+}$-independent control

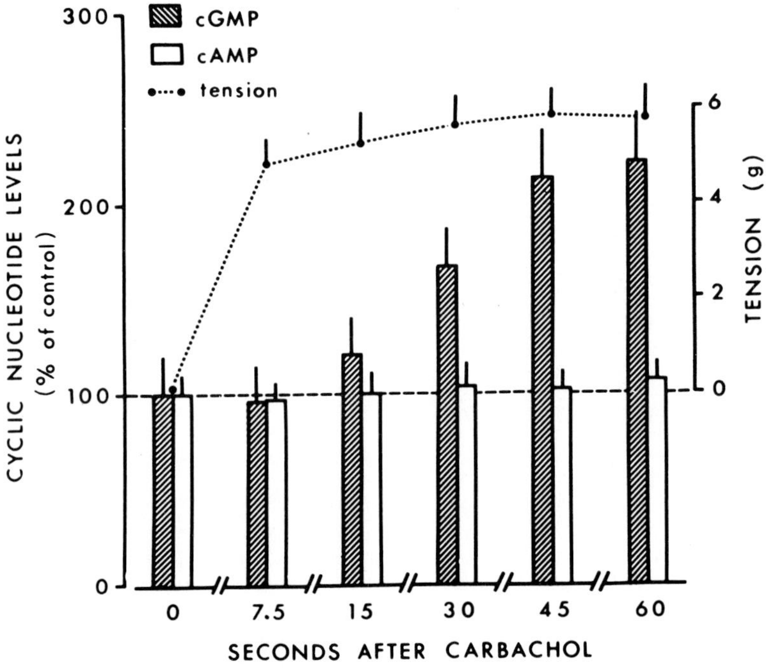


**FIGURE 16** Effects of carbachol ($10^{-5}$ M) on tension and cyclic nucleotide levels in estrogen-primed guinea pig uterus. Bars and points represent means ± SE of five to nine myometrial strips. Cyclic GMP levels are significantly different from controls ($P < 0.05$) at 30, 45, and 60 sec after carbachol administration. (From J. Diamond [117], Evidence for dissociation between cyclic nucleotide levels and tension in smooth muscle. In *The Biochemistry of Smooth Muscle*. Edited by N. L. Stephens. Baltimore, University Park Press, 1977, pp. 343-360.)

mechanisms of guanylate cyclase activity must be reconsidered. Moreover, the discrepancy between cyclic GMP levels and smooth muscle tone may result from hydrolysis of cyclic GMP by $Ca^{2+}$-dependent phosphodiesterase (see Sec. II.C) [152, 180].

**Strontium** This ion can replace $Ca^{2+}$ in the response of cyclic GMP or smooth muscle tone. For example, when $Sr^{2+}$ was used in a concentration twice the usual $Ca^{2+}$ concentration, acetylcholine increased tone and cyclic GMP of rat ductus deferens comparable to effects observed with $Ca^{2+}$ [44].

**Manganese** $Mn^{2+}$ increases concentrations of cyclic GMP in smooth muscle, but inhibits contractile effects of diverse agonists. When rat ductus deferens was incubated in a $Ca^{2+}$-free medium, basal cyclic GMP was decreased; when

$Mn^{2+}$ was added, cyclic GMP increased several-fold [108], but cyclic AMP concentrations were unchanged. Acetylcholine or norepinephrine in the presence of $Mn^{2+}$ (with or without $Ca^{2+}$) causes increased cyclic GMP without increased smooth muscle tone. This $Mn^{2+}$-dependent increase in cyclic GMP may be due to an effect of the neurotransmitter on the permeability of the membrane, or to some direct effect on guanylate cyclase activity [189].

### Effects of Oxygen

The increased cyclic GMP in human umbilical arteries caused by hormones and calcium depends on oxygen [45]. The effect of $O_2$ on hormone- and calcium-induced increases in concentrations of cyclic GMP in other tissues is not well defined, but decreased $O_2$ increased cyclic GMP in peripheral lung of dog and guinea pig (Barnett and Gold, unpublished observations).

### Agonists That Prevent Smooth Muscle Contraction

Recently, marked increases in cyclic GMP have been reported to occur in the presence of oxidants [48-50]. These agonists can also dilate vascular smooth muscle and, at higher concentrations, rat ductus deferens [189].

In rat ductus deferens, hydroxylamine increased the concentration of cyclic GMP 20- to 50-fold without changing the concentration of cyclic AMP [189]. Nitroglycerol increased concentrations of cyclic GMP in rat myometrium [186], canine femoral artery [188], and relaxed these tissues without changing concentrations of cyclic AMP. Furthermore, a derivative of verapamil (D-600), a "calcium antagonist," increased cyclic GMP concentrations and prevented contraction. Similarly, small concentrations of sodium nitroprusside (a potent smooth muscle relaxant in many tissues, including blood vessels), increased concentrations of cyclic GMP 50-fold without changing cyclic AMP or tone of the ductus deferens [190]. In contrast to hormones and neurotransmitters, these agonists increased cyclic GMP independently of extracellular calcium ion or change in smooth muscle tone, often at least one order of magnitude more than agonists which increased cyclic GMP and caused changes in smooth muscle tone. Most of these agents appear to stimulate guanylate cyclase directly [48-54]. More recently, Katsuki and Murad showed that $NaN_3$, $NH_2OH$, $NaNO_2$, and nitroglycerin (1 $\mu$M to 5 mM) increased cyclic GMP 5- to 20-fold and relaxed bovine tracheal smooth muscle without changes in cyclic AMP or dependence on $Ca^{2+}$; increased cyclic GMP induced by carbamylcholine or histamine followed the onset of tension and required $Ca^{2+}$ [191].

### Influences on Guanylate Cyclase

Guanylate cyclase has not been studied extensively in smooth muscle. As described previously, it occurs in soluble and particulate forms, but no direct effects of hormones or neurotransmitters which affect cyclic GMP in intact tissues have been demonstrated on either form of the enzyme.

Divalent cations appear to have potent effects on guanylate cyclase activity [43]. Manganese is more potent than $Mg^{2+}$, $Ca^{2+}$, or $Sr^{2+}$, and other divalent cations in vitro, but present evidence is inconclusive concerning the role played by $Mn^{2+}$ with guanylate cyclase in vivo.

The effect of $Ca^{2+}$ on both soluble and particulate guanylate cyclase has been studied extensively. Concentrations of $Ca^{2+}$ required for stimulation of the soluble enzyme fraction are large relative to the intracellular concentrations assumed to occur in cells stimulated by hormones. As reviewed above, some of the agonists that increase concentrations of cyclic GMP independently of $Ca^{2+}$ can stimulate guanylate cyclase in cell-free preparations from several tissues. Hydroxylamine stimulates soluble and particulate guanylate cyclase from rat ductus deferens; sodium nitroprusside also stimulates soluble guanylate cyclase from the rat ductus deferens.

### *Effects of Exogenous Cyclic GMP and Synthetic Cyclic GMP*

Despite many attempts [14], there are few reports that contractile effects of hormones on smooth muscle can be reproduced by cyclic GMP or its derivatives applied exogenously to intact tissues. In large concentrations, cyclic GMP or its 8-bromo derivatives applied to isolated tissues caused relaxation of smooth muscle (e.g., guinea pig trachea [192,193] and ileum). Some contractile responses have been observed, but these were blocked by atropine, suggesting they were indirect and involved release of endogenous acetylcholine [192]. In careful studies, 8-bromo-cyclic GMP inhibited the contractile response of rat ductus deferens and rat aorta to norepinephrine without altering the intracellular concentration of cyclic AMP [108]. These important studies suggest that cyclic GMP may act to reduce smooth muscle excitability, rather than induce increased tension.

### *Cyclic GMP and Cellular Function*

Little is known about cellular mechanisms controlled by cyclic GMP in smooth muscle. There are cyclic GMP-dependent protein kinases in a variety of mammalian tissues, but none has been demonstrated in smooth muscle. Increased phosphorylation of proteins in smooth muscle membrane by cyclic GMP has been reported, but the physiological significance of this finding is uncertain [169]. Cyclic GMP inhibits the binding of $Ca^{2+}$ by a microsomal fraction from rabbit intestinal smooth muscle [8,116], but this has not been confirmed elsewhere.

### *Biologic Role of Cyclic GMP*

There is considerable circumstantial evidence that cyclic GMP mediates some of the effects of agonists which contract and relax smooth muscle, although the cellular mechanisms regulated by this chemical are not defined. Early reports that increased smooth muscle tone was correlated with increased cyclic GMP appear invalid. Considerable evidence has been accumulated that agonists which relax smooth muscle also increase cyclic GMP and that small concentrations of 8-bromo-cyclic GMP inhibit contractile responses [8,116,151]. Schultz et al. suggest that cyclic GMP acts as a negative feedback inhibitor of the excitation process induced by hormones and neurotransmitters [44,108]. Cyclic GMP probably does not act by inhibiting $Ca^{2+}$ influx into the cytoplasm. Since sodium nitroprusside may cause a marked increase in cyclic GMP without affecting smooth muscle tone, it is also unjustified to assume that "calcium antagonists" and other vasodilators cause relaxation solely on the basis of increasing the concentration of cyclic GMP in smooth muscle. As suggested at the outset of this review, the function of cyclic GMP probably differs even among smooth muscles; the exact function still remains to be defined [108]. Many of these relationships are illustrated in Figure 6.

## C. Immunocytochemical Studies of Muscle

Some of the problems in evaluating the biologic role of cyclic nucleotides in smooth muscle may be solved by immunocytochemical methods. This approach has provided useful clues concerning the roles played by these chemicals in cardiac and skeletal muscle.

Distinct staining patterns for cyclic AMP and cyclic GMP have been observed in rat cardiac and skeletal muscle [194]. Antibody to cyclic AMP is found in the area of the sarcoplasmic reticulum and the sarcolemma in both cardiac and skeletal muscle. This pattern is consistent with biochemical data which have identified a cyclic AMP-dependent protein kinase in microsomal fractions of both cardiac and slow skeletal muscle [195,196]. Staining for cyclic AMP was also located at the intercalated disks of cardiac muscle, and in longitudinal sections of this muscle, faint staining was seen in cross bands corresponding to I and A bands.

Analysis of the concentration of cyclic AMP and binding capacities of the principal proteins of the contractile elements should help to determine whether the nucleotide is associated with the sarcoplasmic reticulum which ensheathes both bands or is associated with structural proteins present in both bands of the myofibrils. Biochemical studies suggest a role of cyclic AMP in phosphorylation of troponin I in cardiac muscle, so association of the nucleotide with proteins of the troponin-tropomyosin complex, which is associated with the thin filaments, would be of particular interest.

The pattern of staining with anti-cyclic GMP antibody is completely different from the staining for cyclic AMP. Cyclic GMP appears to be localized in bands in both tissues with a periodicity of 1.2 to 2.5 $\mu$m. Staining is most marked in skeletal muscle, particularly in contracted rather than in relaxed regions. Intercalated disks in cardiac muscle also stain intensely. Neither sarcoplasmic reticulum nor sarcolemma stain in either skeletal or cardiac muscle. Matched polarization and fluorescence photographs show that cyclic GMP is localized in the anisotropic bands, indicating cyclic GMP is present in A bands (containing myosin). Absence of cyclic GMP fluorescence in the I band suggests that the nucleotide is not bound to receptors in actin, troponin, or tropomyosin, at least in concentrations sufficient for cytochemical detection.

The distinct and different localization of the two cyclic nucleotides suggests diverse roles in regulation of muscle contraction. These studies support biochemical data indicating that cyclic AMP plays a role in regulating uptake of calcium by sarcoplasmic reticulum [195,196]. Binding of cyclic GMP antibody in the region of the A band suggests that cyclic GMP may play a role in regulating a function of myosin. A protein kinase sensitive to calcium which phosphorylates the myosin light chain component (molecular weight 18,500) from white and red skeletal muscle and from cardiac muscle has been described. Cyclic AMP does not appear to regulate this protein kinase, with or without calcium ion. Conceivably, cyclic GMP controls phosphorylation by this light-chain kinase or dephosphorylation of the light chain by a phosphatase. Cyclic GMP might also modulate cation binding in the components of myosin since there appears to be a close interrelationship between changes in concentration of cyclic GMP and uptake of calcium in other tissues [9,44,116]. Cyclic GMP might also be involved in regulating the structural integrity of myosin in some other manner.

Ong and Steiner have suggested that these findings may have wider application. Actin and myosin are found in association with plasma membrane and other intracellular organelles which may regulate intracellular rearrangement, in addition to their role in contraction of muscle [194]. Moreover, cyclic nucleotides are postulated to play a role in modulating the surface of the cell and cytoskeletal movement. Hopefully, these techniques can be applied to study airway smooth muscle and other contractile elements in tissues, in addition to cardiac and skeletal muscle.

### D. Cyclic Nucleotides and Calcium Metabolism

Calcium ion plays a critical role in the regulation of contraction and relaxation in smooth muscle [197] as well as in striated and cardiac muscle. $Ca^{2+}$ activates the contractile proteins in the muscle fiber [197]. To understand the regulation of the mechanical behavior of smooth muscle by cyclic nucleotides, it is necessary to understand the manner in which $Ca^{2+}$ is regulated in smooth muscle. Current investigations are concerned with the localization of pools of $Ca^{2+}$ that serve as sources of mobilizable $Ca^{2+}$, localization of depots within the cell and outside the cell that function as reservoirs for the $Ca^{2+}$ removed from the cytoplasm, and the characterization [198] of the cellular mechanisms that regulate movement of $Ca^{2+}$ in and out of the cytoplasm.

Numerous physiological experiments on diverse types of smooth muscle indicate there are two different sources of $Ca^{2+}$ that can be mobilized for contraction [198]: (1) a tightly bound pool of $Ca^{2+}$ sequestered in some intracellular location or locations in the muscle fiber, and (2) a pool of $Ca^{2+}$ in the extracellular fluid or loosely bound to superficial sites in the muscle fiber. Both these pools may not play equally important roles in all types of smooth muscle. In smooth muscles such as rabbit pulmonary artery [199] or rabbit aorta, a tightly bound intracellular $Ca^{2+}$ pool appears to be most important; in other muscle such as rabbit colon [199], this pool is less important; and in other muscles, such as the longitudinal muscle of guinea pig ileum [198], a tightly bound intracellular $Ca^{2+}$ pool is of negligible importance in supporting mechanical activity.

There are three different sites within smooth muscle cells where $Ca^{2+}$ can be concentrated: the endoplasmic reticulum, the mitochondria, and the plasma membrane. These loci may serve as sources or sinks for calcium flux associated with contractile activity.

Andersson and coworkers [8,116] have studied calcium binding by different subcellular fractions of smooth muscles. Cyclic AMP increased $Ca^{2+}$ binding in microsomal fractions (portions of plasma membrane) of rabbit colon, but had no effect on the mitochondrial fraction. Isoproterenol increased $Ca^{2+}$ binding in microsomal fraction (plasma membrane) and stimulated adenylate cyclase activity in this fraction; it was ineffective in the portion of plasma membrane containing surface vesicles and adjoining sarcotubular system. Carbamylcholine caused release of $Ca^{2+}$ from the microsomal fraction of plasma membrane and decreased adenylate cyclase activity in it, but had a smaller effect on the fraction containing surface vesicles and adjoining sarcotubular system. Carbamylcholine also caused sufficient $Ca^{2+}$ release from the microsomal fraction of plasma membrane to contract glycerinated smooth muscle fibers, proving that extracellular calcium is not required for calcium-dependent contraction in certain smooth muscles, particularly if their stores of cytoplasmic calcium are large.

There are two different mechanisms by which stimuli induce the movement of $Ca^{2+}$ from storage sites to the cytoplasm. One mechanism is poorly defined but is independent of any change in membrane potential [200]; the other mechanism involves generation of action potentials [201] or, in some cases, a sustained depolarization of the membrane [197]. The $Ca^{2+}$ transport system (which is activated directly or indirectly by an excitatory drug and which moves calcium ion from an extracellular or superficial site to the cytoplasm) appears to possess the characteristics of a saturable system [198]. Little is known about the transport system which is actuated by excitatory drugs and which releases firmly bound calcium ions from intracellular sites.

Removal of $Ca^{2+}$ from the cytoplasm and the initiation of relaxation probably involve energy-dependent calcium transport systems [8,116,198]. These systems have been demonstrated in isolated mitochondria, and in isolated cell fragments derived from the plasma membrane and the endoplasmic reticulum [8,198]. This suggests the possibility that calcium pumps operating in the surface membrane, mitochondrial membrane, and membranes of the endoplasmic reticulum may be responsible for the movement of $Ca^{2+}$ from the cytoplasm to the extracellular fluid or to storage pools in intracellular organelles, or both.

Current knowledge does not permit a detailed description of the sequence of events from the point when the excitatory drug complexes with specific receptors in the tissue to the point when cytoplasmic $Ca^{2+}$ is taken up and stored; further clarification is also required of the manner in which drugs which relax smooth muscle alter $Ca^{2+}$ flux within it. Many of these relationships are illustrated in Figure 6.

### E. Cyclic Nucleotides and Carbohydrate Metabolism*

Little direct information is available concerning airway smooth muscle. Present evidence suggests that increased cyclic AMP following contraction depends on calcium ion; activation of phosphorylase during contraction also depends on calcium ion, but the effect on calcium ion may be mediated in part by cyclic AMP. The increase in cyclic AMP also appears to depend on prostaglandins since it can be prevented by indomethacin.

Although controversy exists concerning the role of cyclic AMP during relaxation, activation of carbohydrate metabolism and relaxation are probably partially parallel effects of increased cyclic AMP. Activation of carbohydrate metabolism probably provides energy necessary for binding calcium ion within the cell or pumping the ion out of the cell.

## VII. Summary

The role of cyclic nucleotides in smooth muscle is controversial and uncertain. Apparently conflicting results have been obtained by different authors using a

*See Chapter 2.

variety of assays and preparations obtained from diverse species. Very little work has been done in airway smooth muscle itself. Therefore, I have reviewed the current status of our knowledge concerning cyclic nucleotide metabolism in the lung in general, and in two specific cells found in lung (mast cell and smooth muscle) in particular. Although considerably more work is required, it appears that both cyclic AMP and cyclic GMP act to inhibit smooth muscle tone or excitability, in part by their effect on calcium pools within the muscle cell.

## References


1. Austen, K. F., and R. P. Orange, Bronchial asthma: The possible role of the chemical mediators of immediate hypersensitivity in the pathogenesis of subacute chronic disease, *Am. Rev. Respir. Dis.*, **112**:423-436 (1975).
2. Kaliner, M., Human lung tissue and anaphylaxis. I. The role of cyclic GMP as a modulator of the immunologically induced secretory process, *J. Allergy Clin. Immunol.*, **60**:204-211 (1977).
3. Sutherland, E. W., and T. W. Rall, The relation of adenosine-3′-5′-phosphate and phosphorylase to the actions of catecholamines and other hormones, *Pharmacol. Rev.*, **12**:265-299 (1960).
4. Robison, G. A., R. W. Butcher, and E. W. Sutherland, Adenyl cyclase as an adrenergic receptor, *Ann. N.Y. Acad. Sci.*, **139**:703-723 (1967).
5. Amer, S., Studies with cholecystokinin in vitro. III. Mechanism of the effect of the isolated rabbit gall bladder strips, *J. Pharmacol. Exp. Ther.*, **183**:527-534 (1972).
6. Lee, T. P., J. F. Kuo, and P. Greengard, Role of muscarinic cholinergic receptors in regulation of guanosine 3′,5′-cyclic monophosphate content in mammalian brain, heart muscle, and intestinal smooth muscle, *Proc. Natl. Acad. Sci. USA*, **69**:3287-3291 (1972).
7. Andersson, K. E., R. Andersson, and P. Hedner, Cholecystokinetic effect and concentration of cyclic AMP on gallbladder muscle in vitro, *Acta Physiol. Scand.*, **85**:511-516 (1972).
8. Andersson, R., K. Nilsson, J. Wikberg, S. Johansson, E. Mohme-Lundholm, and L. Lundholm, Cyclic nucleotides and the contraction of smooth muscle. In *Advances in Cyclic Nucleotide Research*, Vol. 5. Edited by G. I. Drummond, P. Greengard, and G. A. Robinson. New York, Raven Press, 1975, pp. 491-518.
9. Gillespie, J. S., K. E. Creed, and T. C. Muir, The mechanics of action of neurotransmitters, *Philos. Trans. R. Soc. Lond. [Biol.]*, **265**:95-106 (1973).
10. Andersson, R., and E. Mohme-Lundholm, Studies on the relaxing actions mediated by stimulation of adrenergic α- and β-receptors in taenia coli of the rabbit and guinea pig, *Acta Physiol. Scand.*, **77**:372-384 (1969).
11. Brody, T. N., and J. Diamond, Blockade of the biochemical correlates of contraction and relaxation in uterine and intestinal smooth muscle, *Ann. N.Y. Acad. Sci.*, **139**:772-779 (1967).
12. Lee, C. Y., Adrenergic receptors in the intestine. In *Smooth Muscle.* Edited

by E. Bülbring, A. F. Brading, A. W. Jones, and T. Tomita, London, E. Arnold Ltd., 1970, pp. 549-557.
13. Takagi, K., I. Takayanagi, and Y. Tsuchida, The effects of caffeine and imidazole on the actions of beta- and alpha-adrenergic stimulants papaverine and cyclic 3′,5′-AMP, *Jpn. J. Pharmacol.,* **22**:403-409 (1972).
14. Paton, W. D. M., and M. Aboo Zar, The origin of acetylcholine released from guinea-pig intestine and longitudinal muscle strips, *J. Physiol. (Lond.),* **194**:13-33 (1968).
15. Andersson, R., Cyclic AMP and calcium ions in mechanical and metabolic responses of smooth muscles; influences of some hormones and drugs, *Acta Physiol. Scand.,* **87**(Suppl. 382):1-59 (1972).
16. Nadel, J. A., Neurophysiologic aspects of asthma. In *Asthma: Physiology, Immunopharmacology, and Treatment.* Edited by K. F. Austen and L. M. Lichtenstein. New York and London, Academic, 1973, pp. 29-38.
17. Bouhuys, A., Action and interaction of pharmacological agents on airway smooth muscle. In *The Biochemistry of Smooth Muscle.* Edited by N. L. Stephens. Baltimore, University Park Press, 1977, pp. 703-722.
18. Goldberg, N. D., M. K. Haddox, S. E. Nicol, D. B. Glass, C. H. Sanford, F. A. Kuehl, and R. Estensen, Biological regulation through opposing influences of cyclic GMP and cyclic AMP: The yin yang hypothesis, *Adv. Cyclic Nucleotide Res.,* **5**:307-330 (1975).
19. Angles d'Auriac, G., and M. Worcel, Variations in cGMP and cAMP levels in rat uterine smooth muscle induced by carbachol, $P6F_{2a}$ and changes in ionic composition, *Br. J. Pharmacol.,* **54**:236-237 (1975).
20. Diamond, J., and D. K. Hartle, Cyclic nucleotide levels during carbachol-induced smooth muscle contractions, *Pharmacologist,* **16**:273 (1974).
21. Steiner, A. L., S. Ong, and H. J. Wedner, Cyclic nucleotide immunochemistry, *Adv. Cyclic Nucleotide Res.,* **7**:116-155 (1976).
22. Earp, H. S., and A. L. Steiner, Compartmentalization of cyclic nucleotide-mediated hormone action, *Ann. Rev. Pharmacol. Toxicol.,* **18**:431-459 (1978).
23. Bourne, H. R., P. Coffino, and G. M. Tomkins, Selection of a variant lymphoma cell deficient in adenylate cyclase, *Science,* **187**:750-751 (1975).
24. Orly, J., and M. Schramm, Coupling of catecholamine receptor from one cell with adenylate cyclase from another cell by cell fusion, *Proc. Natl. Acad. Sci. USA,* **73**:4410-4414 (1976).
25. Zenser, T. V., V. J. Petrella, and F. Hughes, Spin-labeled sterates as probes for microenvironment of murine thymocyte adenylate cyclase-cyclic adenosine 3′:5′-monophosphate system, *J. Biol. Chem.,* **251**:7431-7436 (1976).
26. Perkins, J. P., Adenyl cyclase, *Adv. Cyclic Nucleotide Res.,* **3**:1-56 (1973).
27. Cuatrecasas, P., Membrane receptors, *Ann. Rev. Biochem.,* **43**:169-214 (1974).
28. Catt, K. J., and M. L. Dufau, Peptide hormone receptors, *Ann. Rev. Physiol.,* **39**:529-557 (1977).
29. Williams, L. T., R. J. Lefkowitz, A. M. Watanabe, D. R. Hathaway, and H.

R. Besch, Thyroid hormone regulation of β-adrenergic receptor number, *J. Biol. Chem.*, **252**:2787-2789 (1977).

30. Limbird, L. E., and R. J. Lefkowitz, Resolution of β-adrenergic receptor binding and adenylate cyclase activity by gel exclusion chromatography, *J. Biol. Chem.*, **252**:799-802 (1977).
31. Haga, T., K. Haga, and A. G. Gilman, Molecular sizes of putative β-adrenergic receptor and adenylate cyclase, *Fed. Proc.*, **36**:685 (1977).
32. Dufau, M. L., K. Hayashi, G. Sala, A. Baukal, and K. J. Catt, Gonadal LH receptors and adenylate cyclase: Transfer of functional lipid-associated receptors to adrenal fasiculata cells, *Clin. Res.*, **26**:491A (1978).
33. Londos, C., Y. Salomon, M. C. Lin, J. P. Harwood, M. Schramm, J. Wolff, and M. Rodbell, 5′-guanylylimidodiphosphate; a potent activator of adenylate cyclase systems in eukaryotic cells, *Proc. Natl. Acad. Sci. USA*, **71**:3087-3090 (1974).
34. Aurbach, G. D., A. M. Spiegel, and J. D. Gardner, β-Adrenergic receptors, cyclic AMP and ion transport in the avian erythrocyte, *Adv. Cyclic Nucleotide Res.*, **5**:117-132 (1975).
35. Lefkowitz, R. J., D. Mullikin, M. G. Caron, Regulation of β-adrenergic receptors by guanyl-5′:imidiphosphate and other purine nucleotides, *J. Biol. Chem.*, **251**:4686-4692 (1976).
36. Sayers, G., R. J. Beall, and S. Seelig, Isolated adrenal cells: Adrenocorticotrophic hormone, calcium, steroidogenesis, and cyclic adenosine monophosphate, *Science*, **175**:1131-1133 (1972).
37. Brostrom, C. O., Y. C. Huang, B. M. Breckenridge, and D. J. Wolff, Identification of a calcium-binding protein as a calcium dependent regulator of brain adenylate cyclase, *Proc. Natl. Acad. Sci. USA*, **72**:64-68 (1975).
38. Mickey, J., R. Tate, and R. J. Lefkowitz, Supersensitivity of adenylate cyclase and decreased β-adrenergic receptor binding after chronic exposure to (-)-isoproterenol in vitro, *J. Biol. Chem.*, **250**:5727-5729 (1975).
39. Su, Y. F., L. Cubeddu, J. P. Perkins, Regulation of adenosine 3′:5′-monophosphate content of human astrocytoma cells: Desensitization to catecholamines and prostaglandins, *J. Cyclic Nucleotide Res.*, **2**:257-270 (1976).
40. Ishikawa, E., S. Ishikawa, J. W. Davis, and E. W. Sutherland, Determination of guanosine 3′:5′-monophosphate in tissues and guanyl cyclase in rat intestine, *J. Biol. Chem.*, **244**:6371-6376 (1969).
41. Kimura, H., and F. Murad, Two forms of guanylate cyclase in mammalian tissues and possible mechanisms for their regulation, *Metabolism*, **24**:439-445 (1975).
42. Kimura, H., and F. Murad, Evidence for two different forms of guanylate cyclase in rat heart, *J. Biol. Chem.*, **249**:6910-6916 (1974).
43. Chrisman, T. D., D. L. Garbers, M. A. Parks, and J. G. Hardman, Characterization of particulate and soluble guanylate cyclases from rat lung, *J. Biol. Chem.*, **250**:374-381 (1975).
44. Schultz, G., J. G. Hardman, K. Schultz, C. E. Baird, and E. W. Sutherland,

The importance of calcium ions for the regulation of guanosine 3′:5′-cyclic monophosphate levels, *Proc. Natl. Acad. Sci. USA,* **70**:3889-3893 (1973).
45. Clyman, R. I., A. S. Blaksin, V. C. Manganiello, and M. Vaughan, Oxygen and cyclic nucleotides in human umbilical artery, *Proc. Natl. Acad. Sci. USA,* **72**:3883-3887 (1975).
46. Garbers, D. L., J. G. Hardman, and F. B. Rudolph, Kinetic analysis of sea urchin sperm guanylate cyclase, *Biochemistry,* **13**:4166-4171 (1974).
47. Earp, H. S., P. Smith, S. H. Ong, and A. L. Steiner, Regulation of hepatic nuclear guanylate cyclase, *Proc. Natl. Acad. Sci. USA,* **74**:946-950 (1977).
48. Kimura, H., C. K. Mittal, and F. Murad, Activation of guanylate cyclase from liver and other tissues by sodium azide, *J. Biol. Chem.,* **250**:8016-8022 (1975).
49. Mittal, C. K., H. Kimura, and F. Murad, Purification and properties of a protein required for sodium azide activation of guanylate cyclase, *J. Biol. Chem.,* **252**:4384-4390 (1977).
50. Miki, N., M. Nagano, and K. Kuriyama, Catalase activates cerebral guanylate cyclase in the presence of sodium azide, *Biochem. Biophys. Res. Commun.,* **72**:952-959 (1976).
51. Arnold, W. P., R. Aldred, and F. Murad, Cigarette smoke activates guanylate cyclase and increases 3′,5′-monophosphate in tissues, *Science,* **198**:934-936 (1977).
52. Katsuki, S., W. V. Arnold, C. Mittal, and F. Murad, Stimulation of guanylate cyclase by sodium nitroprusside, nitroglycerin and nitric oxide in various tissue preparations and comparison to the effects of sodium azide and hydroxylamine, *J. Cyclic Nucleotide Res.,* **3**:23-35 (1977).
53. DeRubertis, F. R., and P. A. Craven, Calcium-independent modulation of cyclic GMP and activation of guanylate cyclase by nitrosamines, *Science,* **193**:897-899 (1976).
54. White, A. A., K. M. Crawford, C. S. Patt, and P. J. Lad, Activation of soluble guanylate cyclase from rat lung by incubation or by hydrogen peroxide, *J. Biol. Chem.,* **251**:7304-7312 (1976).
55. Glass, D. B., W. Frey, D. W. Carr, and N. D. Goldberg, Stimulation of human platelet guanylate cyclase by fatty acids, *J. Biol. Chem.,* **252**:1279-1285 (1977).
56. Wallach, D., and I. Pastan, Stimulation of guanylate cyclase of fibroblasts by free fatty acids, *J. Biol. Chem.,* **251**:5802-5809 (1976).
57. Asakawa, T., I. Scheinbaum, and R. J. Ho, Stimulation of guanylate cyclase activity by several fatty acids, *Biochem. Biophys. Res. Commun.,* **73**:141-148 (1976).
58. Murad, F., C. K. Mittal, and J. M. Braughler, Cyclic AMP formation by guanylate cyclase, a new pathway for its synthesis, *Clin. Res.,* **26**:531A (1978).
59. Spruill, W. A., A. L. Steiner, and H. S. Earp, Testicular guanylate cyclase: Correlation between tissue cGMP levels and soluble guanylate cyclase activity (GCA), *Fed. Proc.,* **36**:347 (1977).

60. Appleman, M. M., W. J. Thompson, and T. R. Russell, Cyclic nucleotide phosphodiesterases, *Adv. Cyclic Nucleotide Res.*, **3**:65-98 (1973).
61. Cheung, W. Y., Cyclic 3′:5′-nucleotide phosphodiesterase: Evidence for and properties of a protein activator, *J. Biol. Chem.*, **246**:2859-2869 (1971).
62. Russell, T. R., W. C. Terasaki, and M. M. Appleman, Separate phosphodiesterases for the hydrolysis of cyclic AMP and cyclic GMP in rat liver, *J. Biol. Chem.*, **248**:1334-1340 (1973).
63. Pichard, A. L., and W. Y. Cheung, Cyclic 3′:5′-nucleotide phosphodiesterase: Interconvertible multiple forms and their effects on enzyme activity and kinetics, *J. Biol. Chem.*, **251**:5726-5737 (1976).
64. Gnegy, M. E., E. Costa, and P. Uzunov, Regulation of transsynaptically elicited increase of 3′:5′-cyclic AMP by endogenous phosphodiesterase activator, *Proc. Natl. Acad. Sci. USA*, **73**:352-355 (1976).
65. Loten, E. G., and J. G. T. Syned, An effect of insulin on adipose-tissue adenosine 3′:5′-cyclic monophosphate phosphodiesterase, *Biochem. J.*, **120**:187-193 (1970).
66. Kono, T., F. W. Robinson, and J. N. Sarver, Insulin-sensitive phosphodiesterase: Its location, hormonal stimulation and oxidative stabilization, *J. Biol. Chem.*, **250**:7826-7835 (1975).
67. Leichter, S. B., and J. W. Anderson, The insulin-like effects of cyclic GMP, *Clin. Res.*, **26**:426A (1978).
68. Corbin, J. D., S. L. Keely, and C. R. Park, The distribution and dissociation of cyclic adenosine 3′:5′-monophosphate-dependent protein kinases in adipose, cardiac, and other tissues, *J. Biol. Chem.*, **250**:218-225 (1975).
69. Walsh, D. A., C. D. Ashby, C. Gonzalez, D. Calkins, E. H. Fischer, and E. G. Krebs, Purification and characterization of a protein inhibitor of adenosine 3′:5′-monophosphate-dependent protein kinase, *J. Biol. Chem.*, **246**: 1977-1985 (1971).
70. Sala, G., M. L. Dufau, and K. J. Catt, Concomitant stimulation of receptor-bound cAMP and steroidogenesis during hormone action in adrenal and luteal cells, *Clin. Res.*, **26**:312A (1978).
71. Szmigielski, A., A. Guidotti, and E. Costa, Endogenous protein kinase inhibitors: Purification, characterization and distribution in different tissues, *J. Biol. Chem.*, **252**:3848-3853 (1977).
72. Palmer, W. K., M. Castagna, and D. A. Walsh, Nuclear protein kinase activity on glucagon-stimulated perfused rat livers, *Biochem. J.*, **143**:469-471 (1974).
73. Costa, E., A. Kurosawa, and A. Guidotti, Activation and nuclear translocation of protein kinase during transsynaptic induction of tyrosine 3-monooxygenase, *Proc. Natl. Acad. Sci. USA*, **73**:1058-1062 (1976).
74. Jungmann, R. A., P. C. Hiestand, and J. S. Schweppe, Mechanism of action of gonadotropin. IV. Cyclic adenosine monophosphate-dependent translocation of ovarian cytoplasmic cyclic adenosine monophosphate-binding protein and protein kinase to nuclear acceptor sites, *Endocrinology*, **94**: 168-183 (1974).

75. Steiner, A. L., Y. Koide, H. S. Earp, P. J. Bechtel, and J. A. Beavo, Compartmentalization of cyclic nucleotides and cyclic AMP-dependent protein kinases in rat liver. Immunocytochemical demonstration, *Adv. Cyclic Nucleotide Res.,* **9**:691-705 (1978).
76. Kuo, J. F., M. Shoji, and W.-N. Kuo, Molecular and physiopathologic aspects of mammalian cyclic GMP-dependent protein kinase, *Ann. Rev. Pharm. Toxicol.,* **18**:341-355 (1978).
77. Gill, G. N., K. E. Holdy, G. M. Walton, and C. B. Kanstein, Purification and characterization of 3′:5′-cyclic GMP-dependent protein kinase, *Proc. Natl. Acad. Sci. USA,* **73**:3918-3922 (1976).
78. Rose, B., and W. R. Loewenstein, Calcium ion distribution in cytoplasm visualized by acquorin. Diffusion in cytosol restricted by energized sequestering, *Science,* **190**:1204-1206 (1975).
79. Van Cauter, E., J. G. Hardman, and J. E. Dumont, Implications of cross inhibitory interactions of potential mediators of hormone and neurotransmitter action, *Proc. Natl. Acad. Sci. USA,* **73**:2982-2986 (1976).
80. Murad, F., A simple, sensitive protein-binding assay for guanosine 3′:5′-monophosphate, *Proc. Natl. Acad. Sci. USA,* **68**:736-739 (1971).
81. Kuo, J. F., T. P. Lee, P. L. Reyes, K. G. Walton, T. E. Donnelly, Jr., and P. Greengard, Cyclic nucleotide-dependent protein kinases, *J. Biol. Chem.,* **247**:16-22 (1972).
82. Murad, F., T. W. Rall, and M. Vaughan, Conditions for the formation, partial purification and assay of an inhibitor of adenosine 3′:5′-monophosphate, *Biochim. Biophys. Acta,* **192**:430-445 (1969).
83. Kimura, H., E. Thomas, and F. Murad, Effects of decapitation, ether, pentobarbital on guanosine 3′:5′-phosphate and adenosine 3′:5′-phosphate levels in rat tissues, *Biochim. Biophys. Acta,* **343**:519-528 (1974).
84. Barrett-Bee, K. J., and L. R. Green, The relationship between prostaglandins release and lung cyclic AMP during anaphylaxis in the guinea-pig, *Prostaglandin,* **10**:589-597 (1975).
85. Polson, J. B., J. J. Krzanowski, and A. Szetivanyi, Histamine induced changes in pulmonary guanosine-3′,5′-cyclic monophosphate (cGMP) and adenosine-3′,5′-cyclic monophosphate (cAMP) levels in mice following sensitization by *Bortella pertussis* and/or propranolol, *Res. Commun. Chem. Pathol. Pharmacol.,* **9**:243-251 (1974).
86. Barnett, D. B., S. E. Chesrown, A. F. Zbinden, M. Nisam, B. R. Reed, H. R. Bourne, K. L. Melmon, and W. M. Gold, Cyclic AMP and cyclic GMP in canine peripheral lung: Regulation in vivo, *Am. Rev. Respir. Dis.,* **118**: 723-733 (1978).
87. Said, S. I., The lung in relation to vasoactive hormones, *Fed. Proc.,* **32**: 1972-1975 (1973).
88. Kaliner, M., The anaphylactic release of prostaglandins from human lung tissue, *Am. Rev. Respir. Dis.,* **115**:60 (1977).
89. Goodman, A. D., A. L. Steiner, and A. S. Pagliara, Effects of acidosis and alkalosis on 3′,5′-GMP and 3′,5′-AMP in renal cortex, *Am. J. Physiol.,* **223**: 620-625 (1972).

90. Butcher, R. W., and C. E. Baird, Effects of prostaglandins on adenosine 3′,5′-monophosphate levels in fats and other tissues, *J. Biol. Chem.,* **243**: 1713-1717 (1968).
91. Duncan, P. E., J. P. Griffin, and S. S. Solomon, Bronchodilator drug efficacy via cyclic AMP, *Thorax,* **30**:192-196 (1975).
92. Palmer, G. C., Characteristics of the hormonal induced cyclic adenosine 3′,5′-monophosphate response in the rat and guinea pig lung in vitro, *Biochim. Biophys. Acta,* **252**:561-566 (1971).
93. Palmer, G. C., Cyclic 3′,5′-adenosine monophosphate response in the rabbit lung—adult properties and development, *Biochem. Pharmacol.,* **21**: 2907-2914 (1972).
94. Kuo, J. F., and W.-N. Kuo, Regulation by β-adrenergic receptor and muscarinic cholinergic receptor activation of intracellular cyclic AMP and cyclic GMP levels in rat lung slices, *Biochem. Biophys. Res. Commun.,* **55**:660-665 (1973).
95. Stoner, J., V. C. Manganiello, and M. Vaughan, Guanosine 3′,5′-monophosphate and guanylate cyclase activity in guinea pig lung: Effect of acetylcholine and cholinesterase inhibitors, *Mol. Pharmacol.,* **10**:155-161 (1974).
96. Stoner, J., V. C. Manganiello, and M. Vaughan, Effects of bradykinin and indomethacin on cyclic GMP and cyclic AMP in lung slices, *Proc. Natl. Acad. Sci. USA,* **70**:3530-3833 (1973).
97. Kaliner, M. A., R. P. Orange, W. J. Koopman, K. F. Austen, and P. J. Laraia, Cyclic adenosine 3′,5′-monophosphate in human lung, *Biochim. Biophys. Acta,* **252**:160-164 (1971).
98. Guidotti, A., B. Weiss, and E. Costa, Adenosine 3′,5′-monophosphate concentrations and isoproterenol-induced synthesis of deoxyribonucleic acid in mouse parotid gland, *Mol. Pharmacol.,* **8**:521-530 (1972).
99. Murad, F., and H. Kimura, Cyclic nucleotide levels in incubations of guinea pig trachea, *Biochim. Biophys. Acta,* **343**:275-286 (1974).
100. Orange, R. P., W. G. Austen, and K. F. Austen, Immunological release of histamine and slow reacting substance of anaphylaxis from human lung. I. Modulation by agents influencing cellular levels of cyclic 3′,5′-adenosine monophosphate, *J. Exp. Med.,* **134**:136s-148s (1971).
101. Tauber, A. I., M. Kaliner, D. J. Stechschulte, and K. F. Austen, Immunological release of histamine and slow reacting substance of anaphylaxis from human lung. V. Effects of prostaglandins on release of histamine, *J. Immunol.,* **111**:27-32 (1973).
102. Kaliner, M., R. P. Orange, and K. F. Austen, Immunologic release of histamine and slow reacting substance of anaphylaxis from human lung. IV. Enhancement by cholinergic and alpha adrenergic stimulation, *J. Exp. Med.,* **136**:556-567 (1972).
103. Haslam, R. J., and A. Taylor, Effects of catecholamines on the formation of adenosine 3′:5′-cyclic monophosphate in human blood platelets, *Biochem. J.,* **125**:377-379 (1971).
104. Triner, L., G. G. Nahas, Y. Vulliemoz, N. I. A. Overweg, M. Verosky, D.

V. Mabif, and S. H. Ngai, Cyclic AMP and smooth muscle function, *Ann. N.Y. Acad. Sci.,* **185**:458-476 (1971).
105. Marquis, N. R., J. A. Becker, and R. L. Vigdahl, Platelet aggregation. III. An epinephrine induced decrease in cyclic AMP synthesis, *Biochem. Biophys. Res. Commun.,* **39**:783-789 (1970).
106. Butcher, F. R., L. Rudich, C. Elmer, and M. Nemerovski, Adrenergic regulation of cyclic nucleotide levels, amylase release, and potassium efflux in rat parotid gland, *Mol. Pharmacol.,* **12**:862-870 (1976).
107. Schultz, G., Possible interrelations between calcium and cyclic nucleotides in smooth muscle. In *Asthma: Physiology, Immunopharmacology, and Treatment.* Edited by L. M. Lichtenstein and K. F. Austen. New York and London, Academic, 1977, pp. 77-91.
108. Schultz, G., and J. G. Hardman, Regulation of cyclic GMP levels in the ductus deferens of the rat, *Adv. Cyclic Nucleotide Res.,* **5**:339-351 (1975).
109. Wojcik, J. D., R. J. Grand, and D. V. Kimberg, Amylase secretion by rabbit parotid gland: Role of cyclic AMP and cyclic GMP, *Biochim. Biophys. Acta,* **411**:250-262 (1975).
110. Malaisse, W., F. Malaisse-Lagae, P. H. Wright, and J. Ashmore, Effects of adrenergic and cholinergic agents upon insulin secretion in vitro, *Endocrinology,* **80**:975-978 (1967).
111. Ignarro, L. J., and W. J. George, Hormonal control of lysosomal enzyme release from human neutrophils. Elevation of cyclic nucleotide levels by autonomic neurohormones, *Proc. Natl. Acad. Sci. USA,* **71**:2027-2031 (1974).
112. Goldberg, N. D., M. K. Haddox, S. E. Nicol, C. H. Sanford, and D. B. Glass, Cyclic GMP and cyclic AMP in biologic regulation: The yin yang hypothesis. In *New Directions in Asthma.* Edited by Myron Stein. American College of Chest Physicians, Illinois, Park Ridge, 1975, pp. 103-124.
113. Brody, M. J., and P. J. Kadowitz, Prostaglandins as modulators of autonomic nervous system, *Fed. Proc.,* **33**:48-60 (1974).
114. Malik, K. U., Prostaglandins—modulation of adrenergic nervous system, *Fed. Proc.,* **37**:203-207 (1978).
115. Mathé, A. A., L. Volicer, and S. K. Puri, Effect of anaphylaxis and histamine, pyrilamine and burimamide on levels of cyclic AMP and cyclic GMP in guinea-pig lung, *Res. Commun. Chem. Pathol. Pharmacol.,* **8**:635-651 (1974).
116. Andersson, R. G. G., and K. B. Nilsson, Role of cyclic nucleotide metabolism and mechanical activity in smooth muscle. In *The Biochemistry of Smooth Muscle.* Edited by N. L. Stephens. Baltimore, University Park Press, 1978, pp. 263-291.
117. Diamond, J., Evidence for dissociation between cyclic nucleotide levels and tension in smooth muscle. In *The Biochemistry of Smooth Muslce.* Edited by N. L. Stephens. Baltimore, University Park Press, 1977, pp. 343-360.

118. Hyman, A. L., E. W. Spannhake, and P. J. Kadowitz, Prostaglandins and the lung, *Am. Rev. Respir. Dis.*, **117**:111-136 (1978).
119. Schmutzler, W., and R. Derwall, Experiments on the role of cyclic AMP in guinea pig anaphylaxis, *Int. Arch. Allergy Appl. Immunol.*, **45**:120-122 (1973).
120. Kaliner, M., The cyclic nucleotide response of human lung tissue to anaphylaxis, *Clin. Res.*, **25**:361A (1977).
121. Lichtenstein, L. M., Mediator release and asthma. In *Asthma: Physiology, Immunopharmacology, and Treatment.* Edited by L. M. Lichtenstein and K. F. Austen. New York and London, Academic, 1977, pp. 93-110.
122. Orange, R. P., Dissociation of the immunologic release of histamine and slow reacting substance of anaphylaxis from human lung using cytochalasins A and B, *J. Immunol.*, **114**:182-186 (1975).
123. Colten, H. R., and K. H. Gabbay, Histamine release from human leukocytes: Modulation by a cytochalasin B-sensitive barrier, *J. Clin. Invest.*, **51**:1927-1931 (1972).
124. Axline, S. G., and E. P. Reaven, Inhibition of phagocytosis and plasma membrane mobility of the cultivated macrophage by cytochalasin B: Role of subplasmalemmal microfilaments, *J. Cell. Biol.*, **62**:647-659 (1974).
125. Orange, R. P., Selective enhancement of the immunologic release of slow reacting substance of anaphylaxis (SRS-A) by cysteine, *Fed. Proc.*, **34**:1046 (1975).
126. Gillespie, E., R. J. Levine, and S. E. Malawista, Histamine release from rat peritoneal mast cells: Inhibition by colchicine and potentiation by deuterium oxide, *J. Pharmacol. Exp. Ther.*, **164**:158-165 (1968).
127. Kaliner, M., Human lung tissue and anaphylaxis. Evidence that cyclic nucleotides modulate the immunologic release of mediators through effects on microtubular assembly, *J. Clin. Invest.*, **60**:951-959 (1977).
128. Goodman, D. B. P., H. Rasmussen, F. DiBella, and C. E. Guthrow, Jr., Cyclic adenosine 3′:5′-monophosphate stimulated phosphorylation of isolated microtubule subunits, *Proc. Natl. Sci. USA*, **67**:652-659 (1970).
129. Lagnado, J. R., C. A. Lyons, M. Waller, and O. Phillipson, The possible significance of adenosine 3′:5′-cyclic monophosphate-stimulated protein kinase activity associated with purified microtubular protein preparations from mammalian brain, *Biochem. J.*, **128**:95P (July 1972).
130. Rappaport, L., J. F. Leterrier, A. Virlon, and J. Nunes, Phosphorylation of microtubule-associated proteins, *Eur. J. Biochem.*, **62**:539-546 (1976).
131. Soiffer, D., Enzymatic activity in tubular preparations: Cyclic AMP dependent protein kinase activity of brain microtubular protein, *J. Newschem.*, **24**:21-33 (1975).
132. Sloboda, R. P., S. A. Rudolph, J. L. Rosenbaum, and P. Greengard, Cyclic AMP-dependent endogenous phosphorylation of a microtubule-associated protein, *Proc. Natl. Acad. Sci. USA*, **72**:177-181 (1975).
133. Lazarus, S. C., S. E. Chesrown, B. R. Reed, M. J. Frey, and W. M. Gold, Experimental canine anaphylaxis: Effects of cyclic AMP (cAMP), cyclic

GMP (cGMP), histamine, and function in the periphery of the lung, *Am. Rev. Respir. Dis.*, **115**:62 (1977).

134. Cutz, E., and R. P. Orange, Mast cells and endocrine (APUD) cells of the lung. In *Asthma: Physiology, Immunopharmacology, and Treatment.* Edited by L. M. Lichtenstein and K. F. Austen. New York and London, Academic, 1977, pp. 51-76.

135. Sullivan, T. J., K. L. Parker, W. Stenson, and C. W. Parker, Modulation of cyclic AMP in purified rat mast cells. I. Responses to pharmacologic, metabolic, and physical stimuli, *J. Immunol.*, **114**:1473-1479 (1975).

136. Sullivan, T. J., K. L. Parker, S. A. Eisen, and C. W. Parker, Modulation of cyclic AMP in purified rat mast cells. II. Studies on the relationship between intracellular cyclic AMP concentrations and histamine release, *J. Immunol.*, **114**:1480-1485 (1975).

137. Goth, A., H. R. Adams, M. Knoohuizen, Phosphatidyl serine: Selective enhancer of histamine release, *Science*, **173**:1034-1035 (1971).

138. Lagunoff, D., The mechanism of histamine release from mast cells, *Biochem. Pharmacol.*, **21**:1889-1896 (1972).

139. Ts'ao, C., R. Patterson, J. M. McKenna, and I. M. Suszko, Ultrastructural identification of mast cells obtained from human bronchial lumens, *J. Allergy Clin. Immunol.*, **59**:320-326 (1977).

140. Boucher, R. C., P. D. Pare, N. J. Gilmore, L. A. Moroz, and J. C. Hogg, Airway mucosal permeability in the *Ascaris suum*-sensitive rhesus monkey, *J. Allergy Clin. Immunol.*, **60**:134-140 (1977).

141. Paterson, N. A. M., S. I. Wasserman, J. W. Said, and K. F. Austen, Release of chemical mediators from partially purified human lung mast cells, *J. Immunol.*, **117**:1356-1362 (1976).

142. Bach, M. K., and J. R. Brashler, In vivo and in vitro production of a slow reacting substance in the rat upon treatment with calcium ionophores, *J. Immunol.*, **113**:2040-2044 (1974).

143. Lewis, R. A., and K. F. Austen, Nonrespiratory functions of pulmonary cells: The mast cell, *Fed. Proc.*, **36**:2676-2683 (1977).

144. Bar, H.-P., Cyclic nucleotides and smooth muscle, *Adv. Cyclic Nucleotide Res.*, **4**:195-237 (1974).

145. Dunham, E. W., M. K. Haddox, and N. D. Goldberg, Alteration of vein cyclic 3′:5′-nucleotide concentrations during changes in contractility, *Proc. Natl. Acad. Sci. USA*, **71**:815-819 (1974).

146. Clyman, R. I., J. A. Sandler, V. Manganiello, M. Vaughan, Guanosine 3′,5′-monophosphate and adenosine 3′,5′-monophosphate content of human umbilical artery, *J. Clin. Invest.*, **55**:1020-1025 (1975).

147. Andersson, K.-E., R. Andersson, P. Hedner, and C. A. Persson, Effect of cholecystokinin on the level of cyclic AMP and on mechanical activity in the isolated sphincter of Oddi, *Life Sci.*, **11**(part 2):723-732 (1972).

148. Robison, G. A., R. W. Butcher, and E. W. Sutherland, *Cyclic AMP.* New York, Academic, 1971.

149. Vulliemoz, Y., M. Verosky, and L. Triner, The cyclic adenosine 3′:5′-monophosphate system in bronchial tissue. In *The Biochemistry of Smooth Muscle.* Edited by N. L. Stephens. Baltimore, University Park Press, 1977, pp. 293-314.

150. Somlyo, A. P., and A. V. Somlyo, Vascular smooth muscle. II: Pharmacology of normal and hypertensive vessel, *Pharmacol. Rev.*, **22**:249-353 (1970).
151. Drummond, G. I., and L. Duncan, Adenylate cyclase in cardiac tissue, *J. Biol. Chem.*, **245**:976-983 (1970).
152. Kakiuchi, S., R. Yamaraki, Y. Teshimo, and K. Uenishi, Regulation of nucleoside cyclic 3′,5′-monophosphate phosphodiesterase activity from rat brain by a modulator and calcium, *Proc. Natl. Acad. Sci. USA*, **70**: 3526-3530 (1973).
153. Selenger, Z., S. Eimerl, and M. Schramm, A calcium ionophore stimulating the action of epinephrine on the α-adrenergic receptor, *Proc. Natl. Acad. Sci. USA*, **71**:128-131 (1974).
154. Schönhöfer, P. S., I. F. Skidmore, J. Forn, and J. H. Fleisch, Adenyl cyclase activity of rabbit aorta, *J. Pharm. Pharmacol.*, **23**:28-31 (1971).
155. Hardman, J. G., J. N. Wells, and P. Hamet, Cyclic nucleotide metabolism in cell-free systems from vascular tissue. In *The Biochemistry of Smooth Muscle.* Edited by N. L. Stephens. Baltimore, University Park Press, 1977, pp. 329-342.
156. Pöch, G., and W. R. Kukovetz, Studies on the possible role of cyclic AMP in drug-induced coronary vasodilation, *Adv. Cyclic Nucleotide Res.*, **1**: 195-211 (1972).
157. Wells, J. N., G. L. Kramer, J. E. Garst, D. L. Garbers, Selective inhibitors of cyclic nucleotide phosphodiesterase, *Fed. Proc.*, **35**:583 (1976).
158. Hidaka, H., T. Asano, and T. Shimamoto, Cyclic 3′,5′-AMP phosphodiesterase of rabbit aorta, *Biochim. Biophys. Acta*, **377**:103-116 (1975).
159. Kukovetz, W. R., and G. Pöch, Inhibition of cyclic 3′,5′-nucleotide-phosphodiesterase as a possible mode of action of papaverine and similarly acting drugs, *Naunyn Schmiedebergs Arch. Pharmacol.*, **267**:189-194 (1970).
160. Weiss, B., R. Fertel, R. Figlin, and P. Uzunov, Selective alteration of the activity of the multiple forms of adenosine 3′,5′-monophosphate phosphodiesterase of rat cerebrum, *Mol. Pharmacol.*, **10**:615-625 (1974).
161. Somlyo, A. P., A. V. Somlyo, and V. Smiesko, Cyclic AMP and vascular smooth muscle, *Adv. Cyclic Nucleotide Res.*, **1**:175-194 (1972).
162. Bueding, E., E. Bülbring, G. Gercken, J. T. Hawkins, and H. Kuriyama, The effect of adrenaline on the adenosinetriphosphate and creatine phosphate content of intestinal smooth muscle, *J. Physiol. (Lond.)*, **193**:187-212 (1967).
163. Burnstock, G., Purinergic nerves, *Pharmacol. Rev.*, **24**:509-581 (1972).
164. Andersson, R., Role of cyclic AMP and $Ca^{++}$ in metabolic and relaxing effects of catecholamines in intestinal smooth muscle, *Acta Physiol. Scand.*, **85**:312-322 (1972).
165. Paton, W. D. M., and E. S. Vizi, The inhibitor action of noradrenaline and adrenaline on acetylcholine output by guinea-pig ileum longitudinal muscle strip, *Br. J. Pharmacol.*, **35**:10-28 (1969).
166. Krebs, E. G., Protein kinases, *Curr. Top. Cell. Regul.*, **5**:99-133 (1972).

167. Walsh, D. A., and C. D. Ashby, Protein kinases: Aspects of their regulation and diversity, *Recent Prog. Horm. Res.*, **29**:329-359 (1973).
168. Sands, H., T. A. Meyer, and H. V. Rickenberg, Adenosine 3′,5′-monophosphate-dependent protein kinase of bovine tracheal smooth muscle, *Biochim. Biophys. Acta,* **302**:267-281 (1973).
169. Casnellie, J. E., and P. Greengard, Guanosine 3′,5′-cyclic monophosphate-dependent phosphorylation of endogenous substrate proteins in mammalian smooth muscle membranes, *Proc. Natl. Acad. Sci. USA,* **71**:1891-1895 (1974).
170. Kroeger, E. A., T. S. Teo, H. Ho, and J. H. Wang, Relaxants, cyclic adenosine 3′:5′-monophosphate, and calcium metabolism in smooth muscle. In *The Biochemistry of Smooth Muscle.* Edited by N. L. Stephens. Baltimore, University Park Press, 1977, pp. 641-652.
171. Kroeger, E. A., and J. M. Marshall, Beta-adrenergic effects on rat myometrium. Role of cyclic AMP, *Am. J. Physiol.,* **226**:1298-1303 (1974).
172. Marshall, J. M., and E. A. Kroeger, Adrenergic influences on uterine smooth muscle, *Philos. Trans. R. Soc. Lond. (Biol.),* **265**:135-148 (1973).
173. Kroeger, E. A., J. M. Marshall, and C. P. Bianchi, Effect of isoproterenol and D-600 on calcium movements in rat myometrium, *J. Pharmacol. Exp. Ther.,* **193**:309-316 (1975).
174. Andersson, R., Relationship between cyclic AMP, phosphodiesterase activity of calcium and contraction in intestinal smooth muscle, *Acta Physiol. Scand.,* **87**:348-358 (1973).
175. Andersson, R., Role of cyclic AMP and $Ca^{++}$ in the mechanical and metabolic events in isometrically contracting vascular smooth muscle, *Acta Physiol. Scand.,* **87**:84-93 (1973).
176. Vane, J. R., Inhibition of prostaglandin synthesis as a mechanism of action of aspirin-like drugs, *Nature (New Biol.),* **231**:232-235 (1971).
177. Jacobs, K. H., K. Schultz, and G. Schultz, Hemmung von Adenyl-Cyclase-Präparationen aus der Ratteniere durch calciumionen und verschiedene Diuretica, *Naunyn Schmiedebergs Arch. Pharmacol.,* **273**:248-266 (1972).
178. Steer, M. L., and A. Levitzki, The control of adenylate cyclase by calcium in turkey erythrocyte ghosts, *J. Biol. Chem.,* **250**:2080-2084 (1975).
179. Rodan, G., and M. B. Feinstein, Interrelationships between $Ca^{2+}$ and adenylate and guanylate cyclases in the control of platelet secretion and aggregation, *Proc. Natl. Acad. Sci. USA,* **73**:1829-1833 (1976).
180. Wells, J. N., C. E. Baird, Y. J. Wu, and J. G. Hardman, Cyclic nucleotide phosphodiesterase activities of pig coronary arteries, *Biochim. Biophys. Acta,* **384**:430-442 (1975).
181. Triner, L., Y. Vulliemoz, M. Verosky, and G. G. Nahas, The effect of catecholamines on adenyl cyclase activity in rat uterus, *Life Sci.,* **9**:707-712 (1970).
182. Harbon, S., and H. Clauser, Cyclic adenosine 3′,5′-monophosphate levels in rat myometrium under the influence of epinephrine, prostaglandins, and oxytocin. Correlations with uterus motility, *Biochem. Biophys. Res. Commun.,* **44**:1496-1503 (1971).

183. Schultz, G., and J. G. Hardman, Possible roles of cyclic nucleotides in the regulation of smooth muscle tonus. In *Eukaryotic Cell Function and Growth: Regulation by Intracellular Cyclic Nucleotides.* Edited by J. E. Dumont, B. L. Broun, and N. J. Marshall. New York, Plenum, 1976, pp. 667-683.
184. Hurwitz, L., and A. Suria, The link between agonist action and response in smooth muscle, *Ann. Rev. Pharmacol.,* **11**:303-326 (1971).
185. Diamond, J., and D. K. Hartle, Cyclic nucleotide levels during carbachol-induced smooth muscle contractions, *J. Cyclic Nucleotide Res.,* **2**:179-188 (1976).
186. Diamond, J., and T. G. Holmes, Effects of potassium chloride and smooth muscle relaxants on tension and cyclic nucleotide levels in rat myometrium, *Can. J. Physiol. Pharmacol.,* **53**:1099-1107 (1975).
187. Diamond, J., and D. K. Hartle, Cyclic nucleotide levels during spontaneous uterine contractions, *Can. J. Physiol. Pharmacol.,* **52**:763-767 (1974).
188. Diamond, J., and K. S. Blisard, Effects of stimulant and relaxant drugs on tension and cyclic nucleotide levels in canine femoral artery, *Mol. Pharmacol.,* **12**:688-692 (1976).
189. Schultz, K. D., K. Schultz, and G. Schultz, $Mn^{++}$ and rat ductus deferens and Ach, *Naunyn Schmiedebergs Arch. Pharmacol.,* in press.
190. Kreye, V. A. W., G. D. Baron, J. B. Lüth, and H. Schmidt-Gayk, Mode of action of sodium nitroprusside on vascular smooth muscle, *Naunyn Schmiedebergs Arch. Pharmacol.,* **288**:381-402 (1975).
191. Katsuki, S., and F. Murad, Cyclic GMP and cyclic AMP levels during contraction and relaxation of bovine tracheal smooth muscle, *Pharmacologist,* **18**:220 (1976).
192. Lewis, A. J., J. S. Douglas, and A. Bouhuys, Biphasic responses to guanosyl nucleotides in two smooth muscle preparations, *J. Pharm. Pharmacol.,* **25**: 1011-1013 (1973).
193. Szaduykis-Szadurski, L., G. Weimann, and F. Berti, Pharmacological effects of cyclic nucleotides and their derivatives on tracheal smooth muscle, *Pharmacol. Res. Commun.,* **4**:63-69(1972).
194. Ong, S. H., and A. L. Steiner, Localization of cyclic GMP and cyclic AMP in cardiac and skeletal muscle: Immunocytochemical demonstration, *Science,* **195**:183-185 (1977).
195. Kirchberger, M. A., M. Tada, D. I. Repke, and A. M. Katz, Cyclic adenosine 3′,5′-monophosphate-dependent protein kinase stimulation of calcium uptake by canine cardiac microsomes, *J. Mol. Cell. Cardiol.,* **4**:673-680 (1972).
196. Kirchberger, M. A., M. Tada, and A. M. Katz, Adenosine 3′:5′-monophosphate dependent protein kinase-catalyzed phosphorylation reaction and its relation to calcium transport in cardiac sarcoplasmic reticulum, *J. Biol. Chem.,* **249**:6166-6173 (1974).
197. Somlyo, A. P., and A. V. Somlyo, Vascular smooth muscle. I. Normal structure, pathology, biochemistry, and biophysics, *Pharmacol. Rev.,* **20**: 197-272 (1968).
198. Hurwitz, L., Calcium metabolism in smooth muscle. In *The Biochemistry*

*of Smooth Muscle.* Edited by N. L. Stephens. Baltimore, University Park Press, 1977, pp. 559-562.

199. Devine, C. E., A. V. Somlyo, and A. P. Somlyo, Sarcoplasmic reticulum and excitation-contraction coupling in mammalian smooth muscles, *J. Cell. Biol.,* **52**:690-718 (1972).
200. Evans, D. H. L., and H. O. Schild, Mechanism of contraction of smooth muscle by drugs, *Nature,* **180**:341-342 (1957).
201. E. Bülbring, Correlation between membrane potential, spike discharge and tension in smooth muscle, *J. Physiol. (Lond.),* **128**:200-221 (1955).

# 4

# Pharmacologic Aspects of Airway Smooth Muscle

*JEROME H. FLEISCH*

Lilly Research Laboratories
Eli Lilly and Company
Indianapolis, Indiana

Many drugs interact with airway smooth muscle [1]. In recent years, new techniques, refined experimental procedures, and novel pharmacologic agents have helped define some of the mechanisms responsible for drug-induced contraction and relaxation. These studies showed a complexity not previously appreciated. In part, this is due to the ability of lung to metabolize various agents [2]. Drugs can also interact with immunologically sensitized cells (i.e., mast cells) in smooth muscle and lung parenchyma. These cells store and manufacture bronchoactive agents that are released upon antigen challenge. Drugs influence airway smooth muscle or sensitized mast cells by acting at one or more of the following locations: pharmacologic receptors on the cell membrane that recognize and unite with selective agonists (stimulants) and antagonists (blocking agents), the membrane itself, or one of the steps in the sequence of events connecting receptor with response mechanism (i.e., adenylate cyclase-cyclic AMP). Additionally, the contractile proteins and autonomic nerve endings of bronchial smooth muscle are potential sites of action. Generally, the interaction of drug with receptor affords the greatest degree of specificity. Thus, one emphasis of current research is toward the development of agents that can predictably react with pharmacologic receptors.

# I. Drug Receptors in Airway Smooth Muscle

## A. General Concepts

Under normal conditions, activation of drug receptors in airway smooth muscle by various endogenous substances probably serves to maintain bronchomotor tone. However, during pathologic states (i.e., obstructive lung disease), stimulation of receptors mediating bronchoconstriction or a decrease in sensitivity of receptors subserving bronchodilation may play a role in airway obstruction.

Within the last decade, it has become clear that receptors of the same class are heterogenous and as such can interact with highly specific agonists and antagonists. Adrenergic receptors represent the classic example. Shortly after the turn of the century, Dale [3] showed that stimulatory but not inhibitory responses to epinephrine and sympathetic nerve stimulation could be decreased by ergot alkaloids. Forty years later, Ahlquist [4] found a difference in the relative potencies of five sympathomimetic amines on various smooth muscles and the heart. He concluded that adrenergic receptors fall into two main classes, $\alpha$ and $\beta$. The dual adrenergic receptor hypothesis was strengthened by Powell and Slater's [5] discovery of dicholoroisoproterenol (DCI), a $\beta$-receptor antagonist and by the subsequent demonstration that DCI selectively reduced $\beta$ receptor-mediated responses of catecholamines [5,6]. The role DCI played in confirming the existence of two adrenergic receptors and, in more recent times, the importance of burimamide, an $H_2$ receptor antagonist [7], in establishing dual histamine receptors ($H_1$ and $H_2$) indicate that, in the final analysis, selective antagonists are necessary to characterize pharmacologic receptors. $pA_2$ and $K_B$ values were introduced by Schild [8], Arunlakshana and Schild [9], and Furchgott [10] to quantitate the relationship between receptor, agonist, and antagonist. They are characteristic of drug receptors and represent the concentration of antagonist necessary to cause a twofold increase in the $ED_{50}$ of the agonist. Furchgott [10,11] used $K_B$ values to postulate that $\beta$ receptors could be divided into subclasses. Lands and coworkers [12] independently came to the same conclusion after comparing the potencies of adrenergic receptor agonists on various tissues. More recently, there have been suggestions of $\alpha$-receptor subclasses [13]. Thus, in 70 years we have gone from the possibility that two adrenergic receptors might exist, to the concept of dual adrenergic receptors, $\alpha$ and $\beta$, with each class being further subdivided. The significance of this cannot be understated. Armed with the knowledge that $\beta$ receptors are heterogenous, medicinal chemists synthesized highly specific agonists and antagonists capable of interacting with $\beta$ receptors located in a select group of organs [14-16]. Agents having a high selectivity for $\beta$ receptors in bronchial smooth muscle are used as bronchodilators in the treatment of asthma [15-19]. In addition to clinical benefits, the new drugs have unmasked basic information on receptor characteristics. Tuttle and Mills [20] chemically modified isoproterenol to reduce chronotropic, arrhythmogenic, and vascular effects. The resultant drug, dobutamine, has profound effects on the heart, but only a small action on $\alpha$- and $\beta$-vascular receptors. At equivalent inotropic doses, this new catecholamine produces less than 25% of the chronotropic response obtained with isoproterenol. This experiments, and others by Dreyer and Offermeier [21] and Tuttle et al. [22], suggested two types of cardiac $\beta$ receptors, one mediating inotropism (force), the other chronotropism (rate).

### B. In Vitro Airway Smooth Muscle Preparations

The presence of specific pharmacologic receptors in airway smooth muscle is readily ascertained with in vitro preparations. Isolated segments of smooth muscle are best suited for determining the direct action of a drug. These preparations do not significantly metabolize agonists or antagonists nor is there a need to consider autonomic reflexes as contributing to a drug's action. Despite these advantages and the inherent simplicity of isolated tissues, the results obtained with such preparations have to be extrapolated cautiously to an intact respiratory system.

An in vitro technique enabling various airway subdivisions to be examined individually would present an ideal situation. Most techniques in use today stem from the early work on tracheal chain by Castillo and DeBeer [23], modified by Akcasu [24], and the spirally cut trachea developed by Patterson [25] (see Fleisch et al. [1] for further references). More recently, Persson and Ekman [26] and Hooker et al. [27] demonstrated the ease by which airways 1 mm in diameter can be studied in vitro. In the procedure of Hooker et al. [27], tissues are slipped onto "L"-shaped supports made from 30-gauge disposable hypodermic needles; responses are recorded on a polygraph via a force-displacement transducer. This modification of existing techniques makes an inexpensive procedure for measuring responses of "small" airways and blood vessels available to most pharmacology and physiology laboratories. Previous attempts by our laboratory and others to measure responses of mouse trachea had resulted in failure. Using the technique of Hooker et al. [27], we successfully recorded responses of several 4- to 5-mm segments from a single mouse trachea. They contracted to carbachol (Fig. 1) and potassium chloride but not to histamine. Mice treated with *Bordetella pertussis* are hypersensitive to various stimuli [28,29]. Pharmacologic experiments comparing trachea from such animals with those from control mice could provide insight into factors contributing to the asthma syndrome.

A new in vitro preparation, the cat lung strip, has been described by Lulich et al. [30]. Drug-induced contractions and relaxations were obtained from a thin strip of cat lung parenchyma suspended in a standard isolated tissue bath. Comparison with cat trachea showed notable differences, i.e., the trachea did

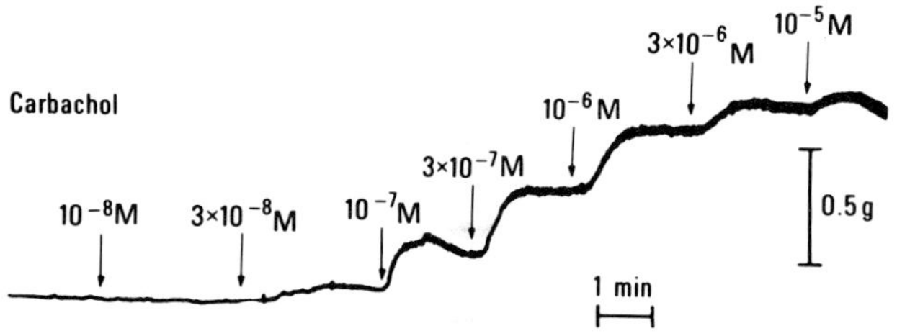


**FIGURE 1** Contractions of mouse trachea to increasing concentrations of carbachol (carbamylcholine). The tissue was set up as described by Hooker et al. [27]. Isometric measurements were made with a force-displacement transducer and recorded on a polygraph as changes in grams of force.

not contract to histamine and prostaglandin $F_{2a}$ ($PGF_{2a}$) whereas the lung strip contracted strongly to these agents. Isoproterenol, epinephrine, and norepinephrine relaxed both preparations. Responses of the lung strip are thought to be due primarily to activation of receptors on peripheral airways. However, the role of pulmonary blood vessels in these responses is unknown. Another new method allows responses of dog tracheal musculature to be measured in situ as changes in pressure of a water-filled cuff inserted into the upper trachea perfused with blood through the cranial thyroid arteries, the main arteries supplying the upper portion of the trachea [31]. Blood flow through these vessels was measured by an electromagnetic flowmeter. Differential effects of drugs, administered intra-arterially, could be seen on tracheal and vascular smooth muscle. For example, acetylcholine increased both intratracheal pressure (constriction) and blood flow (dilation). In contrast, isoproterenol decreased intratracheal pressure and increased blood flow as a result of tracheal dilation and vasodilation.

### C. Pharmacologic Heterogeneity of Trachea and Bronchi: Histamine Receptors

Lack of pharmacologic uniformity in airway smooth muscle is of prime importance when considering the action of drugs on the tracheobronchial tree. This was pointed out as early as 1913 by Golla and Symes [32]. Later on, Brocklehurst [33] reported that trachea and bronchioles respond differently to drugs. The most impressive example of a lack of pharmacologic uniformity can be seen with histamine. Eyre [34] demonstrated that histamine contracts trachea and major bronchi from sheep but relaxes lesser bronchi and bronchioles. The former action was antagonized by an $H_1$ receptor antagonist [34,35], the latter by an $H_2$ blocking agent [35]. Rabbit bronchus was reported by Somlyo and Somlyo

[36] to contract in response to histamine whereas trachea might either relax or contract. Fleisch and Calkins [37] found that histamine contracted the terminal end of the rabbit main bronchus but invariably relaxed rabbit trachea previously contracted with carbamylcholine. Pyrilamine, an $H_1$ receptor antagonist, blocked histamine-induced contraction of the bronchus, but relaxation of the trachea to histamine could not be antagonized by either pyrilamine or $H_2$ antihistamines. Studies by Maengwyn-Davies [38] and Eyre [35] showed cat trachea relaxed by histamine. Unlike rabbit trachea, histamine-induced relaxation of cat trachea appears to be mediated by both $H_1$ and $H_2$ receptors and to some extent by a release of endogenous catecholamines [35,38]. High concentrations of histamine, 2-methylhistamine ($H_1$ agonist), and 4-methylhistamine ($H_2$ agonist) relaxed carbachol-contracted cat bronchial strips [39]. Relaxant responses to histamine were not antagonized by $H_1$ and $H_2$ blocking agents, $\beta$-receptor blockade, or prostaglandin synthesis inhibition. A number of interpretations can account for the results obtained with histamine on rabbit trachea [37] and cat bronchus [39]. Higher concentrations of antagonists might have been necessary to block the histamine-induced relaxation. Another might be that histamine releases a nonadrenergic, nonprostaglandin mediator which causes relaxation. A third suggests that these tissues contain a class of histamine receptors not heretofore appreciated. Large and small airways from guinea pig, dog, and human have been reported to contract to histamine [26]. More information on the pharmacology and biochemistry of histamine can be obtained from recent reviews by Beaven [40,41].

Additionally, we demonstrated that rabbit trachea and bronchus relaxed similarly to papaverine and aminophylline but the trachea relaxed more completely to isoproterenol, bradykinin, and $PGE_2$ [37]. Acetylcholine and congeners produce surprisingly uniform contractions within various levels of bronchial smooth muscle from all species. Nevertheless, as a general rule, every drug has the potential for marked species variations in addition to quantitative and qualitative differences within airway subdivisions.

### D. $\alpha$-Adrenergic Receptors

Based on a survey of the literature, we previously concluded that a paucity of $\alpha$ receptors subserving bronchoconstriction exists in the tracheobronchial tree [1]. A number of additional studies, including those of Adolphson et al. [42], Anthracite et al. [43], Prime et al. [44], Hiratsuka et al. [45], Himori and Taira [31], and Lulich et al. [30], support this concept although others dispute this claim [46]. Perhaps the most interesting combination of in vivo and in vitro experiments were carried out by Simonsson et al. [47]. $\alpha$-receptor stimulation during $\beta$-receptor blockade caused bronchoconstriction in 8 of 15 patients suffering from airway obstruction. Phenylephrine, an $\alpha$-receptor stimulant, in the presence of sotalol, a $\beta$-receptor antagonist, caused a small contraction of isolated bronchi obtained from patients undergoing resection for lung carcinoma. After addition of *Escherichia coli* endotoxin to the bathing medium, the contractile effect of phenylephrine increased 2 to 10 times in tissues obtained from patients free of abstructive lung disease but the endotoxin potentiated this $\alpha$ receptor-mediated contraction more than 1000 times in a tissue from a patient with chronic obstructive bronchitis. This finding has far reaching implications but must be verified before any positive statements can be made.[1] Nevertheless, it is interesting to note a number of documented cases in which $\alpha$-receptor blockade has lessened the symptoms associated with asthma [48-51]. This treatment looks promising for certain asthmatic patients. Available evidence does not distinguish between an action of the $\alpha$-receptor antagonists on $\alpha$ receptors in the airway or on those present in sensitized mast cells (see below).

### E. $\beta$-Adrenergic Receptors

In contrast to $\alpha$ receptors, there is an abundance of $\beta$-adrenergic receptors in the tracheobronchial tree. As indicated above, $\beta$ receptors are heterogenous and can be subdivided into different classes depending upon their interaction with various agonists and antagonists [10-12]. Lands et al. [12] originally proposed two major classes of $\beta$ receptors, $\beta_1$ subserving lipolysis and cardiac stimulation and $\beta_2$ mediating bronchodilation and vasodepression. Additional experiments now suggest the possibility of further subdivisions [11]. The situation became more complicated with the discovery by Furchgott and colleagues [52] that guinea pig trachea contains $\beta_1$ and $\beta_2$ receptors and the ratio of $\beta_1:\beta_2$ varied in trachea from different animals. A similar idea was proposed by Ablad et al. [53] in connection with the pharmacologic analysis of metopolol, a selective $\beta_1$ receptor antagonist. Ultimately, we may have to consider differences in the $\beta_1:\beta_2$ ratio at various levels of airway smooth muscle.

Activation of $\beta$ receptors by norepinephrine released from sympathetic nerves and by epinephrine and norepinephrine derived from the adrenal medulla modulates bronchoconstriction resulting both from vagal nerve stimulation (parasympathetic) and circulating bronchoconstrictor substances [54-56]. Likewise, exogenously administered $\beta$-receptor agonists cause a pronounced bronchodilation that temporarily reverses the decreased conductance associated with obstructive airways. In experiments where efferent sympathetic nerve activity was interrupted by guanethidine, an adrenergic neuronal blocking agent, histamine-induced bronchoconstriction in guinea pigs and dogs was potentiated [55,56].

[1] Kneussl and Richardson (*Am. Rev. Respir. Dis.*, **117**, Suppl. 70, 1978) demonstrated the existence of alpha receptors in isolated human airways. Bronchial tissue from people with respiratory disorders showed significantly higher alpha receptor activity.

A similar phenomenon was also seen in animals pretreated with β-receptor antagonists (i.e., propranolol) [55,56]. In fact, guanethidine and propranolol are contraindicated in patients with asthma. Bronchoconstriction in asthmatic patients caused by a β-receptor antagonist can be relieved with atropine but not by phentolamine, indicating a prominent cholinergic mechanism with no apparent α-receptor component [57].

### β-Receptor Activity as a Function of Age

In some tissues, β-receptor activity is age dependent [58]. Relaxation of rabbit and rat arteries mediated by the β-receptor system decreases with increasing age [59-66]. This relationship was not found in rabbit or rat portal vein [66] or in rabbit renal vein [67], suggesting a difference in the manner by which arteries and veins age. Aging influences pharmacologic responses of other tissues. Lakatta et al. [68] demonstrated diminished inotropic responses to catecholamines but not to $Ca^{2+}$ in aged myocardium. An age-related reduction in sensitivity to isoproterenol was seen in rat and guinea pig trachea during the first months of life [69]. Other relaxant agonists were not examined to determine if this phenomenon was confined to the β-receptor system. Since trachea and bronchi can react differently to drugs, it would be interesting to know whether β-receptor activity in small airways is age dependent.

### β-Receptor Desensitization

Tolerance or desensitization (tachyphylaxis) is an interesting feature of β-receptor agonists. Coret and Van Dyke [70] injected large amounts of isoproterenol into cats and found subsequent blood pressure responses to small doses of isoproterenol blocked. Walz et al. [71,72] and Butterworth [73] then described "isoproterenol reversal," a phenomenon characterized by a change in the action of isoproterenol from vasodepressor (β-receptor mediated) to vasopressor (α-receptor mediated) after prior addition of either large amounts of isoproterenol or various other sympathomimetic amines [71]. Isoproterenol reversal was also demonstrated in isolated rat aortic strips [74]. A diverse group of organic substances, including phentolamine, bromo-LSD, tetracaine, papaverine, nitroglycerin, and aminophylline, prevented isoproterenol reversal and converted isoproterenol-induced contractions into relaxations [74]. That isoproterenol-induced contractions, mediated through α receptors [59,73] are not tachyphylactic suggests a fundamental difference between the two adrenergic receptor systems. It would be of great interest to determine the variations and subtypes of α and β receptors with respect to tolerance.

β-Receptor agonists are widely used as bronchodilators. The extent to which their tolerance is responsible for mortality associated with the treatment of asthma has been the subject of much debate. Conolly et al. [75] reported resistance to the chronotropic actions of isoproterenol after prolonged exposure of human and dog to isoproterenol. They also demonstrated an increased mortality to histamine in guinea pigs pretreated with one of three β-receptor stimulants, isoproterenol, terbutaline, or salbutamol, suggesting a decreased ability of the β-receptor system to compensate for the powerful histamine-induced bronchoconstriction. The latter experiments with isoproterenol were confirmed by Douglas et al. [76]. Minatoya and Spilker [77] were unable to produce tachyphylaxis to the cardiac or bronchodilator effects of isoproterenol in dogs. Spilker and Tyll [78] then demonstrated an increased mortality to histamine in guinea pigs after minoxidil, a drug that lowers blood pressure. From these experiments they concluded that the ability of isoproterenol to lower blood pressure and not its pulmonary action is responsible for the increased mortality to histamine.

Isoproterenol desensitization has been extensively studied in isolated airway smooth muscle. Fleisch and Titus [74] could not produce tolerance to isoproterenol in rat trachea as they had done in aorta with a single concentration of isoproterenol at a constant time interval. However, by incubating guinea pig trachea in either isoproterenol, norepinephrine, phosphodiesterase inhibitors, or cyclic nucleotides for 20 min, Douglas et al. [76] were indeed able to desensitize β receptors. Incubation with adenosine, methoxamine, or sodium nitrite did not produce β-receptor desensitization. Pretreatment of tracheas with indomethacin, a prostaglandin synthesis inhibitor, prevented desensitization. Douglas et al. [76] postulated that elevated levels of cyclic AMP and an increased synthesis of prostaglandins may result in a diminished response to β-receptor stimulation. Earlier, Tothill and colleagues [79] demonstrated a biphasic effect of adrenaline on rat uterus. The initial inhibitory action is mediated by β-receptors and the secondary contraction is through the liberation of $PGE_2$ which fits with the postulate of Douglas et al. [76]. Watanabe and colleagues [80] were also successful in establishing β-receptor desensitization of guinea pig trachea. They did so by subjecting the tissue to 200 times the $ED_{50}$ concentration of either isoproterenol or epinephrine. More recently, Lin et al. [81] studied the mechanism of isoproterenol-induced desensitization of spirally cut rat trachea. By comparing $K_B$ values for propranolol in desensitized and normal tissues, they concluded that a pronounced reduction in affinity of the β receptor for isoproterenol is one demonstrable change that occurred as a result of β-receptor desensitization.

Anderson and Lees [82] pretreated guinea pigs with epinephrine or salbutamol for 5 or 12 days and compared β receptor-mediated responses of atria, trachea, and ileum from these animals with tissues from saline-treated controls. Only in trachea from guinea pigs pretreated for 12 days with epinephrine was desensitization to epinephrine evident. Cross tolerance to isoproterenol or salbutamol was not present. Tracheas from animals pretreated with salbutamol were not desensitized to either salbutamol, epinephrine, or isoproterenol. In a variation of this procedure, Benoy et al. [83] treated guinea pigs with either isoproterenol or epinephrine for various times. Lungs were excised from the animals and perfused through the trachea with Krebs solution; bronchoconstriction reduced the flow, bronchodilation increased the flow. Tolerance was noted to the bronchodilator action of isoproterenol and epinephrine. Cross tolerance was observed between aminophylline and the catecholamines.

Lichterfeld and Lollgen [84] repeatedly administered isoproterenol to 12 patients with obstructive lung disease. No decrease in bronchospasmolytic or heart rate effects was demonstrated after 35- to 40-min infusions of isoproternol. Svedmyr et al. [85] treated asthmatic patients with terbutaline and tested them periodically with isoproterenol. Again, there was no evidence of resistance to β-receptor stimulation. In contrast, normal subjects showed desensitization to large doses of salbutamol when a change in airway conductance was used as an index of β-receptor stimulation [86]. The bronchodilator activity of salbutamol was fully restored after intravenous administration of hydrocortisone.

β-Receptor desensitization appears easier to induce in vascular smooth muscle (see above), frog erythrocytes [87,88], and human fibroblasts [89,90] than in airway smooth muscle. Thus, although β-receptor desensitization may contribute to mortality associated with the treatment of asthma, other factors, including excess secretions, mucosal edema, and cardiovascular toxicity of certain bronchodilators, should be given prime consideration. This presupposes that a decrease in sensitivity of the bronchial β-receptor system does not occur just prior to the onset of status asthmaticus.

### F. Prostaglandin Receptors

Prostaglandin are a family of 20-carbon unsaturated lipid acids active on the lung [91,92]. In general, $PGF_{2a}$ causes bronchoconstriction whereas prostaglandins of the E series produce relaxation [92-94]. Exceptions are found in rabbit trachea and bronchus which relax in response to $PGE_2$ but do not respond to $PGF_{2a}$ [37]. Cat bronchi also relax to $PGE_2$; $PGF_{2a}$ either has no effect or elicits an occasional contraction [95]. Responses of isolated guinea pig trachea to prostaglandins are dependent on resting tone. After the tissue is relaxed with indomethacin, both $PGF_{2a}$ and $PGE_2$ cause contraction [96].

Lung tissue can synthesize and metabolize prostaglandins [97]. In concert with these observations, Aiken and Waddell [98] reported that arachidonic acid, a precursor of prostaglandins, relaxed previously contracted rabbit and guinea pig trachea. This relaxation was specifically antagonized by agents that inhibited prostaglandin synthesis, suggesting that airway smooth muscle can convert arachidonic acid to prostaglandins.

Not only do prostaglandins exert their own effect, but they are involved in the action of other bronchoactive agents. Orehek et al. [99,100] used thin-layer chromatography and bioassay to show that $PGE_2$ and $PGF_{2a}$ are released from guinea pig trachea during contractions elicited by histamine or acetylcholine. Grodzinska et al. [101] found a PGE-like material released from histamine superfused guinea pig trachea but their bioassay did not detect a PGF-like material. Furthermore, maximal tracheal relaxation by isoproterenol was not accompanied by the elaboration of a PG-like substance. These results led Grodzinska et al. [101] to postulate that release of PGE from tracheal smooth muscle is a negative feedback mechanism employed by the tissue to offset powerful contractions. Turker and Ercan [102] recently described relaxation of superfused cat trachea in response to angiotensin I, angiotensin II, and bradykinin. These responses were antagonized by aspirin, an inhibitor of prostaglandin synthesis. In the same experiment, aspirin did not influence relaxation elicited by $PGE_2$, norepinephrine, or histamine. In addition, relaxation of rabbit trachea by bradykinin is blocked by indomethacin [98]. These studies indicate a relationship between contraction and relaxation of airway smooth muscle and prostaglandin synthesis. This is not exclusive for bronchial smooth muscle. For example, bradykinin-induced and angiotensin-induced relaxations of isolated rabbit celiac artery were shown to be specifically antagonized by inhibitors of prostaglandin synthesis [103]. Also of interest is the work of Okpako [104] who found that responses to $PGE_2$ and $PGF_{2a}$ on rat colon and stomach, guinea pig ileum, and rat blood pressure have an age-dependent component [104]. Perhaps examination of prostaglandin effectiveness on various levels of airway smooth muscle from different aged animals is warranted.

Suggestions that prostaglandins play a role in asthma are based on the actions just described as well as on the demonstration of their release from lung tissue upon antigen challenge [105,106]. However, Smith [107] found symptoms of asthmatic patients unchanged after suppression of prostaglandin biosynthesis with indomethacin (200 mg/day) casting doubt upon the hypothesis that prostaglandins play a major role in human bronchial asthma. Studies by Szczeklik et al. [108] on asthmatic patients with a history of aspirin-induced obstruction of airflow indicated that "aspirin-like drugs" precipitated asthmatic attacks by virtue of their ability to inhibit prostaglandin biosynthesis. Thus, at least in this population, endogenous prostaglandins may act to maintain patent airways.

Current prostaglandin research centers around the physiology, pharmacology, and biochemistry of the newly discovered thromboxanes and prostacyclin. The reader is referred to the recent review by Hyman et al. [109] on prostaglandins and the lung for significant details.

### G. Actions of Other Drugs on Airway Smooth Muscle

Guinea pig trachea, treated with agents known to interfere with adrenergic nerve function and adrenergic receptors, relaxes to electrical field stimulation [110-112]. A similar phenomenon can also be found in human airways [113]. Burnstock and colleagues [114,115] demonstrated such a system in the intestine and suggested a purine nucleotide, most likely ATP, as the neurotransmitter. Richardson and Bouchard [112] found ATP capable of relaxing guinea pig trachea. Kamikawa and Shimo [116] showed this response to be antagonized by indomethacin, aspirin, or polyphloretin phosphate, a prostaglandin receptor antagonist. Subsequently, they demonstrated that neither indomethacin nor polyphloretin phosphate decreased tracheal relaxation caused by field stimulation [117]. This nonadrenergic, nonprostaglandin inhibitory response and the relaxation induced by ATP were thus thought to be different. More studies are needed to characterize the inhibitory transmitter which might function as a bronchodilator. The subject of nonadrenergic inhibition of airway smooth muscle will be discussed in Chapter 1, Morphology of the Airways.

Notwithstanding the above discussion, activation of a drug receptor system is unnecessary to contract or relax smooth muscle. Cations like $K^+$ or $Ba^{2+}$ contract many smooth muscles by increasing the movement of $Ca^{2+}$ intracellularly with a resultant shortening of the contractile proteins [118]. Other agents, i.e., nitroglycerin and sodium nitroprusside, are thought to relax smooth muscle by inhibiting $Ca^{2+}$ influx and/or by activating a process that sequesters $Ca^{2+}$ away from the contractile apparatus [118,119]. Smooth muscle pharmacology received a boost with the discovery that A23187, a carboxylic acid antibiotic, transports $Ca^{2+}$ across biologic membranes [120]. This ionophore increases cardiac contractility [121] and contracts such smooth muscles as guinea pig ileal longitudinal muscle [122,123] and isolated stomach muscularis cells of Bufo marinus [124]. Figure 2 shows a contraction of an isolated guinea pig main bronchus to A23187. Preliminary experiments indicated that this relatively "all or none" response is increased by $10^{-6}$ M indomethacin.

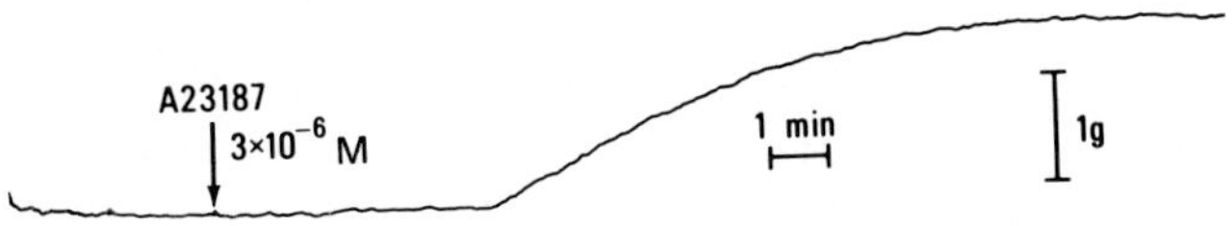


**FIGURE 2** Contraction of guinea pig main bronchus to $3 \times 10^{-6}$ M A23187 in the presence of $10^{-6}$ M indomethacin. Note 5-min latent period. The tissue was prepared by the method of Hooker et al. [27]. Isometric measurement was made with a force-displacement transducer and recorded on a polygraph as changes in grams of force.

## II. Antigen-Induced Mediator Release

### A. SRS-A Receptor

The presence of a specific pharmacologic receptor in smooth muscle for slow-reacting substance of anaphylaxis (SRS-A) has taken many years to confirm. As early as 1940, Kellaway and Trethewie [125] discovered that histamine and a substance causing a slow contraction of guinea pig gut were released from guinea pig lung during anaphylactic reactions. With the advent of antihistamines, Brocklehurst [126] pharmacologically separated histamine from this slow-reacting substance which he termed SRS-A "to identify it as separate from other 'lipid soluble acids' or totally uncharacterized gut contracting agents" [127]. Much time and energy has been expended defining this mysterious substance. As of this writing, some physicochemical and pharmacological characteristics are known, but the exact chemical structure has resisted analysis [128,129]. Documentation of an SRS-A receptor came from the work of Augstein et al. [130]. These investigators developed FPL 55712, a highly selective SRS-A antagonist capable of blocking the action of SRS-A on guinea pig ileum and on both human bronchial strips and guinea pig tracheal tubes (P. Sheard, personal communication, 1976).

There appears to be a differential sensitivity of airway smooth muscle to SRS-A. Bovine bronchus contracts to lower concentrations of bovine SRS-A than does trachea [131]. The same SRS-A contracts cat bronchus but not cat trachea [39]. Drazen et al. [132] studied the effects of histamine and SRS-A on guinea pig tracheal strips (central airways) and parenchymal strips (peripheral airways). Histamine contracted both tissues; SRS-A had a substantially greater action on the parenchymal strips. Although SRS-A does not appear to significantly contract tracheal smooth muscle, Wanner et al. [133] suggested that SRS-A released upon antigen challenge might decrease the velocity of tracheal mucous secretions in experimental canine asthma.

### B. Mediator Release: General Considerations

As indicated before, sensitized mast cells associated with airway smooth muscle or lung parenchyma are potential sources of bronchoactive agents (SRS-A, histamine, prostaglandins, bradykinin, and so on). Antigen-induced release of these mediators of anaphylaxis are thought to be responsible for the bronchospasm noted in extrinsic asthma [134].

Following the lead of Kellaway and Trethewie [125] and Brocklehurst [126], Austen and colleagues thoroughly investigated mediator release from fragmented human lung tissue. This work has been the subject of excellent reviews [128,129,134-136]. Although many substances are liberated from the lung upon antigen challenge, emphasis has been placed on histamine and SRS-A. An intimate association between release of mediators elicited by antigen challenge and intracellular levels of cyclic nucleotides has been demonstrated [136]. Increasing tissue levels of cyclic AMP by β-receptor agonists, prostaglandins, or phosphodiesterase inhibitors reduce mediator generation and/or release. Conversely, a decrease in cyclic AMP levels, by α-receptor stimulation, is reflected as an increased release of mediators. Increasing levels of cyclic GMP, by cholinergic stimulation, also results in an enhanced release of chemical mediators. Human basophils and rat mast cells are among other cell types that release pharmacologic mediators via an antigen-IgE antibody reaction [137,138]. The biochemical events governing mediator release from these cells appear similar, at least in some respects, to the lung, although agents active in lung are not necessarily active in mast cells and vice versa.

### C. Drugs That Inhibit Mediator Release

Curbing potentially harmful biogenic substances from being released into the airway milieu has generally been achieved experimentally with agents that increase intracellular levels of cyclic AMP. Interestingly, histamine, a primary mediator of anaphylaxis, raises cyclic AMP levels in human basophils [139]. Histamine released from one basophil is thought to prevent release of histamine from neighboring cells although it is incapable of a negative feedback in the originating cell [137]. $H_2$ but not $H_1$ antagonists block this action of histamine [140]. $K_B$ values for burimamide and metiamide on $H_2$ receptors in human basophils are the same order of magnitude as those described for guinea pig atria and rat uterus suggesting a similarity among these receptors [141].

The antianaphylactic action of epinephrine was reported by Schild in 1936 [142]. Due to the prominent action of catecholamines on bronchial and vascular smooth muscle, it was not until 30 years later, when Lichtenstein and Margolis observed that epinephrine and isoproterenol suppressed histamine release from human basophils, that this additional effect of epinephrine was appreciated [143]. An important question raised by these observations is whether β receptors that modulate mediator release are similar to other β receptors. Three laboratories using different techniques analyzed this problem on actively sensitized guinea pig lungs [144-146]. Assem and Schild [144] concluded that antianaphylactic β receptors differ from those in heart and smooth muscle. Malter and Raper [145] found differences between these receptors and those in guinea pig atria and trachea. Sorenby's [146] results suggested that β receptors mediating inhibition of antigen-induced histamine release are more related to those in trachea than those associated with cardiac stimulation. Clearly, then, β receptors in heart differ from those on lung mast cells. β-receptor activation decrease histamine release from all sensitized mast cell preparations. Histamine release from bovine granulocytes is potentiated by β-receptor stimulation and inhibited by activation of α receptors [147].

Ever since Schultz [148] and Dale [149] described their classic studies on the anaphylactic reaction of smooth muscle, isolated segments of gut or airways from sensitized animals have been used as models of antigen-induced mediator release. The antigen, usually ovalbumin, has no effect on tissues from control animals. However, it produces a marked contraction of tissues obtained from animals previously sensitized to ovalbumin. Mediators released from tissue mast cells are presumably responsible for this response. Recently, we described a sensitive Schultz-Dale reaction [150]. Guinea pigs were sensitized with 2 mg of ovalbumin in 50% complete Freunds adjuvant on day 1 and day 5; the animals were used on day 21 or later. Concentrations of ovalbumin as low as 1 ng/ml contracted guinea pig main bronchus. Nearly maximal responses could be elicited every 45 to 60 min with little to no desensitization. During a series of experiments to ascertain whether some water-insoluble compounds could inhibit the Schultz-Dale reaction, we found that relatively low concentrations of ethanol and propylene glycol, the solvents used to dissolve these agents, inhibited contractions of guinea pig bronchi caused by ovalbumin. This property was shared by two other aliphatic alcohols, propanol and butanol. Contractions of the same tissues to $PGF_{2\alpha}$ were either not influenced or only slightly reduced by the four alcohols. Ovalbumin-induced mediator release from chopped guinea pig lung was also reduced by the alcohols. In an extension of this work, we found that release of histamine and SRS-A from passively sensitized guinea pig lung was related to the donor animal's age [151]. Lung from 1- and 2-month-old guinea pigs released less mediators than lung from 1-week-old animals. A reduced tissue content of histamine and SRS-A and a smaller percentage of total release of these mediators from the older guinea pig lungs was responsible for this decline.

Many compounds inhibit mediator release from lung [152,153]. Most are not useful clinically due to toxicity or a lack of specificity. An exception is disodium cromoglycate [154-156]. Knowledge that pharmacologic receptors can differ from organ to organ, and that various forms of the same enzyme (isoenzymes) exist with slightly different biochemical properties, should enable drugs to be designed with increasing degrees of specificity. Highly specific agents will have fewer side effects and greatly facilitate treatment of obstructive airway diseases such as asthma.

## III. Alteration of Drug-Receptor Systems in Disease

Finally, we come to a question difficult to answer: Do changes in pharmacologic receptor systems of airway smooth muscle contribute to airway obstruction?

Szentivanyi [157] hypothesized a relationship between asthma and a reduced responsiveness of the β-receptor system. Reed [158,159] considered such a defect responsible, in part, for excessive airway irritability since a loss of this component would leave airways vulnerable to constriction by various factors. In addition to Szentivanyi's experiments, Kirkpatrick and Keller [160] found less mobilization of fatty acids after epinephrine in people with asthma. Makino et al. [161] reported that hyperresponsiveness of bronchi to acetylcholine in people with varying degrees of asthma correlated with the decreased amount of hyperglycemia, hyperlacticacidemia, and eosinopenia induced by epinephrine. Logsdon et al. [162] and Parker and Smith [163] demonstrated a decreased ability of isoproterenol to increase cyclic AMP in leukocytes from asthmatic patients. After similar experiments, Gillespie et al. [164] concluded that responses of cells from normal and asthmatic individuals overlap and thus an actual defect in the β receptor is unlikely. Sokol and Beall [165] could not find a substantial difference in epinephrine binding to leukocytes from asthmatic and normal patients. Kalisker and colleagues reexamined responses of mononuclear leukocytes from normal subjects and asthmatic children to isoproterenol [166]. Previous contact of the cells with isoproterenol (in vitro) or with terbutaline, a β-receptor stimulant, administered orally prior to collection of the cells, decreased the magnitude of the in vitro response to isoproterenol. Kalisker et al. [166] concluded that treatment of asthmatic patients with sympathomimetic agents and not the asthma was responsible for the presumed β-receptor defect. Another factor for consideration is that β-receptor blockade in normal individuals does not produce an asthmalike syndrome. Thus, if a loss in β-receptor activity is associated with asthma, it is most likely secondary to the disease and not the cause. We must also keep in mind that extrapolation from β receptors on lymphocytes, or on another cell, to those in bronchial smooth muscle is very difficult. Numerous factors, including pH and hormonal balance, can alter responsivity of drug receptors in smooth muscle. Whether such changes occur in airway disease remains a promising field of research.

## Acknowledgments

Most of the literature search for this manuscript was completed in December 1976. The author expressed appreciation to Ms. Hendretta Reagan for expert assistance with the literature search, to Ms. Patricia Steward and Ms. Kathleen Edwards for help with preparing the manuscript, and to Ms. Mildred Burton and Ms. Linda Hendrickson for typing the manuscript. The author also thanks Drs. Marlene Cohen and Irwin Slater for their helpful comments and suggestions.

## References

1. Fleisch, J. H., K. M. Kent, and T. Cooper, Drug receptors in smooth muscle. In *Asthma: Physiology, Immunopharmacology, and Treatment.* Edited by K. F. Austen and L. M. Lichtenstein. New York, Academic, 1973, pp. 139-167.
2. Gillis, C. N., and J. A. Roth, Pulmonary disposition of circulating vasoactive hormones, *Biochem. Pharmacol.,* **25**:2547-2553 (1976).
3. Dale, H. H., On some physiological actions of ergot, *J. Physiol. (London),* **34**:163-206 (1906).
4. Ahlquist, R. P., Study of the adrenotropic receptors, *Am. J. Physiol.,* **153**: 586-600 (1948).
5. Powell, C. E., and I. H. Slater, Blocking of inhibitory adrenergic receptors by a dichloro analogue of isoproterenol, *J. Pharmacol. Exp. Ther.,* **122**: 480-488 (1958).
6. Moran, N. C., and M. E. Perkins, Adrenergic blockade of the mammalian heart by a dichloro analogue of isoproterenol, *J. Pharmacol. Exp. Ther.,* **124**:223-237 (1958).
7. Black, J. W., W. A. M. Duncan, C. J. Durant, C. R. Ganellin, and E. M. Parsons, Definition and antagonism of histamine $H_2$-receptors, *Nature (London),* **236**:385-390 (1972).
8. Schild, H. O., pA, A new scale for the measurement of drug antagonism, *Br. J. Pharmacol. Chemother.,* **2**:189-206 (1947).
9. Arunlakshana, O., and H. O. Schild, Some quantitative uses of drug antagonists, *Br. J. Pharmacol. Chemother.,* **14**:45-58 (1959).
10. Furchgott, R. F., The pharmacological differentiation of adrenergic receptors, *Ann. N.Y. Acad. Sci.,* **139**:553-570 (1967).
11. Furchgott, R. F., The classification of adrenoceptors (adrenergic receptors). An evaluation from the standpoint of receptor theory. In *Handbook of Experimental Pharmacology,* Vol. 33. Edited by O. Eichler, A. Farah, H. Herken, and A. D. Welch. New York, Springer-Verlag, 1972, pp. 283-335.
12. Lands, A. M., A. Arnold, J. P. McAuliffe, F. P. Luduena, and T. G. Brown, Jr., Differentiation of receptor systems activated by sympathomimetic amines, *Nature (London),* **214**:597-598 (1967).
13. Altura, B. M., Comparative studies on adrenergic receptors in different rat blood vessels. In *Microcirculation 1: Blood Vessel Interactions; Systems in Special Tissues.* Edited by J. Grayson and W. Zingy. New York, Plenum, 1976.
14. Wasserman, M. A., and B. Levy, Selective beta adrenergic receptor antagonism in the anesthetized dog, *J. Pharmacol. Exp. Ther.,* **188**:357-367 (1973).
15. Jack, D., Selectively acting β-adrenoreceptor stimulants in asthma. In *Asthma: Physiology, Immunopharmacology, and Treatment.* Edited by K. F. Austen and L. M. Lichtenstein. New York, Academic, 1973, pp. 251-266.

16. Brittain, R. T., C. M. Dean, and D. Jack, Sympathomimetic bronchodilator drugs, *Pharmacol. Ther. B.,* **2**:423-462 (1976).
17. Wardell, J. R., D. F. Collela, A. Shetzline, and P. J. Fowler, Studies on carbuterol (SKF 40383-A), a new selective bronchodilator agent, *J. Pharmacol. Exp. Ther.,* **189**:167-184 (1973).
18. Giles, R. E., J. C. Williams, and M. P. Finkel, The bronchodilator and cardiac stimulant effects of Th1165A, salbutamol and isoproterenol, *J. Pharmacol. Exp. Ther.,* **186**:472-481 (1973).
19. Bowman, W. C., and C. Raper, Sympathomimetic bronchodilators and animal models for assessing their potential value in asthma, *J. Pharm. Pharmacol.,* **28**:369-374 (1976).
20. Tuttle, R. R., and J. Mills, Development of a new catecholamine to selectively increase cardiac contractility, *Circ. Res.,* **36**:185-196 (1975).
21. Dreyer, A. C., and J. Offermeier, Indications for the existence of two types of cardiac β-adrenergic receptors, *Pharmacol. Res. Commun.,* **7**:151-161 (1975).
22. Tuttle, R. R., C. C. Hillman, and R. E. Toomey, Differential β-adrenergic sensitivity of atrial and ventricular tissue assessed by chronotropic, inotropic, and cyclic AMP responses to isoprenaline and dobutamine, *Cardiovasc. Res.,* **10**:452-458 (1976).
23. Castillo, J. C., and E. J. DeBeer, The tracheal chain, I. A preparation for the study of antispasmodics with particular reference to bronchodilator drugs, *J. Pharmacol. Exp. Ther.,* **90**:104-109 (1947).
24. Akcasu, A., The physiologic and pharmacologic characteristics of the tracheal muscle, *Arch. Int. Pharmacodyn. Ther.,* **122**:201-207 (1959).
25. Patterson, R., The tracheal strip: Observations on the response of tracheal muscle, *J. Allergy,* **29**:165-172 (1958).
26. Persson, C. G. A., and M. Ekman, Contractile effects of histamine in large and small respiratory airways, *Agents and Actions,* **6**:389-393 (1976).
27. Hooker, C. S., P. J. Calkins, and J. H. Fleisch, On the measurement of vascular and respiratory smooth muscle responses *in vitro,* Blood Vessels, **14**:1-11 (1977).
28. Kind, L. S., The altered reactivity of mice after inoculation with bordetella pertussis vaccine, *Bact. Rev.,* **22**:173-182 (1958).
29. Szentivanyi, A., Effect of bacterial products and adrenergic blocking agents on allergic reactions. In *Immunological Diseases I.* Edited by M. Samter. Boston, Little Brown, 1971, pp. 356-374.
30. Lulich, K. M., H. W. Mitchell, and M. P. Sparrow, The cat lung strip as an in vitro preparation of peripheral airways: A comparison of β-adrenoceptor agonists, autacoids and anaphylactic challenge on the lung strip and trachea, *Br. J. Pharmacol.,* **58**:71-79 (1976).
31. Himori, N., and N. Taira, A method for recording smooth muscle and vascular responses of the blood-perfused dog trachea in situ, *Br. J. Pharmacol.,* **56**:293-299 (1976).
32. Golla, F. L., and W. L. Symes, The reversible action of adrenaline and some

kindred drugs on the bronchioles, *J. Pharmacol. Exp. Ther.*, **5**:87-103 (1913).
33. Brocklehurst, W., The action of 5-hydroxytryptamine on smooth muscle. In *5-Hydroxytryptamine.* Edited by G. P. Lewis. London, Pergamon, 1958, pp. 172-176
34. Eyre, P., The pharmacology of sheep tracheobronchial muscle: A relaxant effect of histamine on the isolated bronchi, *Br. J. Pharmacol.*, **36**:409-417 (1969).
35. Eyre, P., Histamine $H_2$-receptors in the sheep bronchus and cat trachea: The action of burimamide, *Br. J. Pharmacol.*, **48**:321-323 (1973).
36. Somlyo, A. P., and A. V. Somlyo, Biophysics of smooth muscle excitation and contraction. In *Airway Biodynamics: Physiology and Pharmacology.* Edited by A. Bouhuys. Springfield, Illinois, Charles C. Thomas, 1970, pp. 209-227.
37. Fleisch, J. H., and P. J. Calkins, Comparison of drug-induced responses of rabbit trachea and bronchus, *J. Appl. Physiol.*, **41**:62-66 (1976).
38. Maengwyn-Davies, G. D., The dual mode of action of histamine in the cat isolated tracheal chain, *J. Pharm. Pharmacol.*, **20**:572-573 (1968).
39. Chand, N., and P. Eyre, Atypical (relaxant) response to histamine in cat bronchus, *Agents Actions,* **7**:183-190 (1977).
40. Beaven, M. A., Histamine (Part I), *N. Engl. J. Med.*, **294**:30-36 (1976).
41. Beaven, M. A., Histamine (Part II), *N. Engl. J. Med.*, **294**:320-325 (1976).
42. Adolphson, R. L., S. B. Abern, and R. G. Townley, Human and guinea pig respiratory smooth muscle—Demonstration of alpha adrenergic receptors, *J. Allergy,* **47**:110-111 (1971).
43. Anthracite, R. F., L. Vachon, and P. L. Knapp, Alpha-adrenergic receptors in the human lung, *Psychosom. Med.*, **33**:481-489 (1971).
44. Prime, F. J., S. Bianco, P. L. Griffin, and P. L. Kamburoff, The effects on airways conductance of alpha-adrenergic stimulation and blocking, *Bull. Physiopathol. Respir., (Nancy),* **8**:99-109 (1972).
45. Hiratsuka, K., K. Wakaboyashi, T. Mayahara, and S. Yamado, Effect of adrenaline derivatives on isolated tracheal muscle of guinea pig, *Folia Pharmacol. Jpn.*, **70**:199-205 (1974).
46. Stone, D. J., T. K. Sarkar, and H. Keltz, Effect of adrenergic stimulation and inhibition on human airways, *J. Appl. Physiol.*, **34**:624-627 (1973).
47. Simonsson, B. G., N. Svedmyr, B. E. Skoogh, R. Andersson, and N. P. Bergh, In vivo and in vitro studies on alpha-receptors in human airway. Potentiation with bacterial endotoxine, *Scand. J. Respir. Dis.*, **53**:227-236 (1972).
48. Marcelle, R., and B. Laurent, Reactivite des bronches humaines in vitro, *Arch. Int. Physiol. Biochim.*, **81**:901-920 (1973).
49. Gross, G. N., J. F. Souhrada, and R. S. Farr, The longterm treatment of an asthmatic patient using phenotolamine, *Chest,* **66**:397-401 (1974).
50. Bianco, S., J. P. Griffin, P. L. Kamburoff, and F. J. Prime, Prevention of exercise-induced asthma by indoramin, *Br. Med. J.*, **4**:18-20 (1974).

51. Patel, K. R., and J. W. Kerr, Alpha-receptor blocking drugs in bronchial asthma, *Lancet,* **1**:348-349 (1975).
52. Furchgott, R. F., T. D. Wakade, R. A. Sorace, and J. S. Stollak, Occurrence of both $beta_1$ and $beta_2$ receptors in guinea pig tracheal smooth muscle and variation of the $beta_1$:$beta_2$ ratio in different animals, *Fed. Proc.,* **34**:794 (1975).
53. Ablad, B., K. O. Borg, E. Carlsson, E. Lars, G. Johnsson, T. Malmfors, and C. G. Regardh, A survey of the pharmacological properties of metoprolol in animals and man, *Acta Pharmacol. Toxicol. [Suppl. V] (Kbh.),* **36**:7-23 (1975).
54. Cabezas, G. A., P. D. Graf, and J. Nadel, Sympathetic versus parasympathetic nervous regulation of airways in dogs, *J. Appl. Physiol.,* **31**:651-655 (1971).
55. Douglas, J. S., M. W. Dennis, P. Ridgeway, and A. Bouhuys, Airway constriction in guinea pigs: Interaction of histamine and autonomic drugs, *J. Pharmacol. Exp. Ther.,* **184**:169-179 (1973).
56. Diamond, L., Potentiation of bronchomotor responses by beta adrenergic antagonists, *J. Pharmacol. Exp. Ther.,* **181**:434-445 (1972).
57. Gayrard, P., J. Orehek, and J. Charpin, Effects of various bronchodilator agents on airway conductance in asthma, after beta adrenergic blockade, *Bull. Physiopathol. Respir. (Nancy),* **8**:625-640 (1972).
58. Fleisch, J. H., Pharmacology of the aorta: A brief review, *Blood Vessels,* **11**:193-211 (1974).
59. Fleisch, J. H., H. M. Maling, and B. B. Brodie, Beta-receptor activity in aorta. Variations with age and species, *Circ. Res.,* **26**:151-162 (1970).
60. Fleisch, J. H., Further studies on the effect of ageing on $\beta$-adrenoceptor activity of rat aorta, *Br. J. Pharmacol.,* **42**:311-313 (1971).
61. Gulati, O. D., B. P. Methew, H. M. Parikh, and V. S. R. Krishnamurty, Beta adrenergic receptor of rabbit thoracic aorta in relation to age, *Jpn. J. Pharmacol.,* **23**:259-268 (1973).
62. Cohen, M. L., and B. A. Berkowitz, Age-related changes in vascular responsiveness to cyclic nucleotides and contractile agonists, *J. Pharmacol. Exp. Ther.,* **191**:147-155 (1974).
63. Cohen, M. L., and B. A. Berkowitz, Differences between the effects of dopamine and apomorphine on rat aortic strips, *Eur. J. Pharmacol.,* **34**: 49-58 (1975).
64. Ericsson, E., and L. Lundholm, Adrenergic beta-receptor activity and cyclic AMP metabolism in vascular smooth muscle; variations with age, *Mech. Ageing Dev.,* **4**:1-6 (1975).
65. Cohen, M. L., A. S. Blume, and B. A. Berkowitz, Vascular adenylate cyclase: Role of age and guanine nucleotide activation, *Blood Vessels,* **14**:25-42 (1977).
66. Fleisch, J. H., and C. S. Hooker, The relationship between age and relaxation of vascular smooth muscle in the rabbit and rat, *Circ. Res.,* **38**:243-249 (1976).

67. Hooker, C. S., P. J. Calkins, and J. H. Fleisch, A simple and inexpensive method for measuring responses of circular smooth muscle in small blood vessels and airways, *Fed. Proc.,* **35**:286 (1976).
68. Lakatta, E. G., G. Gestenblith, C. S. Angell, N. W. Shock, and M. L. Weisfeldt, Diminished inotropic response of aged myocardium to catecholamines, *Circ. Res.,* **36**:262-269 (1975).
69. Åberg, G., G. Adler, and E. Ericsson, The effect of age on beta-adrenoceptor activity in tracheal smooth muscle, *Br. J. Pharmacol.,* **47**:181-182 (1973).
70. Coret, I. A., and H. B. Van Dyke, The altered blood-pressure response after adrenolytic drugs and large doses of sympathomimetic amines, *J. Pharmacol. Exp. Ther.,* **95**:415-420 (1949).
71. Walz, D. T., T. Koppanyi, and G. D. Maengwyn-Davies, Isoproterenol vasomotor reversal by sympathomimetic amines, *J. Pharmacol. Exp. Ther.,* **129**: 200-207 (1960).
72. Walz, D. T., and G. D. Maengwyn-Davies, The mechanism of isoproterenol vasomotor reversal by phenylephrine, *J. Pharmacol. Exp. Ther.,* **129**:208-213 (1960).
73. Butterworth, K. R., The β-adrenergic blocking and pressor actions of isoprenaline in the cat, *Br. J. Pharmacol.,* **21**:378-392 (1963).
74. Fleisch, J. H., and E. Titus, The prevention of isoproterenol desensitization and isoproterenol reversal, *J. Pharmacol. Exp. Ther.,* **181**:425-433 (1972).
75. Conolly, M. E., D. S. Davies, C. T. Dollery, and C. F. George, Resistance to β-adrenoceptor stimulants (a possible explanation for the rise in asthma deaths), *Br. J. Pharmacol.,* **43**:389-402 (1971).
76. Douglas, J. S., A. J. Lewis, P. Ridgeway, C. Brink, and A. Bouhuys, Tachyphylaxis to beta-adrenoceptor agonists in guinea pig airway smooth muscle in vivo and in vitro, *Eur. J. Pharmacol.,* **42**:195-205 (1977).
77. Minatoya, H., and B. A. Spilker, Lack of cardiac or bronchodilator tachyphylaxis to isoprenaline in the dog, *Br. J. Pharmacol.,* **53**:333-340 (1975).
78. Spilker, B., and J. Tyll, On the question of tachyphylaxis to isoproterenol in guinea pigs, *Eur. J. Pharmacol.,* **36**:283-288 (1976).
79. Tothill, A., L. Rathbone and E. Willman, Relation between prostaglandin $E_2$ and adrenaline reversal in the rat uterus, *Nature (London),* **233**:56-57 (1971).
80. Watanabe, M., Y. Ohno, and Y. Kasuya, Desensitization of guinea pig tracheal muscle preparation to beta-adrenergic stimulants by a preceding exposure to a high dose of catecholamines, *Jpn. J. Pharmacol.,* **26**:191-199 (1976).
81. Lin, C. S., L. Hurwitz, J. Jenne, and B. P. Avner, Mechanism of isoproterenol-induced desensitization of tracheal smooth muscle, *J. Pharmacol. Exp. Ther.,* **202**:12-22 (1977).
82. Anderson, A. A., and G. M. Lees, Investigation of occurrence of tolerance to bronchodilator drugs in chronically pretreated guinea pigs, *Br. J. Pharmacol.,* **56**:331-338 (1976).

83. Benoy, C. J., M. S. El-Fellah, R. Schneider, and O. L. Wade, Tolerance to sympathomimetic bronchodilators in guinea pig isolated lungs following chronic administration in vivo, *Br. J. Pharmacol.*, **55**:547-554 (1975).
84. Lichterfeld, A., and H. Lollgen, Investigation into isoprenaline resistance in patients with obstructive lung disease, *Eur. J. Clin. Pharmacol.*, **7**:347-351 (1974).
85. Svedmyr, N., A. L. Larsson, and G. K. Thiringer, Development of "resistance" in beta adrenergic receptors of asthmatic patients, *Chest*, **69**:479-483 (1976).
86. Holgate, S. T., C. J. Baldwin, and A. E. Tattersfield, Beta-adrenergic agonist resistance in normal human airways, *Lancet*, **2**:375-377 (1977).
87. Mukherjee, C., M. G. Caron, and R. J. Lefkowitz, Catecholamine-induced subsensitivity of adenylate cyclase associated with loss of β-adrenergic receptor binding sites, *Proc. Natl. Acad. Sci. USA*, **72**:1945-1949 (1975).
88. Mickey, J., R. Tate, and R. J. Lefkowitz, Subsensitivity of adenylate cyclase and decreased β-adrenergic receptor binding after chronic exposure to (-)-isoproterenol in vitro, *J. Biol. Chem.*, **250**:5727-5729 (1975).
89. Franklin, T. J., and S. J. Foster, Hormone-induced desensitization of hormonal control of cyclic AMP levels in human diploid fibroblasts, *Nature [New Biol.]*, **246**:146-148 (1973).
90. Franklin, T. J., W. P. Morris, and P. A. Twose, Desensitization of beta-adrenergic receptors in human fibroblasts in tissue culture, *Mol. Pharmacol.*, **11**:485-491 (1975).
91. Smith, A. P., Role of prostaglandins in the pathogenesis and treatment of asthma. In *Asthma: Physiology, Immunopharmacology, and Treatment.* Edited by K. F. Austen and L. M. Lichtenstein. New York, Academic, 1973, pp. 267-277.
92. Fanburg, B. L., Prostaglandins and the lung, *Am. Rev. Respir. Dis.*, **108**: 482-489 (1973).
93. Sweatman, W. J. F., and H. O. J. Collier, Effects of prostaglandins on human bronchial muscle, *Nature (London)*, **217**:69 (1968).
94. Gardiner, P. J., The effects of some natural prostaglandins on isolated human circular bronchial muscle, *Prostaglandins*, **10**:607-616 (1975).
95. Joiner, P. D., L. Minor, L. B. Davis, P. J. Kadowitz, and A. L. Hyman, Studies of pharmacology of canine intrapulmonary bronchi, *Pharmacologist*, **17**:191 (1975).
96. Lambley, J. E., and A. P. Smith, The effects of arachidomic acid, indomethacin and SC-19220 of guinea-pig tracheal muscle tone, *Eur. J. Pharmacol.*, **30**:148-153 (1975).
97. Anggard, E., and B. Samuelsson, The metabolism of prostaglandins in lung tissue. In *Prostaglandins*, Nobel Symposium 2. Edited by S. Bergstrom and B. Samuelsson. Stockholm, Almquist and Wiksell, 1966, pp. 97-105.
98. Aiken, J. W., and J. E. Waddell, Relaxation of isolated tracheal smooth muscle produced by prostaglandin precursors and bradykinin: Antagonism by aspirin-like drugs, *Fed. Proc.*, **35**:803 (1976).

99. Orehek, J., J. S. Douglas, A. J. Lewis, and A. Bouhuys, Prostaglandin regulation of airway smooth muscle tone, *Nature [New Biol.]*, **245**:84-85 (1973).
100. Orehek, J., J. S. Douglas, and A. Bouhuys, Contractile responses of the guinea pig trachea in vitro: Modification by prostaglandin synthesis-inhibiting drugs, *J. Pharmacol. Exp. Ther.*, **194**:554-563 (1975).
101. Grodzinska, L., B. Panczenko, and R. J. Gryglewski, Generation of prostaglandin E-like material by the guinea-pig trachea contracted by histamine, *J. Pharm. Pharmacol.*, **27**:88-91 (1975).
102. Turker, R. K., and Z. S. Ercan, The effects of angiotensin I and angiotensin II on the isolated tracheal muscle of the cat, *J. Pharm. Pharmacol.*, **28**:298-301 (1976).
103. Aiken, J. W., Inhibitors of prostaglandin synthesis specifically antagonize bradykinin and angiotensin-induced relaxations of the isolated celiac artery from rabbit, *Pharmacologist*, **16**:295 (1974).
104. Okpako, D. T., Effects of animal maturity on smooth muscle and blood pressure responses to prostaglandins $E_2$ and $F_{2a}$, *J. Pharm. Pharmacol.*, **28**:613-616 (1976).
105. Piper, P. J., and J. R. Vane, Release of additional factors in anaphylaxis and its antagonism by anti-inflammatory drugs, *Nature (London)*, **223**:29-35 (1969).
106. Liebig, R., W. Bernauer, and B. A. Peskar, Release of prostaglandins, a prostaglandin metabolite, slow-reacting substance and histamine from anaphylactic lungs, and its modifications by catecholamines, *Naunyn-Schmiedebergs Arch. Pharmacol.*, **284**:279-293 (1974).
107. Smith, A. P., Effect of indomethacin in asthma: Evidence against a role for prostaglandins in its pathogenesis, *Br. J. Clin. Pharmacol.*, **2**:307-309 (1975).
108. Szczeklik, A., R. J. Gryglewski, and G. Czerniawska-Mysik, Clinical patterns of hypersensitivity to nonsteroidal anti-inflammatory drugs and their pathogenesis, *J. Allergy Clin. Immunol.*, **60**:276-284 (1977).
109. Hyman, A. L., E. W. Spannhake, and P. J. Kadowitz, Prostaglandins and the lung, *Am. Rev. Respir. Dis.*, **117**:111-136 (1978).
110. Coburn, R. F., and T. Tomita, Evidence for nonadrenergic inhibitory nerves in the guinea pig trachealis muscle, *Am. J. Physiol.*, **224**:1072-1080 (1973).
111. Coleman, R. A., and G. P. Levy, A non-adrenergic inhibitory nervous pathway in guinea-pig trachea, *Br. J. Pharmacol.*, **52**:167-174 (1974).
112. Richardson, J. B., and T. Bouchard, Demonstration of a nonadrenergic inhibitory nervous system in the trachea of the guinea pig, *J. Allergy Clin. Immunol.*, **56**:473-480 (1975).
113. Richardson, J. B., and J. Beland, A non-adrenergic inhibitory nervous system in human airways, *J. Appl. Physiol.*, **41**:764-771 (1976).
114. Burnstock, G., Purinergic nerves, *Pharmacol. Rev.*, **24**:509-581 (1972).
115. Burnstock, G., Purinergic receptors, *J. Theor. Biol.*, **62**:491-503 (1976).

116. Kamikawa, Y., and Y. Shimo, Mediation of prostaglandin $E_2$ in the biphasic response to ATP of the isolated tracheal muscle of guinea-pigs, *J. Pharm. Pharmacol.,* **28**:294-297 (1976).
117. Kamikawa, Y., and Y. Shimo, Pharmacological differences of nonadrenergic inhibitory response and of ATP-induced relaxation in guinea-pig tracheal strip-chains, *J. Pharm. Pharmacol.,* **28**:854-855 (1976).
118. Somlyo, A. P., and A. V. Somlyo, Vascular smooth muscle II. Pharmacology of normal and hypertensive vessels, *Pharmacol. Rev.,* **22**:249-353 (1970).
119. Kreye, V. A. W., G. D. Baron, J. B. Tuth, and H. Schmidt-Gayk, Mode of action of sodium nitroprusside on vascular smooth muscle, *Naunyn-Schmiedebergs Arch. Pharmackol.,* **288**:381-402 (1975).
120. Wong, D. T., J. R. Wilkinson, R. L. Hamill, and J. S. Horng, Effects of antibiotic ionophore, A23187, on oxidative phosphorylation and calcium transport of liver mitochondria, *J. Biochem. Biophys.,* **156**:578-585 (1973).
121. Holland, D. R., M. I. Steinberg, and W. McD. Armstrong, A23187: A calcium ionophore that directly increases cardiac contractility, *Proc. Soc. Exp. Biol. Med.,* **148**:1141-1145 (1975).
122. Swamy, V. C., M. Ticku, C. R. Triggle, and D. J. Triggle, The action of the ionophores X-537A and A-23187, on smooth muscle, *Can. J. Physiol. Pharmacol.,* **53**:1108-1114 (1975).
123. Triggle, C. R., W. F. Grant, and D. J. Triggle, Intestinal smooth muscle contraction and the effects of cadmium and A23187, *J. Pharmacol. Exp. Ther.,* **194**:182-190 (1975).
124. Murray, J. J., P. W. Reed, and F. S. Fay, Contraction of isolated smooth muscle cells by ionophore A23187, *Proc. Natl. Acad. Sci. USA,* **72**:4459-4463 (1975).
125. Kellaway, C. H., and E. R. Trethewie, The liberation of a slow-reacting smooth muscle stimulating substance in anaphylaxis, *Q. J. Exp. Physiol.,* **30**:121-145 (1940).
126. Brocklehurst, W. E., The release of histamine and formation of a slow-reacting substance (SRS-A) during anaphylactic shock, *J. Physiol. (London),* **151**:416-435 (1960).
127. Brocklehurst, W. E., Many facts, but insufficient knowledge: The story of asthma, *J. Pharm. Pharmacol.,* **28**:361-368 (1976).
128. Austen, K. F., and R. P. Orange, Bronchial asthma: The possible role of the chemical mediators of immediate hypersensitivity in the pathogenesis of subacute chronic disease, *Am. Rev. Respir. Dis.,* **112**:423-436 (1975).
129. Lewis, R. A., and K. F. Austen, Nonrespiratory functions of pulmonary cells: The mast cell, *Fed. Proc.,* **36**:2676-2684 (1977).
130. Augstein, J., J. B. Farmer, T. B. Lee, P. Sheard, and M. L. Tattersall, Selective inhibitor of slow reacting substance of anaphylaxis, *Nature [New Biol.],* **245**:215-217 (1973).
131. Burka, J. F., and P. Eyre, Effect of bovine SRS-A on bovine respiratory

tract and lung vasculature in vitro, *Eur. J. Pharmacol.,* **44**:169-177 (1977).

132. Drazen, J. M., R. A. Lewis, S. I. Wasserman, and K. F. Austen, Effects of histamine and slow reacting substance of anaphylaxis (SRS-A) on central and peripheral airway function in vitro, *Am. Rev. Respir. Dis.,* **117**:Suppl. 63 (1978).
133. Wanner, A., S. Zarzecki, J. Hirsch, and S. Epstein, Tracheal mucous transport in experimental canine asthma, *J. Appl. Physiol.,* **39**:950-957 (1975).
134. Austen, K. F., A review of immunological, biochemical and pharmacological factors in the release of chemical mediators from human lung. In *Asthma: Physiology, Immunopharmacology, and Treatment.* Edited by K. F. Austen and L. M. Lichtenstein. New York, Academic, 1973, pp. 109-122.
135. Austen, K. F., Reaction mechanisms in the release of mediators of immediate hypersensitivity from human lung, *Fed. Proc.,* **33**:2256-2262 (1974).
136. Kaliner, M., and K. F. Austen, Immunologic release of chemical mediators from human tissue, *Ann. Rev. Pharmacol.,* **15**:177-189 (1975).
137. Lichtenstein, L. M., The control of IgE-mediated histamine release: Implications for the study of asthma. In *Asthma: Physiology, Immunopharmacology, and Treatment.* Edited by K. F. Austen and L. M. Lichtenstein. New York, Academic, 1973, pp. 91-107.
138. Sullivan, T. J., K. L. Parker, S. A. Eisen, and C. W. Parker, Modulation of cyclic AMP in purified rat mast cells II. Studies on the relationship between intracellular cyclic AMP concentrations and histamine release, *J. Immunol.,* **114**:1480-1485 (1975).
139. Bourne, H. R., K. L. Melmon, and L. M. Lichtenstein, Histamine augments leukocyte adenosine 3′,5′-monophosphate and blocks antigenic histamine release, *Science,* **173**:743-745 (1971).
140. Lichtenstein, L. M., and E. Gillespie, Inhibition of histamine release by histamine controlled by $H_2$ receptor, *Nature,* **244**:287-288 (1973).
141. Lichtenstein, L., and E. Gillespie, The effects of the $H_1$ and $H_2$ antihistamines on "allergic" histamine release and its inhibition by histamine, *J. Pharmacol. Exp. Ther.,* **192**:441-450 (1975).
142. Schild, H. O., Histamine release and anaphylactic shock in isolated lungs of guinea pigs, *Q. J. Exp. Physiol.,* **26**:165-179 (1936).
143. Lichtenstein, L. M., and S. Margolis, Histamine release in vitro: Inhibition by catecholamines and methylxanthines, *Science,* **161**:902-903 (1968).
144. Assem, E. S. K., and H. O. Schild, Beta adrenergic receptors concerned with the anaphylactic mechanism, *Int. Arch. Allergy,* **45**:62-69 (1973).
145. Malta, E., and C. Raper, Beta-adrenoceptors involved in inhibition of histamine release from sensitized guinea-pig lung, *Eur. J. Pharmacol.,* **30**:79-85 (1975).
146. Sorenby, L., The beta-adrenoceptors of the lung mediating inhibition of antigen-induced histamine release, *Eur. J. Pharmacol.,* **30**:140-147 (1975).

147. Holroyde, M. C., and P. Eyre, Immunological release of histamine from bovine leucocytes. Unusual adrenergic modulation, *Immunology,* **31**: 167-170 (1976).
148. Schultz, W. H., Physiological studies in anaphylaxis. I. The reaction of smooth muscle of the guinea pig sensitized with horse serum, *J. Pharmacol. Exp. Ther.,* **1**:549-567 (1910).
149. Dale, H. H., The anaphylactic reaction of plain muscle in the guinea pig, *J. Pharmacol. Exp. Ther.,* **4**:167-223 (1913).
150. Fleisch, J. H., P. J. Calkins, T. C. Troxell, and C. S. Hooker, Inhibition of antigen-induced mediator release from guinea pig lung by alcohols, *Am. Rev. Respir. Dis.,* **114**:1107-1112 (1976).
151. Fleisch, J. H., P. J. Calkins, and C. S. Hooker, Reduction in antigen-induced release of histamine and slow reacting substance of anaphylaxis from guinea pig lung with increasing age, *Biochem. Pharmacol.,* **27**:2119-2122 (1978).
152. Mongar, J. L., and H. O. Schild, Inhibition of the anaphylactic reaction, *J. Physiol. (London),* **135**:301-319 (1957).
153. Mongar, J. L., and H. O. Schild, Cellular mechanisms in anaphylaxis, *Physiol. Rev.,* **42**:226-270 (1962).
154. Cox, J. S. G., Disodium cromoglycate (FPL670) (INTAL): A specific inhibitor of reaginic antibody-antigen mechanisms, *Nature,* **216**:1328-1329 (1967).
155. Kusner, E. J., B. Dubnick, and D. J. Herzig, The inhibition by disodium cromoglycate in vitro of anaphylactically induced histamine release from rat peritoneal mast cells, *J. Pharmacol. Exp. Ther.,* **184**:41-46 (1973).
156. Pepys, J., Disodium cromoglycate in clinical and experimental asthma. In *Asthma: Physiology, Immunopharmacology, and Treatment.* Edited by K. F. Austen and L. M. Lichtenstein. New York, Academic, 1973, pp. 279-294.
157. Szentivanyi, A., The beta adrenergic theory of the atopic abnormality in bronchial asthma, *J. Allergy,* **42**:203-232 (1968).
158. Reed, C. E., Abnormal autonomic mechanisms in asthma, *J. Allerg. Clin. Immunol.,* **53**:34-41 (1974).
159. Reed, C. E., The pathogenesis of asthma, *Med. Clin. North Am.,* **58**:55-63 (1974).
160. Kirkpatrick, C. H., and C. Keller, Impaired responsiveness to epinephrine in asthma, *Am. Rev. Respir. Dis.,* **96**:692-699 (1967).
161. Makino, S., J. J. Ouellette, C. E. Reed, and C. Fishel, Correlation between increased bronchial response to acetylcholine and diminished metabolic and eosinopenic responses to epinephrine in asthma, *J. Allergy,* **46**:178-189 (1970).
162. Logsdon, P. J., E. Middleton, Jr., and R. G. Coffey, Stimulation of leukocyte adenyl cyclase by hydrocortisone and isoproterenol in asthmatic and nonasthmatic subjects, *J. Allerg. Clin. Immunol.,* **50**:45-56 (1972).
163. Parker, C. W., and J. W. Smith, Alterations in cyclic adenosine monophosphate metabolism in human bronchial asthma. I. Leukocyte responsiveness to $\beta$-adrenergic agents, *J. Clin. Invest.,* **52**:48-58 (1973).

164. Gillespie, E., M. D. Valentine, and L. M. Lichtenstein, Cyclic AMP metabolism in asthma: Studies with leukocytes and lymphocytes, *J. Allerg. Clin. Immunol.,* **53**:27-33 (1974).
165. Sokol, W. N., and G. N. Beall, Leukocytic epinephrine receptors of normal and asthmatic individuals, *J. Allerg. Clin. Immunol.,* **55**:310-324 (1975).
166. Kalisker, A., H. E. Nelson, and E. Middleton Jr., Drug-induced changes of nonasthmatic subjects, *J. Allerg. Clin. Immunol.,* **60**:259-265 (1977).

# 5

# Autonomic Regulation of Airway Smooth Muscle

*JAY A. NADEL*

University of California, San Francisco
School of Medicine
San Francisco, California

## I. Parasympathetic Nervous System

### A. General Considerations

The anatomy of the parasympathetic nervous system is reviewed in Chapter 1. and the pharmacology is reviewed in Chapter 4. Burnstock has provided evidence that the cholinergic excitatory function in the lungs was transferred from the sympathetic to the parasympathetic outflow at some evolutionary stage higher than the Amphibia [1]. Although some relatively recent articles suggest that parasympathetic control of airway smooth muscle is weak [2], present evidence indicates that the vagus nerves play an important role in regulating airway smooth muscle. The parasympathetic efferent nerve supply to the airways is by way of the vagus nerves. Electrical stimulation of the distal ends of the cut cervical vagus nerves causes bronchoconstriction [3-9], and this response is present when tested shortly after birth [10]. The bronchoconstrictor response to vagal stimulation is potentiated by cholinesterase inhibitors [3,4] and blocked by atropine [3]. During vagal stimulation, airflow resistance increases within 1 sec and reaches a maximum value within 6 sec in cats [4]. Reflex bronchoconstriction during irritation of the airways has a similar time course [11,12]. The rapid rates of these responses and of their reversibility suggest that they are due to contraction of smooth muscle, rather than mucosal edema or obstruction of the airway lumen by mucus. This impression is confirmed by bronchographic visualization of the airways in dogs which eliminated mucus as the cause of the airway narrowing [9], and by rapid freezing of the airways in the open thorax in cats which showed muscle contraction but no edema or excessive mucus [4]. Vagal stimulation appears to cause bronchoconstriction at a lower threshold than that at which mucus production can be detected [4], but this may depend on the sensitivity of the methods. The constriction produced by vagal stimulation occurs from the trachea to large bronchioles. Maximum constriction occurs in bronchi of intermediate size [7,9], the sites of most of the resistance to airflow [13,14]. Although vagal stimulation produces diffuse bronchoconstriction, physiologic studies suggest that the relative contribution of large and small airways may vary among animals [7,15,16]. Alveolar ducts and terminal bronchioles are unaffected [4,9,17]. The location of airway constriction corresponds to the distribution of cholinergic innervation [18-20]. During unilateral vagosympathetic nerve stimulation, the increase in resistance was mainly limited to the homolateral lung [4]. When the bronchomotor responses were potentiated by administration of cholinesterase inhibitors, a small increase in resistance could usually be demonstrated in the nonstimulated lung, indicating that a small degree of motor nerve crossover to the opposite lung exists [4]. These studies confirm earlier observations based on indirect measurements of resistance [21,22] and histologic studies of rabbits and mice after unilateral vagotomy and subsequent degeneration of nerve fibers [23,24], which suggested that motor innervation is largely to the homolateral lung. One or two electrical impluses per second in the vagus nerves of cats causes a measurable increase in airflow resistance, and approximately 12 impulses/sec causes a maximal response [4]. These responses are similar to those in autonomic nerves to other organs in animals [25-28] and in humans [29, 30]. In cats, electrical stimulation of the peripheral ends of the cut cervical vagi at a frequency of 4/sec restored resistance to prevagotomy values [4]. This is the same as the normal frequency of firing in these nerves [31].

Another method of stimulating the parasympathetic nerves is with field stimulation of isolated muscle. Field stimulation of tracheal smooth muscle caused contraction which was prevented by tetrodotoxin [32], indicating that nervous elements were involved in the response, or by atropine, indicating that postganglionic cholinergic pathways were involved [32,33]. Electrical stimulation of the isolated guinea pig trachea also caused muscle contraction which was potentiated by cholinesterase inhibitors and abolished by atropine but not by hexamethonium, suggesting that the contraction was due to stimulation of postganglionic cholinergic nerve fibers [33].

An early study [34] showed that vagal stimulation in guinea pigs caused a substance resembling acetylcholine to appear in the perfusion fluid. Using guinea pig ileum or rabbit trachea and appropriate blocking agents for the bioassays [35], Carlyle showed that the guinea pig trachea released acetylcholine, approximately 0.06 mg/min, at rest. After cholinesterase inhibitors, transmural stimulation of the trachea resulted in well-sustained contractions and caused acetylcholine to be released, most of which came from the muscle rather than the cartilage or mucosa [35]. Stimulation of the vagus nerves causes the release of acetylcholine by the nerve endings from electron-transparent or agranular vesicles into the junctional cleft by a process of partial exocytosis. Released acetylcholine interacts with postjunctional receptors to produce an effect that is usually terminated by local hydrolysis by postjunctional acetylcholinesterase. Thus, isolated perfused dog lungs rapidly inactivated large amounts of acetylcholine [36]. Thus, acetylcholine is normally an extremely important local, but not circulating, hormone. With blockade of acetylcholinesterase by drugs [37] or by toxins (e.g., ozone [38]), the effects of acetylcholine are potentiated.

Anatomical studies suggest that the vagal efferent fibers entering the lungs are preganglionic [39,40], and neurophysiologic studies of conduction velocities in these nerves are consistent with the fibers being preganglionic [31]. Bronchoconstrictor nerves completely reinnervated the bronchi 3 to 6 months after excision and reimplantation of one lung in dogs [41]. The rapid restitution of function is explained by the fact that preganglionic, rather than postganglionic, nerves were cut [42], and because regenerating fibers probably had to grow only a few centimeters to contact cholinergic ganglia. This rapid reinnervation is one reason surgical pulmonary vagal denervation is not likely to be an effective surgical procedure for decreasing vagal efferent activity [43]. Preganglionic vagal efferent nervous activity has been studied by recording action potentials in fibers traveling to the airways; these studies have demonstrated the effects of various interventions [44] and have been important in the characterization of airway reflexes [45].

The vagal ganglia are located within the airways themselves [46,47]. Study of these neural elements has been neglected, probably due to the fact that they are located posteriorly in large airways [46] and are difficult to identify. They are found randomly during sectioning of stained tissue but are not identified easily in live tissue. Anatomical descriptions of "pericellular baskets" formed by preganglionic axons suggest a complex arrangement but do not indicate the intimate relationships of the ganglion cells to cholinergic, monaminergic, small intensely fluorescent (SIF) cells, and other elements. Synaptic interaction producing inhibitory and facilitatory mechanisms within ganglia has been shown in other tissues, and these modulate the output to effector tissues [48-51]. In some species, catechol-containing varicosities exist in cholinergic ganglia of the airways [20,52,53], and small dense-core vesicles are found in axon profiles within ganglia in human airways [54]. Thus, sympathetic neurotransmitters could modulate cholinergic ganglionic transmission. A considerable deficiency in knowledge of motor mechanisms in the lungs derives from a lack of information concerning the physiology of the neurons. Microelectrode studies of single-unit activity in Auerbach's plexus have provided important information concerning the nervous regulation of the gut [55], and similar studies are possible in the lungs. Another approach is the selective damaging of neurons and observation of subsequent physiologic changes. Selective neural lesions of the brain have been produced by local injections of kainic acid [56], and destruction of ganglionic cells in the colon has been produced by ischemia with subsequent changes in colonic motility [57]. It would be of interest to examine the effects of ganglion cell destruction in the lungs.

Postganglionic cholinergic nervous activity has not been studied because of relative inaccessibility. Studies in isolated airway tissue indicate that both cholinergic and adrenergic nerves influence airway smooth muscle tone [32,33], but it is not known whether they simply summate at the smooth muscle cell or whether they interact presynaptically. Catecholamines depress the evoked release of acetylcholine from the guinea pig ileum [58] and a similar effect is suggested in the feline urinary bladder [59]. In cats, electrical stimulation of the sympathetic nerves inhibited bronchomotor tone induced by the vagus but not by histamine [22], suggesting a specific inhibitory role of the sympathetic nerves on vagal nervous output. Electrical stimulation of canine bronchi in vitro causes the release of norepinephrine which inhibits bronchoconstriction produced by stimulation of the cholinergic nerves [60], and this effect could be due to effects similar to the ileum and bladder. In addition to adrenergic inhibition of cholinergic neurotransmission, acetylcholine causes a marked inhibition of transmitter release during sympathetic nerve stimulation in canine blood vessels [61,62]. Similarly, acetylcholine inhibits the release of norepinephrine from nerve endings in canine airway smooth muscle [63].

The anatomy of the nerve endings also suggests that reciprocal inhibitory actions of adrenergic and cholinergic neurotransmitters could play an important role in the regulation of airway smooth muscle: varicosities of presumed adrenergic and cholinergic axons commonly occur within 1 to 5 $\mu$m of each other in the trachealis muscle of cats ([64]; Carol Basbaum, 1979, personal communication), chickens [65], and guinea pigs (Carol Basbaum, 1979, personal communication). This distance is probably short enough to allow neurotransmitter released from one varicosity to influence the excitability of another. Thus, the anatomical substrate for interaction between postganglionic axons exists in some instances. It remains to be demonstrated that postganglionic axons possess adrenergic and cholinergic receptor molecules and also that physiological levels of nerve stimulation can release neurotransmitter in sufficiently large amounts to compensate for concentration decrements which occur.

Serotonin facilitates vagal tone in canine airways via an action on efferent vagal pathways [66]; the effect could be due to actions on ganglia, postganglionic pathways or on the muscle itself. Serotonin has an effect on nervous structures [48,51], on cholinergic receptors [67], and at intracellular levels [68]. In the gastrointestinal tract, serotonin acts on both neural elements [69-71] and on smooth muscle [72,73]. The effects of serotonin could be physiologically significant if serotonergic axons exist. In the gastrointestinal tract, serotonergic axons [74] have been found to contain morphologically distinct synaptic vesicles which has assisted in their ultrastructural differentiation from other autonomic axons [75]. Since the gastrointestinal tract is related embryologically to the lungs, similar axons may exist in the lungs.

Pharmacologic techniques for studying the release of norepinephrine and acetylcholine from airway smooth muscle, studies of adrenergic and cholinergic receptors, and anatomical methods for studying recycling of axon varicosities [76] could be applied to these problems.

The airways of animals and healthy humans are tonically constricted, and this tone is maintained by vagal efferent nervous activity [31]. Thus, cutting or cooling the vagus nerves in animals [3-6,77-79] or administration of atropine in animals [77] and in humans [45,77-84] causes bronchodilation. The degree of tonic activity appears to differ among species. Thus, cutting the vagus nerves decreases resistance to airflow markedly in cats [4], less in dogs [6,78], and only slightly in rabbits [5]. This difference in the degree of vagal tone may explain why anticholinesterase drugs produce early and severe bronchoconstriction in cats, but only slight bronchoconstriction in rabbits [85]. When the vagus nerves are cut, sympathetic nerve stimulation has little or no effect on airway size in vivo [6,22,86,87]. In isolated guinea pig tracheal muscle, no significant change in inherent tone occurred after inhibition of cholinesterase [35,88]. Hyosine or atropine did not affect the muscle tone in vitro in concentrations which abolished the action of acetylcholine [35,88-90]. Thus, it appears that parasympathetic nerve terminals are generally not active spontaneously at rest. This differs from the guinea pig ileum where significant contraction occurs after cholinesterase inhibition [91]. From these studies, it is concluded that nervous impulses carried from the central nervous system by way of the vagus nerves maintain the normal airway tone. This is confirmed by recordings of action potentials which show that irregular firing occurs normally at rest in vagal efferent nerve fibers innervating the trachea and bronchi of cats and dogs [31,44].

### B. Reflex Control of Airway Smooth Muscle

Demonstration of reflex bronchoconstriction requires the determination of the pathways. Multiple receptors have been shown to affect bronchomotor tone

[92], including the nose [12,93,94], larynx [93,95,96], lungs [11,12,45,97-103], central and peripheral chemoreceptors [78,104], and baroreceptors [78]. Bronchoconstriction associated with intravenous injection of hypertonic sodium chloride causes bronchoconstriction that is abolished by vagotomy, but the exact pathway is unknown [105]. Possible reflex effects of stimulation of receptors in many areas of the body (e.g., gastrointestinal tract) on bronchomotor tone are untested.

Little is known about the central nervous connections of these afferent pathways and the reflex organization of bronchomotor tone. The efferent pathways are mainly by way of the vagus nerves; bronchoconstrictor reflexes are associated with increased vagal efferent activity to the airways and bronchodilator reflexes are associated with decreased vagal efferent activity [31,93,106]. The role of the sympathetic nerves in bronchomotor reflexes is less clear, and possible interaction with parasympathetic nervous regulation has not been explored in detail.

The study of bronchomotor reflexes requires methods which can detect changes in airway dimensions sensitively and accurately. Because of the relative inaccessibility of the airways, early methods which measured mechanical impedance could not distinguish bronchial from nonbronchial effects [107]. Recently, sensitive methods have been developed and applied to the study of bronchomotor reflexes [108]. Since the airways are "tethered" to the lungs, changes in lung volume (e.g., with breathing) may have profound effects on airway dimensions, especially when increased bronchomotor tone exists [109]. The apparent increased sensitivity of airway resistance compared to other methods of evaluating bronchomotor tone [110,111] may be due to the fact that the other methods require a prior deep breath, a respiratory maneuver that temporarily decreases bronchomotor tone [112]. Respiratory maneuvers may also have different effects in healthy individuals and patients. Thus, a deep breath temporarily decreases airway smooth muscle tone in healthy subjects [112], but may cause bronchoconstriction in asthmatic subjects [113]. In some experiments designed to discover possible bronchomotor reflexes, local anesthetics [114], atropine premedication [114], and general anesthetics [115-118], or the fact that the study was performed in vitro [119], may have prevented a reflex response. In addition to blocking afferent nervous pathways, local anesthetics may have multiple other effects on the airway neuromuscular system which might interfere with reflex bronchomotor responses [120-122]. General anesthetics not only depress smooth muscle and vagal efferent pathways [10,116,118], but also affect the activity of pulmonary receptors [123]. Hydrogen ion concentration has a selective effect on drug-induced contraction of airway smooth muscle, affecting serotonin-induced contraction more than acetylcholine-induced contraction [124,125]. There is evidence that neural control of airway smooth muscle also varies with physiologic state. Thus, in dogs, airway smooth muscle tone decreases with progression of sleep through the nonrapid eye movement stages, and during rapid eye movement sleep, tracheal smooth muscle tone fluctuates markedly [126].

Stimuli may have multiple effects on the airways. For example, histamine may have local effects on airway smooth muscle [127], reflex effects [97] by stimulating receptors in the airways [100,101], and effects on the efferent parasympathetic pathways [66]. In addition, stimuli that may affect bronchi also affect laryngeal caliber [128-131]. In spontaneously breathing guinea pigs, measurement of airflow resistance includes the larynx. Effects interpreted as bronchial [132] could be due to effects on the larynx [128]. In humans, the body plethysmograph is used to measure airway resistance; measurements are made during a panting maneuver to abduct the larynx [133]. However, it has not been shown that the panting maneuver prevents laryngeal narrowing during stimulation. This confounding effect needs to be ruled out whenever the larynx is included in the measured resistance (e.g., Ref. 134).

Definitive proof of reflex bronchoconstriction has come from studies where the stimulation of receptors is separated from the effector. For example, $SO_2$ delivered only to the upper airways caused constriction of the lower airway, an effect that could only be due to a reflex [11]. Similarly, mechanical stimulation of the larynx caused constriction of the lower airways, an effect that was abolished by cutting the sensory nerves from the larynx [93]. Inflation of the lungs dilated a segment of cervical trachea that was isolated mechanically from the lungs in dogs [98,104]. Thus, methods exist in vivo and in vitro for determining whether a specific mechanism exists. The reader is referred to a detailed discussion of methods used in the study of airway smooth muscle [108]. The more difficult problem is the assessment of the integration and importance of different factors in regulating airway smooth muscle tone in health and disease.

What is the purpose of these bronchomotor reflexes and are they beneficial? Airway caliber balances two conflicting factors, airway volume and airway resistance. A large increase in airway volume may be disadvantageous if the need for increased ventilation of dead space is excessive, and severe bronchoconstriction (e.g., in asthma) produces an undesirable increase in the resistive work of breathing. Nervously mediated airway tone in healthy subjects may represent an optimal relationship between airway resistance and dead space to allow a minimum of respiratory work or respiratory force [135].

Slowly adapting and irritant receptors appear to have reciprocal actions on bronchial smooth muscle: stimulation of irritant receptors causes bronchoconstriction [45], and stimulation of slowly adapting receptors causes bronchodilation [98]. There is evidence in awake dogs that these two groups of receptors also play opposing roles in the normal control of respiration: slowly adapting receptors appear to inhibit and irritant receptors stimulate breathing [136].

Since the sensitivity of the irritant receptors is determined in part by the level of bronchomotor tone, the output from the slowly adapting and irritant receptors may "set" the level of irritant receptor output and thereby serve as an autoregulatory system to adjust the pattern of breathing. Interaction between slowly adapting and irritant receptors could provide the mechanism that adjusts the depth and frequency of breathing to minimize the work of breathing [137] and to minimize the mean force of respiratory muscle contraction [138].

Another possible purpose of reflex bronchoconstriction associated with stimulation of receptors in the large airways may be as a normal part of the cough reflex: the combination of reflex bronchoconstriction, mucus production, and cough may produce effective removal of foreign irritants [139].

Several feedback mechanisms tend to limit the degree of reflex bronchoconstriction. For example, stimulation of chemoreceptors causes reflex bronchoconstriction [78]; this stimulus also increases the rate and depth of breathing, which stimulates slowly adapting stretch receptors and the trachea reflexly dilates [98]. Thus, in paralyzed dogs, stimulation of carotid body chemoreceptors causes only bronchoconstriction [78]. In spontaneously breathing dogs allowed to hyperventilate during carotid body stimulation, the initial bronchoconstriction is followed by considerable dilation, an effect that is abolished by pulmonary denervation [6]. Sensitization of slowly adapting stretch receptors could also limit bronchoconstriction: bronchoconstriction increases the sensitivity of these receptors [140], which then reflexly inhibits vagal efferent activity, thus tending to minimize the effect of the original bronchoconstriction [98]. Simultaneous stimulation of sympathetic and parasympathetic nervous activity may also limit a reflex effect. Thus, mechanical irritation of the larynx produces reflex bronchoconstriction by increasing vagal efferent nervous activity. This stimulus also increases discharge in sympathetic efferent fibers to the airways [93], an effect that tends to decrease bronchomotor tone.

In addition to "negative feedback loops," there are mechanisms that tend to augment reflex bronchoconstriction. Thus, stimulation of the airways causes reflex bronchoconstriction [45]; bronchoconstriction, in turn, stimulates the airway receptors [100]. This type of "positive feedback loop" could be important in bronchospastic diseases and may explain, at least in part, the effect of atropine in dilating airways in asthma [141-149] and in bronchitis [150-153].

In the natural environment, inhaled stimuli may stimulate various receptors, depending on factors such as particle size and solubility of the irritant (see Chapter 6). Different types of receptors are likely to be stimulated simultaneously and the effects depend on the interaction of the various inputs.

There is no evidence that the bronchomotor reflexes are under voluntary control. The pathways for conditioned reflexes exist, but studies designed to test whether reflex conditioning is possible have not been performed. In asthma, the role of emotions on airways is assumed to be expressed through the parasympathetic nervous system [154,155]. A significant number of asthmatic subjects respond to psychological stimuli with bronchoconstriction [156-160]. That this bronchoconstriction is abolished by cholinergic antagonists suggests that the parasympathetic nervous system plays a role [157].

Although other bronchomotor reflexes have been described, the following review concentrates on receptors in the lungs and airways.

### *Upper Airways*

#### Nose and Pharynx

Kratschmer [161] observed that the respiratory and circulatory reflexes produced by irritant gases applied to the nasal cavities and stimulating the trigeminal nerves differed from the action of these gases in the deeper respiratory passages. Subsequent studies have shown that nasal irritation causes vagal bradycardia, peripheral sympathetic vasoconstriction, and apnea [12,93]. Many studies on bronchomotor tone suggested that nasal stimulation caused bronchoconstriction [21,162,163]. However, the results of these experiments are difficult to interpret because of the inexact methods and poor localization of the stimulus. For example, Rall and coworkers [162] claimed that stimulation of the nose in dogs caused reflex bronchoconstriction. The state of airway "tone" was evaluated by measuring pressure in an inflated balloon placed in an airway, a method which is sensitive to respiratory artifacts. Furthermore, the study was performed with an open pneumothorax, so the airways being measured were probably collapsed. Using this method, the authors presented evidence that the reflex was not abolished by atropine or vagotomy, but was mediated by inhibition of sympathetic activity. However, present evidence indicates that the vagus nerves are responsible for the tone in airways, and that after vagotomy sympathetic stimulation has no effect on bronchomotor tone in dogs [87]. This makes one question further the validity of Rall's observations. Studies using modern techniques indicate that mechanical or chemical stimulation of the nasal mucosa dilates the airways in cats [12,94]. The effect was intensified when vagal bronchomotor tone was increased. In a previous study, stimulation of the nasal mucosa resulted in slight bronchodilation which was not statistically significant [93]. This could be due to the absence of sufficient bronchomotor tone in the control state. The bronchodilator effect was associated with a decrease in nervous activity in vagal efferent fibers in the trachea and with an increase in activity in cervical sympathetic efferent fibers [12]. The rapidity of onset of the bronchodilator effects suggests that most of the effect was due to inhibition of vagal tone [4], since sympathetic effects occur more slowly [87]. However, further studies are required to establish the roles of vagal bronchoconstrictor fibers, thoracic bronchodilator fibers, and circulating catecholamines. Few studies exist on the effect of nasal stimulation in humans and localization of the stimulus is more difficult. Studies comparing effects of sulfur dioxide inhaled through the mouth or nose suggest that sulfur dioxide causes bronchoconstriction by stimulating receptors in the larynx and bronchi but not the nose [164-166]. Inhalation of sulfur dioxide through the nose decreased the bronchoconstrictor response compared to oral inhalation, presumably because sulfur dioxide was trapped in the nose, so a lower concentration of the gas reached the responsible receptors in the lower airways [165]. Kaufman and Wright [134] showed that aerosols of silica insufflated into the nose during breath-holding resulted in an increase in airway resistance which was abolished by atropine sulfate, suggesting that cholinergic postganglionic pathways were involved in the response. Receptors in the larynx, trachea, and bronchi are stimulated by dust particles and cause potent reflex bronchoconstriction [12,80, 96]. If some of the particles delivered into the nose reached these receptors, the response could have been due to stimulation of cough rather than nasal receptors. An additional problem arises from the fact that nasal stimulation causes reflex narrowing of the larynx [129]. Thus, the increase in airway resistance could have been due to laryngeal, rather than bronchial, narrowing. Further studies are required to determine the role of nasal stimulation in the control of bronchomotor tone.

Recently, a new respiratory reflex has been described, originating in receptors in the epipharynx (the "aspiration reflex"). This reflex, activated by mechanical stimulation of the epipharynx in cats, has its afferent pathway in the glossopharyngeal nerves and results in strong sniff and gasplike inspirations, reflex increase in systemic blood pressure, and reflex bronchodilation [12,94]. The bronchodilator effect of epipharyngeal stimulation was more potent than that produced by nasal stimulation. Like nasal stimulation, stimulation of the epipharynx was associated with a decrease in nervous activity in vagal efferent fibers in the trachea and an increase in activity in cervical sympathetic efferent fibers; the relative contributions of the sympathetic and parasympathetic systems were not studied.

### Larynx

Stimulation of the laryngeal mucosa in cats causes expulsive coughing characterized by potent stimulation of action potentials in the diaphragm and in abdominal muscles, reflex increase in blood pressure, and bronchoconstriction [12,93, 95]. The bronchomotor response began within 2 sec after the onset of stimulation and usually returned to control levels within 1 min after the stimulus was removed [93]. The bronchoconstrictor response could be obtained by mechanical irritation of the larynx [12,93,95], insufflation of dust [163], ammonia vapor [95], or acetic acid vapor [93], or by phenyldiguanide [95], but not by sulfur dioxide, $CO_2$, or histamine [95]. Cooling or cutting the cervical vagosympathetic nerves prevented the bronchoconstriction, suggesting that the efferent pathways were in the vagus nerves [93,95]. This impression was confirmed by the demonstration that laryngeal stimulation increased impulse traffic in vagal efferent fibers to the lungs [31] and to the trachea [12,93]. The afferent path for the reflex is in the superior laryngeal nerves [93,95]. Recordings of action potentials in single afferent fibers from laryngeal mucosal receptors show that at least three types of receptors exist [96], but the role of these different receptors in bronchomotor reflexes is unknown.

### *Lower Airways and Lungs*

#### Cough and "Irritant" Receptors

Although many reflexes have been described which previously were ascribed to different receptors in the lungs and airways, these reflexes now can be explained on the basis of three groups of receptors: (1) rapidly adapting "cough" and "irritant" receptors; (2) slowly adapting "pulmonary stretch" receptors; and (3) type-C receptors [103]. Recently, studies of respiratory receptors have utilized electron microscopy, more comprehensive analysis of receptors by recordings from single afferent nerve fibers, and more detailed studies of reflexes in animals and humans [103]. In spite of extensive investigation, the exact histologic identification of the three groups of receptors has not been accomplished. Newer techniques can be applied to label specific axons and to correlate structure and function. Thus, ganglion cells synthesize [$^3$H]protein from [$^3$H]amino acid precursors [167-169], and autoradiography following injection of [$^3$H]amino acids into the nodose ganglion might be used to determine the structure of individual sensory nerve endings. Horseradish peroxidase (HRP) has been shown to be transported intra-axonally within the airway wall [170]. Pulmonary location [100, 171,172] and the fact that their stimulation leads to hyperpnea rather than cough [172,173] distinguishes cough from irritant receptors. Cough receptors are more rapidly adapting than the intrapulmonary receptors and have a more pronounced "off-effect" to volume changes [172]. Cough receptors appear to be more sensitive to mechanical than to chemical stimuli [172], but the methods used (e.g., touching the mucosa with a catheter) do not permit accurate quantification. Intrapulmonary receptors are purported to be more sensitive to chemical irritants [172] and to histamine [100,173]. Because the intrapulmonary receptors are very sensitive to inhaled dusts, irritating gases, and aerosols, the term "irritant" receptor was coined to describe them and has been used since 1963 [45]. A drawback to this term derives from the fact that lung inflation also stimulates the receptors. In recognition of the rapid adaptation to maintained lung inflation [174], some authors refer to them simply as "rapidly adapting" receptors [101].

The location of the irritant receptor endings has been defined with the aid of a fiber bronchoscope [101]. In dogs, the concentration of these receptors increases from the trachea to the lobar bronchi and then decreases sharply in the smaller airways [175]. Since they are sensitive to inhaled dust, irritant chemicals, and gentle application of a catheter, it has been suggested that the responsible receptors lie within the epithelium [173]. Sant'Ambrogio et al. performed studies of rapidly adapting receptors before and after removal of the mucosa in the receptive field. They concluded that mucosal endings provide sensitivity to light touch and that deeper endings mediate the response to gross mechanical deformation [176]. Sensory nerve fibers branch between cells of the airway epithelium and contain endings that lie immediately beneath tight junctions between epithelial cells [177], and these endings are likely to be the rapidly adapting sensory endings that respond to light touch and perhaps to chemical stimuli [99,100, 103,173]. A single receptor field may be distributed over an area as large as 1 cm; the morphology of a single receptor is unknown [177].

Irritant receptors are located within the thoracic cavity and are therefore affected by changes in elastic recoil [99]. This may explain why they are stimulated by pulmonary congestion, microembolism, atelectasis, and pneumothorax [99]. The reasons for the other physiological differences between cough and irritant receptors are not obvious, since the receptors themselves have no apparent structural differences [103]. However, other differences in the anatomy of the surrounding tissue elements may play a role: differences in the thickness and chemical properties of the mucous layer will affect diffusion and buffering of chemical irritants. The mechanical properties of mucus will affect the ability of deposited materials to deform the subjacent structures. The bronchial epithelium is columnar and the epithelial nerve terminals appear to end between these cells close to the surface [103]. The laryngeal epithelium is squamous and the nerve terminals may be located in a different relation to the surface, although anatomical studies of the nerves in the larynx are not described in sufficient detail to state this with certainty. Additionally, effects of receptors in various locations may possibly be explained by differences in reflex connections.

The exact mechanism of stimulation of the receptors is unknown. In the case of mechanical stimulation with a catheter or insufflation of dust, deformation of the epithelium is presumably required. Careful quantitative studies of the receptors are needed for an understanding of their operation. Studies of pulmonary receptor activity have been performed in vitro, and discharge from rapidly adapting receptors has been demonstrated [178]. Further studies of the localization of mechanical changes required for activation of the receptors and effects of surrounding tissue elements is thus feasible. Such a study, including determination of threshold, rectification, and quantitation, could add to the understanding of receptor activation. This preparation also has the advantage of eliminating cardiovascular effects.

Various types of stimuli stimulate subepithelial airway receptors and cause bronchoconstriction.

**Mechanical Stimulation** Mechanical irritation of the larynx, trachea, and bronchi excites rapidly adapting irregular discharge in cough and irritant receptors [172,173], presumably by deforming the airway in such a way as to depolarize the receptors. It is claimed that receptors in the larger airways (cough receptors) are more sensitive than those in smaller airways (irritant receptors) to mechanical stimulation [172], but present techniques (i.e., introduction of a catheter into the lumen) do not permit quantification. Stimulation of the laryngeal, tracheal, and bronchial mucosa stimulated activity in vagal efferent fibers to the trachea and bronchi [31,44], and caused bronchoconstriction [12,93,95] which was abolished by vagotomy [93,95].

The increase in resistance occurred on the first ventilatory cycle after application of the catheter and usually returned to control levels within 1 min [93], indicating a rapid response and reversal.

The effect of mechanical stimulation of the airway mucosa has been studied in human subjects, and bronchoconstriction was not found [115]. However, local anesthesia and the depressant effects of barbiturate anesthesia may have inhibited a vagal reflex response. The possible importance of such a reflex is suggested by the clinical observation that atropine reduces the occurrence of laryngospasm during general anesthesia [179]. Further study is required to determine whether atropine has its effect, not on the larynx, but on bronchi.

**Insufflation of Dust** Inhalation of chemically inert dust stimulates irregular activity in cough receptors in cats [80] and in irritant receptors in rabbits [100]; it also stimulates activity in vagal efferent fibers to bronchi in cats [80] and increases airflow resistance in cats [80] and in dogs [180]. This bronchoconstriction is abolished by vagotomy [80] or by atropine sulfate [180]. In healthy human subjects, inhalation of chemically inert dust also increases airway resistance [80,110,134,180] and decreases maximal expiratory airflow [181,182]. Isoproterenol prevented the bronchoconstriction [180], suggesting that the effect was due to smooth muscle contraction. The effect was also abolished by atropine [80], suggesting that postganglionic cholinergic pathways were involved in the bronchomotor response to inhaled dust in humans.

Following cessation of inhalation of dust, bronchoconstriction continued for up to one hour [180], in contrast to the bronchoconstriction due to stimulation with a catheter when the response disappeared within 1 min after cessation of stimulation [93]. The sustained response is probably due to the continuing stimulation of receptors by dust particles in the airways before they are cleared by mucociliary activity [182].

Inhalation of cigarette smoke also causes bronchoconstriction in animals [183,184] and in healthy humans [185-191]. Since the effect is not abolished by removal of volatile substances [185], it is likely that the bronchoconstriction is at least partly due to the particles themselves. Some studies suggest that volatile materials present in cigarette smoke also play a role [190]. Cigarette smoke stimulates irritant receptors [100], and the resulting bronchoconstriction is abolished by isoproterenol [185], atropine [183,189,192], or vagotomy [192], suggesting that cigarette smoke causes bronchoconstriction by means of the same pathways as other dusts. Dust particles of different sizes deposit preferentially in airways of different sizes. Thus, it is not surprising that small particles contained in cigarette smoke stimulate preferentially intrapulmonary irritant receptors, whereas receptors in the trachea and larynx are less affected [103]. Similarly, larger particles deposit in the upper airways and stimulate cough receptors [163].

**Chemical Irritants** Inhalation of various chemical irritants stimulates activity in rapidly adapting receptors in the airways [172,173]. Receptors in the lower airways are claimed to be more sensitive to chemical irritants than those in the upper airways [172]. Inhalation of ammonia vapor increased activity in vagal efferent fibers to the trachea and bronchi of cats [31,44]. The response varies with species, since ammonia did not stimulate efferent vagal activity or cough in dogs [31]. Inhalation of sulfur dioxide increased airflow resistance in guinea pigs [193], dogs [194], cats [11], and healthy human subjects [11,195,196]. Constriction of the lower airways occurred when $SO_2$ was delivered only to the upper airways, suggesting that the response was due to a reflex [11]. This was confirmed by the observation that bronchoconstriction following inhalation of $SO_2$ is prevented by blocking conduction in the vagus nerves [11], or by atropine sulfate [11,196]. Other chemical irritants, including ammonia [12,95,197], ozone [198-201], sulfuric acid [202], phosgene [197], aerosols of sorbital and lecithin [82], and chymotrypsin [203] cause bronchoconstriction. Bronchoconstriction occurred when ammonia exposure was limited to the larynx [12,95]. Some chemical irritants, expecially in low concentrations (e.g., $SO_2$), cause only reflex bronchoconstriction with no evidence of local effects, although a few studies suggest the local effects may be important [184]. Thus, resistance to airflow usually increases rapidly during exposure to the irritant and returns to the control state after vagotomy. In the case of other chemicals (e.g., phosgene), in addition to the reflex component, there is a delayed, local effect which remains after vagotomy. In most studies, it appears that the reflex component is large and the direct component small [103], but few careful studies correlating physiologic findings and anatomical changes are available. The rapid onset of the changes suggests that an increase in smooth muscle tone was responsible for the constriction [11,195]. The rapid reversal by atropine sulfate suggests that postganglionic cholinergic pathways were involved in the responses [11,82,196]; it is likely that the subepithelial receptors are also responsible for the reflex bronchoconstrictor response.

**Drugs** The pharmacology of airway smooth muscle is discussed in Chapter 4. Only effects on the autonomic nervous system will be discussed here. Although many drugs have actions which involve cholinergic pathways, two drugs (histamine and serotonin) will serve to discuss various mechanisms.

Histamine has long been known to act locally on airway smooth muscle to cause contraction [90,127], an action that occurs in vitro as well as in vivo. It has often been assumed that its action in vivo is due solely to its local action on bronchial smooth muscle. However, many investigators have reported that the bronchoconstrictor effect of histamine in vivo can be abolished or decreased by hexamethonium [204-206] or by atropine [97,182,204,207,208]. It has been suggested that this effect is due to the stimulation by histamine of cholinergic ganglia that exist in the walls of the airways [204,206]. Histamine has been shown to potentiate the response of the perfused superior cervical ganglion of the cat to submaximal preganglionic stimulation [48]. This possibility could be studied by direct electrical recording of ganglion cell activity in the airway by methods used in the gut [55]. The increased resistance to airflow that occurs when histamine is injected into the bronchial artery [5,97,209], injected IV or ously, or inhaled as an aerosol [210-212] can be diminished or abolished by cervical vagotomy in dogs, cats, and rabbits. Since the smooth muscle and ganglia are not affected by vagotomy, it was suggested that the effect of small doses of histamine was due to a reflex [97]. Furthermore, after vagotomy, effects of histamine aerosol were not affected by atropine but were abolished by isoproterenol, suggesting that the remaining effects were local and not due to ganglionic stimulation [210].

That histamine stimulated reflex bronchoconstriction by way of vagal efferent pathways was further substantiated by the demonstration that histamine increased activity in efferent vagal fibers to bronchi in cats [209]. Injection of histamine into the bronchial artery constricted a bypassed segment of trachea (not perfused by the bronchial artery), and this effect was abolished by pulmonary vagotomy, indicating that the afferent pathways were located in the pulmonary vagi [97]. Dose-response curves showed that bronchial effects of small doses of histamine were abolished completely by vagal blockade, or by atropine, and effects of larger doses were inhibited markedly [5,97]. Cooling the cervical vagus nerves to approximately 7 to 10°C abolished the reflex response to histamine [5,97,211]. This is the range of temperatures at which the irritant receptor fibers are blocked but vagal efferent pathways are intact, so it was suggested that histamine reflexly constricts the airways by stimulating irritant receptors [5,97,212]. The respiratory responses to histamine [97,212,213] are also compatible with the effects of irritant receptor stimulation on respiration [173]. Finally, histamine has been shown to stimulate rapidly adapting pulmonary irritant receptors [100,101,173,214]. The reflex effect of histamine on bronchomotor tone is much greater when histamine is delivered into the bronchial tree than into the pulmonary artery, suggesting that the responsible receptors are located in the bronchi rather than in terminal bronchioles, alveolar ducts, or alveoli [97]. Inhalation of finely dispersed aerosols of histamine produced mainly local constriction of bronchioles [210]. The location of the receptors might be better characterized by use of aerosols of different diameters. It is not clear whether histamine stimulates the receptors directly or by deforming the tissue by contracting the smooth muscle. In favor of the latter is the fact that histamine stimulates intrapulmonary [100,209] and tracheal [103] but not laryngeal [96] receptors; the difference could be due to the fact that the larynx does not contain smooth muscle. The fact that stimulation of irritant receptors by intravenous injection of histamine is decreased by isoproterenol (a drug which relaxes the histamine-induced smooth muscle contractions) is used as further evidence that the effect of histamine is secondary to muscle contraction [100,209]. However, the main effect of intravenous histamine is on the peripheral airways, causing local constriction of terminal bronchioles and alveolar ducts with a resulting decrease in lung compliance [215]. Any condition which decreases lung compliance sensitizes irritant receptors [99], and this effect would be reversed by isoproterenol. In favor of a direct effect of histamine on irritant receptors is the fact that bronchoconstriction due to low doses of histamine is completely abolished by atropine or vagotomy [5,97], and the fact that histamine stimulated irritant receptors of vagotomized animals in concentrations that did not affect resistance or compliance [209]. In addition, locally applied histamine in the vicinity of an irritant receptor increased the rate of receptor discharge, even after isoproterenol [101]. Nevertheless, it is likely that the receptors are also sensitive to the state of airway smooth muscle tone [101]. Histamine causes reflex bronchoconstriction [5] and stimulates irritant receptors in rabbits [100,209], a species whose isolated airways are reported not to respond to histamine [216]. This could be used as evidence of a primary effect on irritant receptors, but other factors (e.g., size of airway affected) have not been eliminated.

Histamine-induced bronchoconstriction in humans is also partially or completely blocked by atropine or by hexamethonium, which suggests a similar vagal mechanism [113,206].

The bronchoconstrictor effect of serotonin can also be decreased or abolished by atropine [66,217], or by vagotomy [66], suggesting that a cholinergic mechanism is involved in this effect of serotonin. However, the fact that atropine prevented the bronchoconstriction caused by serotonin in isolated perfused lungs [218] suggests another, nonreflex cholinergic effect. In vagotomized dogs, doses of serotonin too low to narrow the airways increased markedly the bronchoconstrictor response to stimulation of the peripheral ends of the cut vagus nerves [66], demonstrating a potent effect of serotonin on the efferent vagal pathway. Serotonin has effects on various nervous and muscle elements [48,51,66-75], but the exact mechanism of action in the airways has not been determined.

Some investigators have found a major vagal component to drug-induced bronchoconstriction, while others have found none. In one case, major vagal effects were reported by one group in one study [219] but not in another study [220]. Differences in species, anesthesia, and mode of delivery of the drugs may explain some of the differences. However, in many cases the reasons for the differences are not obvious; their elucidation may contribute to an understanding of the increased responsiveness of the airways that occurs in diseases such as asthma and bronchitis [113].

**Pulmonary Stretch Receptors**

Pulmonary stretch receptors have been characterized by their action potentials. They are stimulated by maintained lung inflation to fire regularly with slow adaptation and usually do not increase their activity on lung deflation [172,221, 222]. Their discharge correlates better with transpulmonary pressure than with lung volume [223], so it is not surprising that they are sensitized by pulmonary congestion, atelectasis, and injection of bronchoactive drugs [140,172]. Present evidence suggests strongly that these sensory endings are located in smooth muscle cells from the trachea to bronchioles [103,224]. Inflation of the lungs inhibits inspiratory activity by the Hering-Breuer inflation reflex, and considerable evidence suggests that stretch receptors are responsible [103,221]. Lung inflation generally increases airway caliber, but this is mainly due to the passive effect of increased traction on the airways by the expanding lung tissue [112,225,226]. However, inflation of the lungs dilated a segment of cervical trachea that was only connected to the lungs by way of nervous pathways [98,104]. The effect was abolished by vagotomy, suggesting that a reflex was involved [98,104]. Small inflations of the lungs inhibit nervous activity in vagal efferent fibers to the trachea and lungs, presumably by stimulating pulmonary stretch receptors [31,44,106], so it appears that lung inflation causes reflex bronchodilation primarily by decreasing vagal efferent nervous activity to airway smooth muscle. Reflex dilation of the cervical trachea during lung inflation was also abolished by pulmonary vagotomy, suggesting that the responsible receptors were located in the lungs [98]. Differential cooling of the cervical vagus nerves until the Hering-Breuer inflation reflex was abolished also prevented the reflex bronchodilation, suggesting that pulmonary stretch receptors were responsible [98]. This was supported by experiments with veratrine, a drug which stimulates pulmonary stretch receptors [227]. Right heart injection of veratrine dilated the cervical trachea, and this response was abolished by pulmonary vagotomy [98].

There is evidence that pulmonary stretch receptor activity inhibits bronchomotor activity during normal breathing. Thus, vagal efferent nerve fibers innervating airways usually decrease their activity during the inspiratory phase of breathing [31,44]. That vagal efferent bronchoconstrictor tone is normally held in check by vagal afferent dilator discharge is supported by the fact that cervical vagotomy greatly increases the activity in efferent vagal fibers to airways [31]. Cutting the pulmonary vagi in dogs resulted in maintained constriction of the cervical trachea, indicating that impulses from the lungs normally inhibit vagal bronchomotor tone [98]. Differential cooling of the cervical vagus nerves to 8 to 10°C to block the Hering-Breuer inflation reflex selectively caused an increase in resistance in cats [98] and rabbits [5].

Anatomically, the pulmonary stretch receptors are located mainly in the walls of the trachea and large bronchi in dogs and cats [172,228]. They appear to be located in the vicinity of airway smooth muscle [103]. Thus, slowly adapting receptor activity continued to be present after the regional mucosa in the area of the receptor had been widely resected, but removal of the smooth muscle layer caused the abrupt cessation of the receptor discharge [229]. Light microscope studies show sensory fibers in the vicinity of the muscle, and electron microscopy shows axons that appear to be sensory [103]. A reconstruction of such a nerve complex has been performed, but there is no direct evidence that it represents a stretch receptor [230]. Studies of segments of canine trachea in vitro have characterized the transduction characteristics of tracheal receptors [231], and the importance of the structure of the cartilaginous and muscle elements have been studied [232]. Tonic stretch receptor discharge is present in humans and increases with lung inflation [233]. Experimentally induced bronchoconstriction is inhibited temporarily after lung inflation in humans and this could be due, in part, to a reflex [112], but this has not been differentiated from stress relaxation in the human studies. The concentration and distribution of c-fiber endings throughout the lungs is still unknown.

**c-Fiber Endings**

Paintal first recorded activity in these small afferent fibers, and he presented evidence that the endings were located close to the pulmonary capillaries (hence, he named them type "J" receptors) [234,235]. Occasional unmyelinated nerve fibers have been found in the alveolar walls which contained inclusions typical of sensory nerves [236,237], and these could represent portions of a c-fiber receptor. No descriptions of such an entire receptor complex exists. Coleridge and associates have described effects on similar small fiber endings (now called c-fibers because of their physiologic characteristics) [238]. They showed that fibers with characteristics similar to the type-J receptors exist in the airways [239] and are responsive to drugs injected into the bronchial circulation [240]. These endings respond to histamine and prostaglandins [241,242]. The importance of these receptors in reflex bronchoconstriction is undetermined; some effects ascribed to "irritant" receptors could be due to stimulation of c-fiber endings.

It is generally assumed that mechanical deformation is the effective stimulus for the receptors. However, lung inflation, a stimulus to c-fiber discharge, also causes the release of prostaglandins [243], mediators known to stimulate lung c-fibers [241,242]. Indomethacin has been shown to block one reflex effect of lung inflation, and this effect of indomethacin could be due to its effect on the release of prostaglandins [244].

## II. Sympathetic Nervous System: General Considerations

The anatomy (Chapter 1) and pharmacology (Chapter 4) of the adrenergic system and the role of cyclic nucleotides (Chapter 3) are discussed in other chapters. The adrenergic system can influence airway smooth muscle both by circulating catecholamines released from chromaffin cells and by direct nervous innervation of the airways. The influence of circulating catecholamines appears to play a more significant role in lower vertebrates; in higher vertebrates, direct nervous control has been more highly developed [1].

In contrast to the parasympathetic nervous system, the sympathetic nerve supply to the airways is not well characterized, and only a few studies of sympathetic nervous regulation exist [245]. The classic studies of sympathetic innervation can be stated as follows: The upper thoracic sympathetic preganglionic fibers terminate in the extrapulmonary stellate ganglia. Conduction velocities of the fibers to the lungs are much slower than in vagal efferent fibers and are compatible with postganglionic fibers [31].

Postganglionic fibers enter the lungs and with parasympathetic postganglionic fibers form a common terminal reticulum of nerve fibers which ramifies throughout the muscle layer as far distally as the respiratory bronchioles [246, 247]. Although it has long been recognized that sympathetic nerves innervate the lungs, it is only since a specific histochemical method has been developed to visualize the adrenergic innervation by fluorescence microscopy that substantive information concerning the distribution of this innervation has been possible. Sympathetic innervation to the airways exists but is sparse [20]. The density of sympathetic innervation appears to be greater in cats and calves than in other species [18,20,64,248]. In the guinea pig, there was less specific fluorescence than in all other tissues examined [249]. In rabbits and rats, the bronchial muscle appeared devoid of fluorescent nerve fibers [18]. It is interesting that in the rabbit airway, the smooth muscle is relatively insensitive [216], and the rat trachea has been reported not to respond to adrenergic agonists [89]. One theory of the pathogenesis of asthma proposes that the disease represents a partial blockade of $\beta$-adrenergic neurotransmitters. The theory is based on two experimental models, one in the guinea pig and the other in mice and rats [250]. It is interesting that these three species have insignificant adrenergic innervation to the bronchi.

In general, in the species with significant adrenergic innervation, some adrenergic fibers can be demonstrated in the tracheal and (perhaps) bronchial muscle [20,32]; in the smaller bronchi and bronchioles, adrenergic fibers may be located only in blood vessels [20]. Adrenergic innervation is conspicuous in the bronchial arteries in several species [251]. Thus, adrenergic innervation, when present in airways, may be mainly to muscle or mainly to bronchial blood vessels. Norepinephrine released from bronchial blood vessels would be expected to constrict the vessels and might thereby limit the access of the mediator to the muscle; narrowing of the vessels from other causes might similarly limit the access of nervously released adrenergic neurotransmitter to the smooth muscle.

Catechol-containing cells are present in the parasympathetic ganglia of the airways in some species [20,52,53,64]. In the rabbit, catechol-containing cells were only present in the ganglia [20], suggesting that the only mechanism by which sympathetic nerve stimulation could dilate the airways is by modulation of cholinergic transmission.

After denervation of a dog's lung by excision and reimplantation, adrenergic bronchodilator activity and the presence of fluorescent adrenergic fibers were not demonstrated after 27 months [41] but were present after 45 months [252]. Reinnervation of the parasympathetic nerves occurs much more rapidly than that of sympathetic nerves [41], possibly because functional restitution takes longer and is less complete after postganglionic (in this case sympathetic) than after preganglionic (in this case parasympathetic) nerve resection [42]. The number of adrenergic fibers necessary to produce a physiologic response is not known, but the bronchodilator response to thoracic sympathetic nerve stimulation was similar in the reimplanted and control lungs, although the density of adrenergic nerves was usually less in the reimplanted lung [252].

There is good evidence for vagal bronchoconstrictor activity in animals and healthy humans, but the role of the sympathetic nerves in the normal regulation of airways is less certain. Cutting the ansa subclavia in a dog caused a slight increase in airflow resistance [8], and cutting the sympathetic nerves resulted in only a small decrease in resistance [6]. These studies suggest that a small degree of sympathetic dilator tone exists in the airways. This is compatible with the finding that sympathetic efferent nerves innervating the trachea and lungs of cats and dogs show a low level of spontaneous activity [31]. The level of sympathetic activity [31] may depend on the type and depth of anesthesia, level of arterial blood gases, and on operative procedures performed.

The usual response of airway smooth muscle to electrical stimulation of the thoracic sympathetic nerves is bronchodilation [6,86,87,253,254]. This effect is abolished by $\beta$-adrenergic antagonists [6,87,237] and is present shortly after birth [10]. The effect of sympathetic nerve stimulation depends on the prior existing level of vagal bronchomotor tone. Thus, in dogs, when the vagi were cut, stimulation of the thoracic sympathetic nerves had no effect on airway dimensions (presumably since airway smooth muscle tone was abolished by vagotomy) [87]. When vagal bronchoconstriction was present, supramaximal sympathetic nerve stimulation inhibited the constriction of airways only in the homolateral lung, indicating that the effect was due to release of sympathetic mediator in nerve endings supplying the airways, and not due to circulating catecholamines. It also indicates that the sympathetic nerve supply is mainly to the homolateral lung. This contradicts the findings of Dixon and Ransom [86], whose results using indirect measurements suggested that in some cases the sympathetic nerve supply was derived from the opposite side. The airway response to sympathetic nerve stimulation remained after adrenalectomy, indicating that the effect was not due to release of catecholamines from the adrenal glands [87]. The sympathetic inhibitory response occurred in all airways constricted by vagal stimulation and was greatest in those airways showing the greatest constriction [87]. The inhibitory effect of sympathetic stimulation was maximal when vagal tone was submaximal, but complete inhibition of vagal constriction was never attained, suggesting that the vagal constrictor pathways to airways are predominant [87]. Eserine potentiated the effects of sympathetic nerve stimulation in cats, presumably by allowing the development of increased cholinergic tone in the muscle [22].

Inhibitory adrenergic nerve fibers have also been demonstrated in isolated airway smooth muscle. Thus, field stimulation of isolated constricted smooth muscle in guinea pigs [32,33,255] and in dogs [256] causes relaxation of muscle tone, an effect that can be abolished with adrenergic blocking agents. However, in human airways [257], a nonadrenergic system appears to be the principal mechanism for relaxing airway smooth muscle. In the guinea pig, both adrenergic and nonadrenergic inhibition have been demonstrated [255,258].

Maximal bronchodilator effects of transmural [33] or sympathetic [87] nerve stimulation occur more slowly than vagal bronchoconstrictor effects, being maximal in approximately 30 sec. Results with electrical stimulation of the sympathetic and vagus nerves is complicated by the fact that, at least in cats, the lower third of the cervical vagi contains sympathetic fibers to lungs, which probably travel up from the stellate ganglion and loop back down the vagi [22]. Thus, during vagal stimulation, some sympathetic fibers could be stimulated along with cholinergic fibers [7,87]. However, midcervical vagotomy does not abolish sympathetic nervous activity in response to stimulation of the stellate ganglion [31], indicating that sympathetic fibers do not loop above the midcervical vagus. Thus, by stimulating the vagi high in the neck investigators have avoided the problem of looping sympathetic fibers [87].

High levels of catecholamines have been found in cat lungs. This was first thought to represent the inhibitory transmitter [259] but was later shown to be of nonnervous origin [260,261]. Since the predominant catecholamine in sympathetically innervated tissues (except the adrenal gland) in mammals is norepinephrine, it is assumed that this is the sympathetic mediator in lungs [1]. Norepinephrine has been found in assays of lungs of the mouse, guinea pig, rat, sheep, human [262], and cow [263]. However, the findings are unusual in several respects. First, levels of epinephrine are either equal to or exceed those of norepinephrine. Second, the absolute levels of norepinephrine are extremely low. For example, in the human, reported values are 1.04 μg/g for heart, 0.54 μg/g for ovary, and 0.04 μg/g for lung [262]. Newer techniques [63] could be applied to examine the release of adrenergic mediators in large and small airways.

The possible presence of sympathetic bronchodilator activity has also been explored by studying the effects of β-adrenergic blocking agents (usually propranolol). This drug has been reported to cause mild constriction of airways in guinea pigs [132,264,265] and in dogs [8,253,266,267] when the vagus nerves are intact. When the vagi are cut, studies in dogs show no significant effects of propranolol [87]. When propranolol did cause bronchoconstriction, it was relieved by vagotomy [266] or by atropine [264], suggesting that the bronchoconstriction was caused by unopposed parasympathetic activity. It is not clear why propranolol has greater effects in the guinea pig than in the cat, rat, or dog [264].

The possible presence of sympathetic bronchodilator activity has also been explored in healthy human subjects by studying the effect of a β-adrenergic blocking agent. Several investigators found no evidence of bronchoconstriction after propranolol [191,268-271]; two studies reported that normal subjects regularly developed mild bronchoconstriction after propranolol [273,274], and other investigators found that occasional healthy subjects developed mild bronchoconstriction after propranolol [266,272]. The differences between these studies could be due to differences in the state of sympathetic activity of the subjects. In none of the studies were plasma or urinary catecholamines measured.

The airway narrowing after propranolol could be due to unopposed bronchoconstrictor activity of the parasympathetic nervous system or unopposed bronchoconstrictor activity of the sympathetic nervous system mediated through α receptors. Since atropine usually antagonized the propranolol effect [266,274-276], it appears that unopposed parasympathetic tone was the main cause of propranolol-induced bronchoconstriction.

Unlike the parasympathetic nervous system, where the blood and tissue contain an enzyme (acetylcholinesterase) which rapidly breaks down the mediator (acetylcholine) released at postganglionic nerve endings, catecholamines released from distal sites may circulate in the blood and have effects on the lungs.

β-Adrenergic effects in lungs could be due to catecholamines released from sympathetic nerve endings distributed to the lungs, or they could be due to effects of circulating catecholamines. Thus, the effects of β-adrenergic blocking drugs demonstrate the presence of sympathetic bronchodilator activity but do not distinguish between nervous and circulating effects. None of the studies report plasma or urinary levels of catecholamines.

There is evidence that the release of catecholamines from the adrenal glands can modify airway smooth muscle reactions. Thus, β-adrenergic blocking agents potentiate the airway constriction caused by histamine [264,277] and bradykinin [278] and by intravenous injection of antigen in sensitized animals [279]. This is not surprising since histamine [280,281], bradykinin [280,282,283], intravenous injections of antigen [280], and possibly SRS-A [283] liberate catecholamines into the circulation in some species. Since most of these catecholamines are derived from the adrenal medulla [280], it is not surprising that adrenalectomy also potentiates the airway constriction due to histamine [277], bradykinin [284], and antigen [279]. Failure of some investigators to demonstrate airway constriction after histamine [285] has been attributed to the release of catecholamines by histamine. In some experiments, β-blocking drugs appeared to be more effective than adrenalectomy in intensifying airway reaction to injected antigen [279] and to histamine [264], suggesting that significant catecholamine release was occurring elsewhere; some experiments suggest that the sympathetic nerves to the airways may be involved, but unfortunately denervation of the thoracic sympathetic nerves was not performed [264].

Very little is actually known about sympathetic reflex control of airway tone. Stimulation of various portions of the respiratory tract (nose, epipharynx, and larynx) enhanced discharge frequencies in efferent sympathetic fibers to airways [12]. Stimulation of the nose and epipharynx cause bronchodilation, but the effect appears to be due mainly to a reduction in vagal constrictor activity rather than to an increase in sympathetic inhibitory activity [94]. Irritation of the larynx or bronchi also stimulates sympathetic efferent activity [12,31,80] but results in bronchoconstriction. This sympathetic activity may limit the degree of bronchoconstriction caused by concomitant stimulation of vagal fibers [7]. The fact that bronchoconstriction due to inhalation of cigarette smoke is exaggerated in healthy subjects by propranolol premedication supports this possibility [191].

## References

1. Burnstock, G., Evolution of the autonomic innervation of visceral and cardiovascular systems in vertebrates, *Pharmacol. Rev.*, **21**:247-324 (1969).

2. Knapp, P. H., The asthmatic and his environment, *J. Nerv. Ment. Dis.*, **149**: 133-151 (1969).
3. Colebatch, H. J. H., and D. F. J. Halmagyi, Effect of vagotomy and vagal stimulation on lung mechanics and circulation, *J. Appl. Physiol.*, **18**:881-887 (1963).
4. Olsen, C. R., H. J. H. Colebatch, P. E. Mebel, J. A. Nadel, and N. C. Staub, Motor control of pulmonary airways studied by nerve stimulation, *J. Appl. Physiol.*, **20**:202-208 (1965).
5. Karczewski, W., and J. G. Widdicombe, The effect of vagotomy, vagal cooling and efferent vagal stimulation on breathing and lung mechanics of rabbits, *J. Physiol. (London)*, **201**:259-270 (1969).
6. Green, M., and J. G. Widdicombe, The effects of ventilation of dogs with different gas mixtures on airway calibre and lung mechanics, *J. Physiol. (London)*, **186**:363-381 (1966).
7. Woolcock, A. J., P. T. Macklem, J. C. Hogg, N. J. Wilson, J. A. Nadel, N. R. Frank, and J. Brain, Effect of vagal stimulation on central and peripheral airways in dogs, *J. Appl. Physiol.*, **26**:806-813 (1969).
8. Woolcock, A. J., P. T. Macklem, J. C. Hogg, and N. J. Wilson, Influence of autonomic nervous system on airway resistance and elastic recoil, *J. Appl. Physiol.*, **26**:814-818 (1969).
9. Nadel, J. A., G. A. Cabezas, J. H. M. Austin, In vivo roentgenographic examination of parasympathetic innervation of small airways: Use of powdered tantalum and a fine focal spot x-ray tube, *Invest. Radiol.*, **6**:9-17 (1971).
10. Schwieler, G. H., J. S. Douglas, and A. Bouhuys, Postnatal development of autonomic efferent innervation in the rabbit, *Am. J. Physiol.*, **219**:391-397 (1970).
11. Nadel, J. A., H. Salem, B. Tamplin, and Y. Tokiwa, Mechanism of bronchoconstriction during inhalation of sulfur dioxide, *J. Appl. Physiol.*, **20**:164-167 (1965).
12. Tomori, Z., and J. G. Widdicombe, Muscular, bronchomotor and cardiovascular reflexes elicited by mechanical stimulation of the respiratory tract, *J. Physiol. (London)*, **200**:25-49 (1969).
13. Macklem, P. T., and J. Mead, Resistance of central and peripheral airways measured by a retrograde catheter, *J. Appl. Physiol.*, **22**:395-401 (1977).
14. Ingram, Jr., R. H., J. J. Wellman, E. R. McFadden, Jr., and J. Mead, Relative contributions of large and small airways to flow limitation in normal subjects before and after atropine and isoproterenol, *J. Clin. Invest.*, **59**: 696-703 (1977).
15. Gardiner, A. J., L. Wood, P. Gayrard, H. Menkes, and P. Macklem, Influence of constriction in central or peripheral airways on maximal expiratory flow rates in dogs, *J. Appl. Physiol.*, **36**:554-560 (1974).
16. Douglas, N. J., M. F. Sudlow, and D. C. Flenley, Effect of an inhaled atropinelike agent on normal airway function, *J. Appl. Physiol.*, **46**:256-262 (1979).

17. Nadel, J. A., Alveolar duct constriction after barium sulfate microembolism. In *Pulmonary Embolic Disease.* Edited by A. A. Sasahara. New York, Grune and Stratton, 1965, pp. 153-161.
18. Hebb, C., Motor innervation of the pulmonary blood vessels of mammals. In *The Pulmonary Circulation and Interstitial Space.* Edited by A. P. Fishman and H. H. Hecht. Chicago, The University of Chicago, 1969, pp. 195-222.
19. Fillenz, M., Innervation of pulmonary and bronchial blood vessels of the dog, *J. Anat.,* **106**:449-461 (1970).
20. Mann, S. P., The innervation of mammalian bronchial smooth muscle: The localization of catecholamines and cholinesterases, *Histochem. J.,* **3**:319-331 (1971).
21. Dixon, W. E., and T. G. Brodie, Contributions to the physiology of the lungs. Part I. The bronchial muscles, their innervation, and the action of drugs upon them, *J. Physiol. (London),* **29**:97-173 (1903).
22. Daly, M. De Burgh, and L. E. Mount, The origin, course and nature of bronchomotor fibres in the cervical sympathetic nerve of the cat, *J. Physiol. (London),* **113**:43-62 (1951).
23. Larsell, O., and M. L. Mason, Experimental degeneration of the vagus nerve and its relation to the nerve terminations in the lung of the rabbit, *J. Comp. Neurol.,* **33**:509-516 (1921).
24. Honjin, R., Experimental degeneration of the vagus, and its relation to the nerve supply of the lung of the mouse, with special reference to the crossing innervation of the lung by the vagi, *J. Comp. Neurol.,* **106**:1-19 (1956).
25. Bronk, D. W., L. K. Ferguson, R. Margaria, and D. Y. Solandt, The activity of the cardiac sympathetic centers, *Am. J. Physiol.,* **117**:237-249 (1936).
26. Van Dorben-Broekema, M., and M. N. J. Dirken, Influence of the sympathetic nervous system on the circulation in the rabbit's ear, *Acta Physiol. Pharmacol. Neerl.,* **1**:584-602 (1950).
27. Folkow, B., Impulse frequency in sympathetic vasomotor fibres correlated to the release and elimination of the transmitter, *Acta Physiol. Scand.,* **25**:49-76 (1952).
28. Girling, F., Vasomotor effects of electrical stimulation, *Am. J. Physiol.,* **170**:131-135 (1952).
29. Folkow, B., and C.-A. Hamberger, Characteristics of sympathetic neuroeffectors in man, *J. Appl. Physiol.,* **9**:268-270 (1956).
30. Carlsten, A., B. Folkow, and C.-A. Hamberger, Cardiovascular effects of direct vagal stimulation in man, *Acta Physiol. Scand.,* **41**:68-76 (1957).
31. Widdicombe, J. G., Action potentials in parasympathetic and sympathetic efferent fibres to the trachea and lungs of dogs and cats, *J. Physiol. (London),* **186**:56-88 (1966).
32. Rikimaru, A., and M. Sudoh, Innervation of the smooth muscle of the guinea pig trachea, *Jap. J. Smooth Muscle Res.,* **7**:35-44 (1971).
33. Foster, R. W., A note on the electrically transmurally stimulated isolated trachea of the guinea pig, *J. Pharm. Pharmacol.,* **16**:125-128 (1964).

34. Thornton, J. W., The liberation of acetylcholine at vagus nerve endings in isolated perfused lungs, *J. Physiol. (London),* **82**:14P (1934).
35. Carlyle, R. F., The mode of action of neostigmine and physostigmine on the guinea pig trachealis muscle, *Br. J. Pharmacol.,* **21**:137-149 (1963).
36. Eiseman, B., L. Bryant, and T. Waltuch, Metabolism of vasomotor agents by the isolated perfused lung, *J. Thorac. Cardiovasc. Surg.,* **48**:798-806 (1964).
37. Koelle, G. B., Anticholinesterase agents. In *The Pharmacologic Basis of Therapeutics,* 3rd ed. Edited by L. S. Goodman and A. Gilman. New York, Macmillan, 1965, pp. 441-463.
38. Goldstein, B. D., B. Pearson, C. Lodi, R. D. Buckley, and O. J. Balchum, The effect of ozone on mouse blood in vivo, *Arch. Environ. Health,* **16**: 648-650 (1968).
39. Daly, M. De Burgh and D. H. L. Evans, Functional and histological changes in the vagus nerve of the cat after degenerative section at various levels, *J. Physiol. (London),* **120**:579-595 (1953).
40. Gabella, G., *Structure of the Autonomic Nervous System.* London, Chapman and Hall, 1976, pp. 133-145.
41. Edmunds, Jr., L. H., P. D. Graf, and J. A. Nadel, Reinnervation of the reimplanted canine lung, *J. Appl. Physiol.,* **31**:722-727 (1971).
42. Guth, L., Regeneration of the mammalian peripheral nervous system, *Physiol. Rev.,* **36**:441-478 (1956).
43. Reinhoff, Jr., W. F., and L. N. Gay, Treatment of intractable bronchial asthma by bilateral resection of the posterior pulmonary plexus, *Arch. Surg.,* **37**:456-469 (1938).
44. Widdicombe, J. G., Action potentials in vagal efferent nerve fibres to the lungs of the cat, *Naunyn-Schmiedeberg's Arch. Exp. Pathol. Pharmacol.,* **241**:415-432 (1961).
45. Nadel, J. A., and J. G. Widdicombe, Reflex control of airway size, *Ann. N.Y. Acad. Sci.,* **109**:712-722 (1963).
46. Larsell, O., The ganglia, plexuses, and nerve-terminations of the mammalian lung and pleura pulmonalis, *J. Comp. Neurol.,* **35**:97-132 (1922).
47. Okamura, C., Die ganglien in der wand der bronchien und alveolen von mammalien und amphibien, *Z. Mikrosk. Anat. Forsch.,* **41**:627-639 (1937).
48. Trendelenburg, U., Modification of transmission through the superior cervican ganglion of the cat, *J. Physiol. (London),* **132**:529-541 (1956).
49. Hamberger, B., K.-A. Norberg, and F. Sjöqvist, Evidence for adrenergic nerve terminals and synapses in sympathetic ganglia, *Int. J. Neuropharmacol.,* **2**:279-282 (1964).
50. Libet, B., Generation of slow inhibitory and excitatory postsynaptic potentials, *Fed. Proc.,* **29**:1945-1956 (1970).
51. Wallis, D. I., and B. Woodward, The facilitatory actions of 5-hydroxytruptamine and bradykinin in the superior cervical ganglion of the rabbit, *Br. J. Pharmacol.,* **51**:521-531 (1974).
52. Blümcke, S., Experimental and morphological studies on the efferent bron-

chial innervation. I. The peribronchial plexus, *Beitr. Pathol. Anat.*, **137**: 239-286 (1968).
53. Jacobowitz, D., K. M. Kent, J. H. Fleisch, and T. Cooper, Histofluorescent study of catecholamine-containing elements in cholinergic ganglia from the calf and dog lung, *Proc. Soc. Exp. Biol. Med.*, **144**:464-466 (1973).
54. Richardson, J., and C. C. Ferguson, The fine structure of the ganglia in human lung, *J. Cell Biol.*, **70**:48a (1976).
55. Wood, J. D., Electrical activity from single neurons in Auerbach's plexus, *Am. J. Physiol.*, **219**:159-169 (1970).
56. Coyle, J. T., M. E. Molliver, and M. J. Kuhar, In situ injection of kainic acid: A new method for selectively lesioning neuronal cell bodies while sparing axons of passage, *J. Comp. Neurol.*, **180**:301-324 (1978).
57. Hukuhara, T., S. Kotani, and G. Sato, Effects of destruction of intramural ganglion cells on colon motility: Possible genesis of congenital megacolon, *Jpn. J. Physiol.*, **11**:635-640 (1961).
58. Paton, W. D. M., and E. S. Vizi, The inhibitory action of noradrenaline and adrenaline on acetylcholine output by guinea pig ileum longitudinal muscle strip, *Br. J. Pharmacol.*, **35**:10-28 (1969).
59. DeGroat, W. C., and W. R. Saum, Sympathetic inhibition of the urinary bladder and of the pelvic ganglionic transmission in the cat, *J. Physiol. (London)*, **220**:297-314 (1972).
60. Vermiere, P. A., and P. M. Vanhoutte, Inhibitory effects of catecholamines in isolated canine bronchial smooth muscle, *J. Appl. Physiol.*, **46**:787-791 (1979).
61. Vanhoutte, P. M., Inhibition by acetylcholine of adrenergic neurotransmission in vascular smooth muscle. In *Physiology of Smooth Muscle*. Edited by E. Bulbring and M. F. Shuba. New York, Raven, 1976, pp. 369-377.
62. Vanhoutte, P. M., Cholinergic inhibition of adrenergic transmission, *Fed. Proc.*, **36**:2444-2449 (1977).
63. Russell, J. A., and S. Bartlett, Inhibition of adrenergic neurotransmission in airway smooth muscle by acetylcholine, *Fed. Proc.*, **38**:1111 (1979).
64. Silva, D. G., and G. Ross, Ultrastructural and fluorescence histochemical studies on the innervation of the tracheo bronchial muscle of normal cats treated with 6-hydroxydopamine, *J. Ultrastruct. Res.*, **47**:310-328 (1974).
65. Cook, R. D., and A. S. King, Observations on the ultrastructure of the smooth muscle and its innervation in the avian lung, *J. Anat.*, **106**:273-283 (1970).
66. Hahn, H. L., A. G. Wilson, P. D. Graf, S. P. Fischer, and J. A. Nadel, Interaction between serotonin and efferent vagus nerves in dog lungs, *J. Appl. Physiol.*, **44**:144-149 (1978).
67. Offermeier, J., and E. J. Ariens, Serotonin. I. Receptors involved in its action, *Arch. Int. Pharmacodyn. Ther.*, **164**:192-215 (1966).
68. Sandler, J. A., J. I. Gallin, and M. Vaughan, Effects of serotonin, carbamylcholine, and ascorbic acid on leukocyte cyclic GMP and chemotaxis, *J. Cell Biol.*, **67**:480-484 (1975).

69. Brownlee, G., and E. S. Johnson, The site of the 5-hydroxytryptamine receptor on the intramural nervous plexus of the guinea pig isolated ileum, *Br. J. Pharmacol.,* **21**:306-322 (1963).
70. Brownlee, G., and E. S. Johnson, The release of acetylcholine from the isolated ileum of the guinea pig induced by 5-hydroxytryptamine and dimethylphenylpiperazinium, *Br. J. Pharmacol.,* **24**:689-700 (1965).
71. Drakontides, A. B., and M. D. Gershon, Studies of the interaction of 5-hydroxytryptamine and the perivascular innervation of the guinea pig caecum, *Br. J. Pharmacol.,* **45**:417-434 (1972).
72. Gaddum, J. H., and Z. P. Picarelli, Two kinds of tryptamine receptor, *Br. J. Pharmacol.,* **12**:323-328 (1957).
73. Paton, W. D. M., and M. Aboo Zar, The origin of acetylcholine released from guinea pig intestine and longitudinal muscle strips, *J. Physiol. (London),* **194**:13-33 (1968).
74. Ross, L. L., and M. D. Gershon, Electron microscopic radioautographic and fluorescence localization of sites of 5-hydroxytryptamine (5-HT) uptake in the myenteric plexus of the guinea pig ileum, *J. Cell Biol.,* **55**:220a (1972).
75. Dreyfus, C. F., D. L. Sherman, and M. D. Gershon, Uptake of serotonin by intrinsic neurons of the myenteric plexus grown in organotypic tissue culture, *Brain Res.,* **128**:109-123 (1977).
76. Basbaum, C. B., and J. E. Heuser, Morphological studies of stimulated adrenergic axon varicosities in the mouse vas deferens, *J. Cell Biol.,* **80**:310-325 (1979).
77. Severinghaus, J. W., and M. Stupfel, Respiratory dead space increase following atropine in man, and atropine, vagal or ganglionic blockade and hypothermia in dogs, *J. Appl. Physiol.,* **8**:81-87 (1955).
78. Nadel, J. A., and J. G. Widdicombe, Effect of changes in blood gas tensions and carotid sinus pressure on tracheal volume and total lung resistance to airflow, *J. Physiol. (London),* **163**:13-33 (1962).
79. Hoppin, Jr., F. C., M. Green, and M. S. Morgan, Relationship of central and peripheral airway resistance to lung volume in dogs, *J. Appl. Physiol.,* **44**:728-737 (1978).
80. Widdicombe, J. G., D. C. Kent, and J. A. Nadel, Mechanisms of bronchoconstriction during inhalation of dust, *J. Appl. Physiol.,* **17**:613-616 (1962).
81. Dautrebande, L., F. W. Lovejoy, Jr., and R. M. McCredie, New studies on aerosols XVIII. Effects of atropine microaerosols on the airway resistance in man, *Arch. Int. Pharmacodyn. Ther.,* **139**:198-211 (1962).
82. Sterling, G. M., and J. C. Batten, Effect of aerosol propellants and surfactants on airway resistance, *Thorax,* **24**:228-231 (1969).
83. deTroyer, A., J.-C. Yernault, and D. Rodenstein, Effects of vagal blockade on lung mechanics in normal man, *J. Appl. Physiol.,* **46**:217-226 (1979).
84. Vincent, N. J., R. Knudson, D. E. Leith, P. T. Macklem, and J. Mead, Factors influencing pulmonary resistance, *J. Appl. Physiol.,* **29**:236-243 (1970).

85. deCandole, C. A., W. W. Douglas, C. L. Evans, R. Holmes, K. E. V. Spencer, R. W. Torrance, and K. M. Wilson, The failure of respiration in death by anticholinesterase poisoning, *Br. J. Pharmacol.*, **8**:466-475 (1953).
86. Dixon, W. E., and F. Ransom, Bronchodilator nerves, *J. Physiol. (London)*, **45**:413-428 (1912).
87. Cabezas, G. A., P. D. Graf, and J. A. Nadel, Sympathetic versus parasympathetic nervous regulation of airways in dogs, *J. Appl. Physiol.*, **31**:651-655 (1971).
88. Carlyle, R. F., The responses to the guinea pig isolated intact trachea to transmural stimulation and the release of an acetylcholine-like substance under conditions of rest and stimulation, *Br. J. Pharmacol.*, **22**:126-136 (1964).
89. Jamieson, D., A method for the quantitative estimation of drugs on the isolated intact trachea, *Br. J. Pharmacol.*, **19**:286-294 (1962).
90. Castillo, J. C., and E. J. deBeer, The tracheal chain. I. A preparation for the study of antispasmodics with particular reference to bronchodilator drugs, *J. Pharm. Exp. Ther.*, **90**:104-109 (1947).
91. Johnson, E. S., A note on the relation between the resting release of acetylcholine and increase in tone of the isolated guinea pig ileum, *J. Pharm. Pharmacol.*, **15**:69-72 (1963).
92. Widdicombe, J. G., Regulation of tracheobronchial smooth muscle, *Physiol. Rev.*, **43**:1-37 (1963).
93. Nadel, J. A., and J. G. Widdicombe, Reflex effects of upper airway irritation on total lung resistance and blood pressure, *J. Appl. Physiol.*, **17**:861-865 (1962).
94. Allison, D. J., T. P. Clay, J. M. B. Hughes, H. A. Jones, and A. Shevis, Effects of nasal stimulation on total respiratory resistance in the rabbit, *J. Physiol. (London)*, **239**:23-24P (1974).
95. Boushey, H. A., P. S. Richardson, and J. G. Widdicombe, Reflex effects of laryngeal irritation on the pattern of breathing and total lung resistance, *J. Physiol. (London)*, **224**:501-513 (1972).
96. Boushey, H. A., P. S. Richardson, J. G. Widdicombe, and J. C. M. Wise, The response of laryngeal afferent fibres to mechanical and chemical stimuli, *J. Physiol. (London)*, **240**:153-175 (1974).
97. DeKock, M. A., J. A. Nadel, S. Swi, H. J. H. Colebatch, and C. R. Olsen, New method for perfusing bronchial arteries: Histamine bronchoconstriction and apnea, *J. Appl. Physiol.*, **21**:185-194 (1966).
98. Widdicombe, J. G., and J. A. Nadel, Reflex effects of lung inflation on tracheal volume, *J. Appl. Physiol.*, **18**:681-686 (1963).
99. Sellick, H., and J. G. Widdicombe, The activity of lung irritant receptors during pneumothorax, hyperpnoea and pulmonary vascular congestion *J. Physiol. (London)*, **203**:359-381 (1969).
100. Sellick, H., and J. G. Widdicombe, Stimulation of lung irritant receptors by cigarette smoke, carbon dust, and histamine, *J. Appl. Physiol.*, **31**:15-19 (1971).

101. Vidruk, E. H., H. L. Hahn, J. A. Nadel, and S. R. Sampson, Mechanisms by which histamine stimulates rapidly adapting receptors in dog lungs, *J. Appl. Physiol.,* **43**:397-402 (1977).
102. Widdicombe, J. G., Studies on afferent airway innervation, *Am. Rev. Respir. Dis.,* **115** (Suppl. 2):99-105 (1977).
103. Fillenz, M., and J. G. Widdicombe, Receptors of the lungs and airways. In *Handbook of Sensory Physiology,* Volume III/1. Edited by E. Neil. New York, Springer-Verlag, 1972, pp. 81-112.
104. Loofbourrow, G. N., W. B. Wood, and I. L. Baird, Tracheal constriction in the dog, *Am. J. Physiol.,* **191**:411-415 (1957).
105. Bruderman, I., and S. Rogel, Changes in ventilation and pulmonary mechanics induced by hypertonic sodium chloride, *J. Appl. Physiol.,* **21**: 383-387 (1966).
106. Vinogradova, M. I., Efferent impulses in the pulmonary nerves, *Ezhegodnik Inst. Eksperim. Med. Akad. Med. Nauk SSSR,* **113** (1955).
107. Konzett, H., and R. Rossler, Versuchsanordnung zu untersuchungen an der bronchialmuskulatur, *Arch. Exp. Pathol. Pharmakol.,* **195**:71-74 (1940).
108. Hahn, H. L., and J. A. Nadel, Methods of study of airway smooth muscle and its physiology. In *International Encyclopedia of Pharmacology and Therapeutics–Respiration Section.* Edited by J. G. Widdicombe. London, Pergamon Press, 1979.
109. Hahn, H. L., P. D. Graf, and J. A. Nadel, Effect of vagal tone on airway diameters and on lung volume in anesthetized dogs, *J. Appl. Physiol.,* **41**: 581-589 (1976).
110. Lloyd, T. C. Jr., and G. W. Wright, Evaluation of methods used in detecting changes of airway resistance in man, *Am. Rev. Respir. Dis.,* **87**:529-537 (1963).
111. Frank, N. R., J. Mead, and J. L. Whittenberger, Comparative sensitivity of four methods for measuring changes in respiratory flow resistance in man, *J. Appl. Physiol.,* **31**:934-938 (1971).
112. Nadel, J. A., and D. F. Tierney, Effect of a previous deep inspiration on airway resistance in man, *J. Appl. Physiol.,* **16**:717-719 (1961).
113. Simonsson, B. G., F. M. Jacobs, and J. A. Nadel, Role of autonomic nervous system and the cough reflex in the increased responsiveness of airways in patients with obstructive airway disease, *J. Clin. Invest.,* **46**:1812-1818 (1967).
114. Arborelius, Jr., M., B. Ekwall, R. Jernerus, G. Lundin, and L. Svanberg, Unilateral provoked bronchial asthma in man, *J. Clin. Invest.,* **41**:1236-1241 (1962).
115. Don, H. F., and J. G. Robson, Effect of mechanical stimulation of the lower airway on respiratory mechanics in apneic anesthetized man, *Anesthesiology,* **27**:284-287 (1966).
116. Hickey, R. F., P. D. Graf, J. A. Nadel, and C. P. Larson, Jr., The effects of halothane and cyclopropane on total pulmonary resistance in the dog, *Anesthesiology,* **31**:334-343 (1969).

117. Jackson, D. M., and I. M. Richards, The effects of pentobarbitone and chloralose anesthesia on the vagal component of bronchoconstriction produced by histamine aerosol in the anesthetized dog, *Br. J. Pharmacol.,* **61**:251-256 (1977).
118. Adriani, J., and E. A. Rovenstein, The effect of anesthetic drugs upon bronchi and bronchioles of excised lung tissue, *Anesthesiology,* **4**:253-262 (1943).
119. Collier, H. O. J., Endogenous broncho-active substances and their antagonism, *Adv. Drug Res.,* **5**:95-107 (1970).
120. Weiss, E. B., W. H. Anderson, and K. P. O'Brien, The effect of a local anesthetic, lidocaine, on guinea pig trachealis muscle in vitro, *Am. Rev. Respir. Dis.,* **112**:393-400 (1975).
121. Fleisch, J. H., and E. Titus, Effect of local anesthetics on pharmacologic receptor systems of smooth muscle, *J. Pharmacol. Exp. Ther.,* **186**:44-51 (1973).
122. Dain, D. S., H. A. Boushey, and W. M. Gold, Inhibition of respiratory reflexes by local anesthetic aerosols in dogs and rabbits, *J. Appl. Physiol.,* **38**:1045-1050 (1975).
123. Coleridge, H. M., J. C. G. Coleridge, J. C. Luck, and J. Norman, The effect of four volatile anaesthetic agents on the impulse activity of two types of pylmonary receptor, *Br. J. Anaesthesiol.,* **40**:484-492 (1968).
124. Sterling, G. M., P. E. Holst, and J. A. Nadel, Effect of $CO_2$ and pH on bronchoconstriction caused by serotonin vs. acetylcholine, *J. Appl. Physiol.,* **32**:39-43 (1972).
125. Duckles, S. P., M. D. Rayner, and J. A. Nadel, Effects of $CO_2$ and pH on drug-induced contractions of airway smooth muscle, *J. Pharmacol. Exp. Ther.,* **190**:472-481 (1974).
126. Sullivan, C. E., N. Zamel, L. F. Kozar, E. Murphy, and E. A. Phillipson, Regulation of airway smooth muscle tone in sleeping dogs, *Am. Rev. Respir. Dis.,* **119**:87-99 (1979).
127. Dale, H. H., and P. P. Laidlaw, The physiological action of β-iminazolylethylamine, *J. Physiol. (London),* **41**:318-344 (1910).
128. Szereda-Przestaszewska, M., and A. Stransky, The effect of changes in bronchial calibre on upper airway calibre, *Bull. Physiopathol. Respir.,* **8**:453-456 (1972).
129. Szereda-Przestaszewska, M., and J. G. Widdicombe, Reflex effects of chemical irritation of the upper airways on the laryngeal lumen in cats, *Respir. Physiol.,* **18**:107-115 (1973).
130. Stransky, A., M. Szereda-Przestaszewska, and J. G. Widdicombe, The effects of lung reflexes on laryngeal resistance and motoneurone discharge, *J. Physiol. (London),* **231**:417-438 (1973).
131. Szereda-Przestaszewska, M., and J. G. Widdicombe, The effect of intravascular injections of veratrine on laryngeal resistance to airflow in cats, *Q. J. Exp. Physiol.,* **58**:379-385 (1973).
132. Douglas, J. S., P. Ridgway, and C. Brink, Airway responses of the guinea pig in vivo and in vitro, *J. Pharmacol. Exp. Ther.,* **202**:116-124 (1977).

133. DuBois, A. B., S. Y. Botelho, and J. H. Comroe, Jr., A new method for measuring airway resistance in man using a body plethysmograph: Values in normal subjects and in patients with respiratory disease, *J. Clin. Invest.*, **35**:327-335 (1956).
134. Kaufman, J., and G. W. Wright, The effect of nasal and nasopharyngeal irritation on airway resistance in man, *Am. Rev. Respir. Dis.*, **100**:626-630 (1969).
135. Widdicombe, J. G., and J. A. Nadel, Airway volume, airway resistance, and work and force of breathing: Theory, *J. Appl. Physiol.*, **18**:863-868 (1963).
136. Nadel, J. A., E. A. Phillipson, N. H. Fishman, and R. F. Hickey, Regulation of respiration by bronchopulmonary receptors in conscious dogs, *Acta Neurobiol. Exp.*, **33**:33-50 (1973).
137. Otis, A. B., W. O. Fenn, and H. Rahn, Mechanics of breathing in man, *J. Appl. Physiol.*, **2**:592-607 (1950).
138. Mead, J., Control of respiratory frequency, *J. Appl. Physiol.*, **15**:325-336 (1960).
139. Nadel, J. A., B. Davis, and R. J. Phipps, Control of mucus secretion and ion transport in airways, *Ann. Rev. Physiol.*, **41**:369-381 (1979).
140. Widdicombe, J. G., The activity of pulmonary stretch receptors during bronchoconstriction, pulmonary oedema, atelectasis, and breathing against a resistance, *J. Physiol. (London)*, **159**:436-450 (1961).
141. Finnegan, J. K., Stramonium cigarettes and powders, *Am. Pharm. Assoc. Bull.*, **18**:131-141 (1950).
142. *Postgraduate Medical Journal*, The place of parasympatholytic drugs in the management of chronic obstructive airways disease. Proceedings of an International Symposium held in Killarney, September 19-21, 1974. Edited by B. I. Hoffbrand.
143. Chamberlain, D. A., D. C. F. Muir, and K. P. Kennedy, Atropine methonitrate and isoprenaline in bronchial asthma, *Lancet*, 1019-1021 (1962).
144. Poppius, H., Y. Salorinne, and A. A. Viljanen, Inhalation of a new anticholinergic drug, Sch 1000, in asthma and chronic bronchitis: Effect on airway resistance, thoracic gas volume, blood gases and exercise-induced asthma, *Bull. Physiopathol. Respir.*, **8**:643-652 (1972).
145. Cropp, G. J. A., The role of the parasympathetic nervous system in the maintenance of chronic airway obstruction in asthmatic children, *Am. Rev. Respir. Dis.*, **112**:599-605 (1975).
146. Storms, W. W., G. A. DoPico, and C. E. Reed, Aerosol Sch 1000, an anticholinergic bronchodilator, *Am. Rev. Respir. Dis.*, **111**:419-422 (1975).
147. Gross, N. J., Sch 1000: A new anticholinergic bronchodilator, *Am. Rev. Respir. Dis.*, **112**:823-828 (1975).
148. Cavanaugh, M. J., and D. M. Cooper, Inhaled atropine sulfate: Dose response characteristics, *Am. Rev. Respir. Dis.*, **114**:517-524 (1976).
149. Chan-Yeung, M., The effect of Sch 1000 and disodium cromoglycate on exercise-induced asthma, *Chest*, **71**:320-323 (1977).

150. Crompton, G. K., A comparison of responses to bronchodilator drugs in chronic bronchitis and chronic asthma, *Thorax,* **23**:46-55 (1968).
151. Poppius, H., and Y. Salorinne, Comparative trial of a new anticholinergic bronchodilator, Sch 1000, and salbutamol in chronic bronchitis, *Br. Med. J.,* **4**:134-136 (1973).
152. Klock, L. E., T. D. Miller, A. H. Morris, S. Watanabe, and M. Dickman, A comparative study of atropine sulfate and isoproterenol hydrochloride in chronic bronchitis, *Am. Rev. Respir. Dis.,* **112**:371-376 (1975).
153. Baigelman, W., and S. Chodosh, Bronchodilator action of the anticholinergic drug, ipratropium bromide (Sch 1000), as an aerosol in chronic bronchitis and asthma, *Chest,* **71**:324-328 (1977).
154. Miller, H., and D. W. Baruch, Recent advances in the psychosomatic concepts of clinical allergy, Proceedings of International Congress of Allergology, Paris, 1958, pp. 323-334.
155. Williams, H. L., A concept of allergy as autonomic dysfunction suggested as an improved working hypothesis, *Am. Acad. Opthalmol. Otolaryngol.,* **55**:123-146 (1950).
156. Luparello, T., H. A. Lyons, E. R. Bleecker, and E. R. McFadden, Jr., Influences of suggestion on airway reactivity in asthmatic subjects, *Psychosomat. Med.,* **30**:819-825 (1968).
157. McFadden, Jr., E. R., T. Luparello, H. A. Lyons, and E. Bleecker, The mechanism of action of suggestion in the induction of acute asthma attacks, *Psychosomat. Med.,* **31**:134-143 (1969).
158. Smith, M. M., H. J. H. Colebatch, and P. S. Clarke, Increase and decrease in pulmonary resistance with hypnotic suggestion in asthma, *Am. Rev. Respir. Dis.,* **102**:236-242 (1970).
159. Spector, S., T. J. Luparello, M. T. Kopetzky, J. Souhrada, and R. A. Kinsman, Response of asthmatics to methacholine and suggestion, *Am. Rev. Respir. Dis.,* **113**:43-50 (1976).
160. Horton, D. J., W. L. Suda, R. A. Kinsman, J. Souhrada, and S. L. Spector, Bronchoconstrictive suggestion in asthma: A role for airways hyperreactivity and emotions, *Am. Rev. Respir. Dis.,* **117**:1029-1038 (1978).
161. Kratschmer, F., Über reflexe von der nesenchlelmhaut auf athmung und krieslauf, *Sber. Akad. Wiss. Wien,* **62**:147-170 (1870).
162. Rall, J. E., N. C. Gilbert, and R. Trump, Certain aspects of the bronchial reflexes obtained by stimulation of the nasopharynx, *J. Lab. Clin. Med.,* **30**:953-956 (1945).
163. Dautrebande, L., E. Robillard, and H. Stone, Effect of sympathomimetic aerosols upon the respiratory reflexes induced by dusting of the supraglottic airways in the dog, *Arch. Int. Pharmacodyn. Ther.,* **129**:455-468 (1960).
164. Frank, N. R., and F. E. Speizer, $SO_2$ effects on the respiratory system in dogs, *Arch. Environ. Health,* **2**:624-634 (1965).
165. Speizer, F. E., and N. R. Frank, A comparison of changes in pulmonary flow resistance in healthy volunteers acutely exposed to $SO_2$ by mouth and by nose, *Br. J. Indust. Med.,* **23**:75-79 (1966).

166. Melville, G. N., Changes in specific airway conductance in healthy volunteers following nasal and oral inhalation of $SO_2$, *West Indian Med. J.,* **19**: 231-235 (1970).
167. Smith, P. G., and E. Mills, Autoradiographic identification of the terminations of petrosal ganglion neurons in the cat carotid body, *Brain Res.,* **113**: 174-178 (1976).
168. Fidone, S. J. P. Zapata, and L. J. Stensaas, Axonal transport of labeled material into sensory nerve endings of cat carotid body, *Brain Res.,* **124**: 9-28 (1977).
169. Bower, A., S. Parker, and V. Molony, An autoradiographic study of the afferent innervation of the trachea, syrinx, and extrapulmonary primary bronchus of *Gallus gallus domesticus, J. Anat.,* **126**:169-180 (1978).
170. Lacey, M., Studies of pulmonary innervation in the rat using horseradish peroxidase as a neuronal marker, *J. Physiol. (London),* **268**:16-18P (1977).
171. Sampson, S. R., Sensory neurophysiology of airways, *Am. Rev. Respir. Dis.,* **115** (Suppl. 2):107-115 (1977).
172. Widdicombe, J. G., Receptors in the trachea and bronchi of the cat, *J. Physiol. (London),* **123**:71-104 (1954).
173. Mills, J. E., H. Sellick, and J. G. Widdicombe, Epithelial irritant receptors in the lungs. In *Breathing: Hering-Breur Centenary Symposium,* a Ciba Foundation Symposium held in London, 1969. Edited by R. Porter. London, Churchill, 1970, pp. 77-92.
174. Widdicombe, J. G., Respiratory reflexes from the trachea and bronchi of the cat, *J. Physiol. (London),* **123**:55-70 (1954).
175. Mortola, J., G. Sant'Ambrogio, and M. G. Clement, Localization of irritant receptors in the airways of the dog, *Respir. Physiol.,* **24**:107-114 (1975).
176. Sant'Ambrogio, G., J. E. Remmers, W. J. De Groot, G. Callas, and J. P. Mortola, Localization of rapidly adapting receptors in the trachea and main stem bronchus of the dog, *Respir. Physiol.,* **33**:359-366 (1978).
177. Widdicombe, J. G., Some experimental models of acute asthma, *J. Roy. Coll. Physicians Lond.,* **11**:141-155 (1977).
178. Bradley, G. W., Pulmonary receptor recording in vitro, *Acta Physiol. Scand.,* **91**:427-429 (1974).
179. Innes, I. R., and M. Nickerson, Drugs inhibiting the action of acetylcholine on structures innervated by postganglionic parasympathetic nerve (antimuscarinic or atropinic drugs). In *The Pharmacological Basis of Therapeutics,* 3rd ed. Edited by L. S. Goodman and A. Gilman. New York, Macmillan, 1965, p. 527.
180. Kessler, G.-F., J. H. M. Austin, P. D. Graf, G. Gamsu, and W. M. Gold, Airway constriction in experimental asthma in dogs: Tantalum bronchographic studies, *J. Appl. Physiol.,* **35**:703-708 (1973).
181. DuBois, A. B., and L. Dautrebande, Acute effects of breathing inert dust particles and of carbachol aerosol on the mechanical characteristics of the lungs in man. Changes in response after inhaling sympathomimetic aerosols, *J. Clin. Invest.,* **37**:1746-1755 (1958).

182. Andersen, I. B., G. R. Lundqvist, D. F. Proctor, and D. L. Swift, Human response to controlled levels of inert dust, *Am. Rev. Respir. Dis.*, **119**: 619-627 (1979).
183. Palacek, F., and D. M. Aviado, Pulmonary effects of tobacco and related substances. II. Comparative effects of cigarette smoke, nicotine, and histamine on the anesthetized cat, *Arch. Environ. Health,* **15**:194-203 (1967).
184. Cho, Y. W., M. Samanek, and D. M. Aviado, Differences in the effects of inhalation of sulfur dioxide and cigarette smoke, *Arch. Environ. Health,* **16**:651-655 (1968).
185. Nadel, J. A., and J. H. Comroe, Jr., Acute effects of inhalation of cigarette smoke on airway conductance, *J. Appl. Physiol.,* **16**:713-716 (1961).
186. Simonsson, B., Effect of cigarette smoking on the forced expiratory flow rate, *Am. Rev. Respir. Dis.,* **85**:534-539 (1962).
187. Zamel, N., H. H. Youssef, and F. J. Prime, Airway resistance and peak expiratory flow-rate in smokers and non-smokers, *Lancet,* **1**:1237-1238 (1963).
188. McDermott, M., and M. M. Collins, Acute effects of smoking on lung airways resistance in normal and bronchitic subjects, *Thorax,* **20**:562-569 (1965).
189. Sterling, G. M., Mechanism of bronchoconstriction caused by cigarette smoking, *Br. Med. J.,* **3**:275-277 (1967).
190. Clarke, B. G., A. R. Guyatt, J. H. Alpers, C. M. Fletcher, and I. D. Hill, Changes in airways conductance on smoking a cigarette. A study of repeatability and of the effect of particulate and vapour phase filters, *Thorax,* **25**:418-422 (1970).
191. Zuskin, E., C. A. Mitchell, and A. Bouhuys, Interaction between effects of beta blockade and cigarette smoke on airways, *J. Appl. Physiol.,* **36**: 449-452 (1974).
192. Aviado, D. M., and M. Samanek, Bronchopulmonary effects of tobacco and related substances. I. Bronchoconstriction and bronchodilation: Influence of lung denervation, *Arch. Environ. Health,* **11**:141-151 (1965).
193. Yokoyama, E., Comparison of the ventilatory effects on guinea pigs of exposure to $SO_2$ and $NO_2$, *Bull. Inst. Publ. Health,* **17**:307-314 (1968).
194. Balchum, O. J., J. Dybicki, and G. R. Meneely, Pulmonary resistance and compliance with concurrent radioactive sulfur distribution in dogs breathing $S^{35}O_2$, *J. Appl. Physiol.,* **15**:62-66 (1960).
195. Frank, N. R., M. O. Amdur, J. Worcester, and J. L. Whittenberger, Effects of acute controlled exposure to $SO_2$ on respiratory mechanics in healthy male adults, *J. Appl. Physiol.,* **17**:252-258 (1962).
196. Yokoyama, E., Y. Matsumura, and T. Suzuki, Effect of atropine and pilocarpine on flow resistance in the lung of healthy subjects exposed to $SO_2$, *Bull. Inst. Publ. Health,* **16**:19-22 (1967).
197. Banister, J., G. Fegler, and C. Bebb, Initial respiratory responses to the intratracheal inhalation of phosgene or ammonia, *Q. J. Exp. Physiol.,* **35**: 233-250 (1949).

198. Goldsmith, J. R., and J. A. Nadel, Experimental exposure of human subjects to ozone, *J. Air Pollution Control Assoc.*, **19**:329-330 (1969).
199. Watanabe, S., R. Frank, and E. Yokoyama, Acute effects of ozone on lungs of cats. I. Functional, *Am. Rev. Respir. Dis.*, **108**:1141-1151 (1973).
200. Hallett, W. Y., Effect of ozone and cigarette smoke on lung function, *Arch. Environ. Health*, **10**:295-302 (1965).
201. Young, W. A., D. B. Shaw, and D. V. Bates, Effect of low concentrations of ozone on pulmonary function in man, *J. Appl. Physiol.*, **19**:765-768 (1964).
202. Sim, V. M., and R. E. Pattle, Effect of possible smog irritants on human subjects, *JAMA*, **165**:1908-1913 (1957).
203. Golberg, L., L. E. Martin, P. Sheard, and C. Harrison, The pharmacology of chymotrypsin administered by inhalation, *Br. J. Pharmacol.*, **15**:304-312 (1960).
204. Herxheimer, H., Bronchoconstrictor agents and their antagonists in the intact guinea-pig, *Arch. Int. Pharmacodyn. Ther.*, **106**:371-380 (1956).
205. Samanek, M., and D. M. Aviado, Bronchopulmonary effects of tobacco and related substances. II. Bronchial arterial injections of nicotine and histamine, *Arch. Environ. Health*, **11**:152-159 (1965).
206. Bouhuys, A., R. Jonsson, S. Lichtneckert, S.-E. Lindell, C. Lundgren, G. Lundin, and T. R. Ringquist, Effects of histamine on pulmonary ventilation in man, *Clin. Sci.*, **19**:79-94 (1960).
207. Wasserman, M. A., Bronchopulmonary responses to prostaglandin $F_{2a}$, histamine and acetylcholine in the dog, *Eur. J. Pharmacol.*, **32**:146-155 (1975).
208. Drazen, J. M., and K. F. Austen, Atropine modification of the pulmonary effects of chemical mediators in the guinea pig, *J. Appl. Physiol.*, **38**:834-838 (1975).
209. Mills, J. E., H. Sellick, and J. G. Widdicombe, Activity of lung irritant receptors in pulmonary microembolism, anaphylaxis and drug-induced bronchoconstrictions, *J. Physiol. (London)*, **203**:337-357 (1969).
210. Nadel, J. A., M. Corn, S. Zwi, J. Flesch, and P. Graf, Location and mechanism of airway constriction after inhalation of histamine aerosol and inorganic sulfate aerosol. In *Inhaled Particles and Vapours II*. British Occupational Hygiene Society, Oxford & New York, Pergamon, 1966, pp. 55-67.
211. Gold, W. M., G.-F. Kessler, and D. Y. C. Yu, Role of vagus nerves in experimental asthma in allergic dogs, *J. Appl. Physiol.*, **33**:719-725 (1972).
212. Mills, J. E., and J. G. Widdicombe, Role of the vagus nerves in anaphylaxis and histamine-induced bronchoconstrictions in guinea-pigs, *Br. J. Pharmacol.*, **39**:724-731 (1970).
213. Bleecker, E. R., D. J. Cotton, S. P. Fischer, P. D. Graf, W. M. Gold, and J. A. Nadel, The mechanism of rapid, shallow breathing after inhaling histamine aerosol in exercising dogs, *Am. Rev. Respir. Dis.*, **114**:909-916 (1976).

214. Sampson, S. R., and E. H. Vidruk, Properties of "irritant" receptors in canine lung, *Respir. Physiol.,* **25**:9-22 (1975).
215. Colebatch, H. J. H., C. R. Olsen, and J. A. Nadel, Effect of histamine, serotonin, and acetylcholine on the peripheral airways, *J. Appl. Physiol.,* **21**:217-226 (1966).
216. McDougal, M. D., and G. B. West, The action of drugs on isolated mammalian bronchial muscle, *Br. J. Pharmacol.,* **8**:26-37 (1953).
217. Islam, M. S., G. N. Melville, and W. T. Ulmer, Role of atropine in antagonizing the effect of 5-hydroxytryptamine (5-HT) on bronchial and pulmonary vascular systems, *Respiration,* **31**:47-59 (1974).
218. Bhattacharya, B. K., A pharmacological study on the effect of 5-hydroxytryptamine and its antagonists on the bronchial musculature, *Arch. Int. Pharmacodyn. Ther.,* **103**:357-369 (1955).
219. Loring, S. H., J. M. Drazen, J. R. Snapper, and R. H. Ingram, Jr., Vagal and aerosol histamine interactions on airway responses in dogs, *J. Appl. Physiol.,* **45**:40-44 (1978).
220. Loring, S. H., J. M. Drazen, and R. H. Ingram, Jr., Canine pulmonary response to aerosol histamine: Direct versus vagal effects, *J. Appl. Physiol.,* **42**:946-952 (1977).
221. Adrian, E. D., Afferent impulses in the vagus and their effect on respiration, *J. Physiol. (London),* **79**:332-358 (1933).
222. Knowlton, G. C., and M. G. Larrabee, A unitary analysis of pulmonary volume receptors, *Am. J. Physiol.,* **147**:100-114 (1946).
223. Davis, H. L., W. S. Fowler, and E. H. Lambert, Effect of volume and rate of inflation and deflation on transpulmonary pressure and response of pulmonary stretch receptors, *Am. J. Physiol.,* **187**:558-566 (1956).
224. Elftman, A. G., The afferent and parasympathetic innervation of the lungs and trachea of the dog, *Am. J. Anat.,* **72**:1-27 (1943).
225. Briscoe, W. A., and A. B. DuBois, The relationship between airway resistance, airway conductance and lung volume in subjects of different age and body size, *J. Clin. Invest.,* **37**:1279-1285 (1958).
226. Butler, J., C. G. Caro, R. Alcala, and A. B. DuBois, Physiological factors affecting airway resistance in normal subjects and in patients with obstructive respiratory disease, *J. Clin. Invest.,* **39**:584-591 (1960).
227. Dawes, G. S., and J. H. Comroe, Jr., Chemoreflexes from the heart and lungs, *Physiol. Rev.,* **34**:167-201 (1954).
228. Miserocchi, G., J. Mortola, and G. Sant'Ambrogio, Localization of the pulmonary stretch receptors in the airways of the dog, *J. Physiol. (London),* **235**:775-782 (1973).
229. Bartlett, Jr., D., P. Jeffery, G. Sant'Ambrogio, and J. C. M. Wise, Location of stretch receptors in the trachea and bronchi of the dog, *J. Physiol. (London),* **258**:409-420 (1976).
230. Düring, M. V., K. H. Andres, and J. Iravani, The fine structure of the pulmonary stretch receptor in the rat, *Z. Anat. Entwicklungsgesch.,* **143**: 215-222 (1974).

231. Bartlett, Jr., D., G. Sant'Ambrogio, and J. C. M. Wise, Transduction properties of tracheal stretch receptors, *J. Physiol. (London)*, **258**:421-432 (1976).
232. Mortola, J. P., and G. Sant'Ambrogio, Mechanics of the trachea and behaviour of its slowly adapting stretch receptors, *J. Physiol. (London)*, **286**:577-590 (1979).
233. Guz, A., and D. W. Trenchard, Pulmonary stretch receptor activity in man: A comparison with dog and cat, *J. Physiol. (London)*, **213**:329-343 (1971).
234. Paintal, A. S., Impulses in vagal afferent fibres from specific pulmonary deflation receptors. The response of these receptors to phenyl diguanide, potato starch, 5-hydroxytryptamine and nicotine and their role in respiratory and cardiovascular reflexes, *Q. J. Exp. Physiol.*, **40**:89-111 (1955).
235. Paintal, A. S., The location and excitation of pulmonary deflation receptors by chemical substances, *Q. J. Exp. Physiol.*, **42**:56-71 (1957).
236. Meyrick, B., and L. Reid, Nerves in rat intra-acinar alveoli: An electron microscopic study, *Respir. Physiol.*, **11**:367-377 (1971).
237. Hung, K.-S., M. S. Hertweck, J. D. Hardy, and C. G. Loosli, Ultrastructure of nerves and associated cells in bronchiolar epithelium of the mouse lung, *J. Ultrastruct. Res.*, **43**:426-437 (1973).
238. Coleridge, H. M., and J. C. G. Coleridge, Afferent vagal C-fibers in the dog lung: Their discharge during spontaneous breathing, and their stimulation by alloxan and pulmonary congestion. In *Krogh Centenary Symposium on Respiratory Adaptations, Capillary Exchange and Reflex Mechanisms.* Edited by A. S. Paintal and P. Gill-Kumar. Delhi:Vallabhbhai Patel Chest Institute, University of Delhi, 1977, pp. 396-406.
239. Coleridge, H. M., J. C. G. Coleridge, and J. C. Luck, Pulmonary afferent fibres of small diameter stimulated by capsaicin and by hyperinflation of the lungs, *J. Physiol. (London)*, **179**:248-262 (1965).
240. Coleridge, H. M., and J. C. G. Coleridge, Impulse activity in afferent vagal C-fibres with endings in the intrapulmonary airways of dogs, *Respir. Physiol.*, **29**:125-142 (1977).
241. Coleridge, H. M., J. C. G. Coleridge, D. G. Baker, K. H. Ginzel, and M. A. Morrison, Comparison of the effects of histamine and prostaglandin on afferent C-fiber endings and irritant receptors in the intrapulmonary airways. In *The Regulation of Respiration During Sleep and Anesthesia.* Edited by R. S. Fitzgerald, H. Gautier, and S. Lahiri. New York, Plenum, 1978, pp. 291-305.
242. Ginzel, K. H., M. A. Morrison, D. G. Baker, H. M. Coleridge, and J. C. G. Coleridge, Stimulation of afferent vagal endings in the intrapulmonary airways by prostaglandin endoperoxide analogues, *Prostaglandins*, **15**:131-138 (1978).
243. Said, S. I., S. Kitamura, and C. Vriem, Prostaglandins: Release from the lung during mechanical ventilation at large tidal volumes, *J. Clin. Invest.*, **51**:83a-84a (1972).
244. Cassidy, S. S., Indomethacin blocks the reflexly mediated cardiovascular depression of lung hyperinflation, *Clin. Res.*, **27**:491A (1979).

245. Richardson, J. B., Nerve supply to the lungs, *Am. Rev. Respir. Dis.*, **119**: 785-802 (1979).
246. Honjin, R., On the nerve supply of the lung of the mouse, with special reference to the structure of the peripheral vegetative nervous system, *J. Comp. Neurol.*, **105**:587-609 (1956).
247. Spencer, H., and D. Leof, The innervation of the human lung, *J. Anat. Lond.*, **98**:599-609 (1964).
248. Dahlström, A., K. Fuxe, T. Hökfelt, and K.-A. Norberg, Adrenergic innervation of the bronchial muscle of the cat, *Acta Physiol. Scand.*, **66**: 507-508 (1966).
249. Hollands, B. C. S., and S. Vanov, Localization of catechol amines in visceral organs and ganglia of the rat, guinea-pig and rabbit, *Br. J. Pharmacol.*, **25**:307-316 (1965).
250. Szentivanyi, A., The beta adrenergic theory of the atopic abnormality in bronchial asthma, *J. Allergy*, **42**:203-231 (1968).
251. Čech, S., Adrenergic innervation of blood vessels in the lung of some mammals, *Acta Anat. (Basel)*, **74**:169-182 (1969).
252. Lall, A., P. D. Graf, J. A. Nadel, and L. H. Edmunds, Jr., Adrenergic reinnervation of the reimplanted dog lung, *J. Appl. Physiol.*, **35**:439-442 (1973).
253. Castro de la Mata, R., M. Penna, and D. M. Aviado, Reversal of sympathomimetic bronchodilation by dichloroisoproterenol, *J. Pharmacol. Exp. Ther.*, **135**:197-203 (1962).
254. Minatoya, H., and F. P. Luduena, Effects of propanolol and guanethidine on the bronchodilation induced by sympathomimetic agents and by stimulation of the stellate ganglia in the anesthetized dog, *Fed. Proc.*, **26**:293 (1967).
255. Richardson, J. B., and T. Bouchard, Demonstration of a nonadrenergic inhibitory nervous system in the trachea of the guinea pig, *J. Allergy Clin. Immunol.*, **56**:473-480 (1975).
256. Suzuki, H., K. Morita, and H. Kuriyama, Innervation and properties of the smooth muscle of the dog trachea, *Jap. J. Physiol.*, **26**:303-320 (1976).
257. Richardson, J., and J. Béland, Nonadrenergic inhibitory nervous system in human airways, *J. Appl. Physiol.*, **41**:764-771 (1976).
258. Coburn, R. F., and T. Tomita, Evidence for nonadrenergic inhibitory nerves in the guinea pig trachealis muscle, *Am. J. Physiol.*, **224**:1072-1080 (1973).
259. Lockett, M. F., The transmitter released by stimulation of the bronchial sympathetic nerves of cats, *Br. J. Pharmacol.*, **12**:86-96 (1957).
260. Eakins, K. E., and M. F. Lockett, The formation of an isoprenaline-like substance from adrenaline, *Br. J. Pharmacol.*, **16**:108-115 (1961).
261. Roberts, D. J., Vasodilation in skeletal muscle produced by an apparent metabolite of adrenaline, *Br. J. Pharmacol.*, **24**:735-741 (1965).
262. Anton, A. H., and D. F. Sayre, A study of the factors affecting the

aluminum oxide-trihydroxyindole procedure for the analysis of catecholamines, *J. Pharmacol. Exp. Ther.*, **138**:360-375 (1962).
263. Von Euler, U. S., and F. Lishajko, Dopamine in mammalian lung and spleen, *Acta Physiol. Pharmacol. Neerlandica*, **6**:295-303 (1957).
264. McCulloch, M. W., C. Proctor, and M. J. Rand, Evidence for an adrenergic homeostatic bronchodilator reflex mechanism, *Eur. J. Pharmacol.*, **2**:214-223 (1967).
265. Herxheimer, H., The bronchoconstrictor action of propranolol aerosol in the guinea pig, *J. Physiol. (London)*, **190**:41P-42P (1967).
266. De Kock, M. A., Mechanism of bronchial obstruction in man. In *Bronchitis III. International Bronchitis Symposium*, 3rd ed. N. G. M. Oriel and R. Vander Linde, editors. Thomas, New York, 1970.
267. Drazen, J. M., Adrenergic influences on histamine-mediated bronchoconstriction in the guinea pig, *J. Appl. Physiol.*, **44**:340-345 (1978).
268. Zaid, G., and G. N. Beall, Bronchial response to beta-adrenergic blockade, *N. Engl. J. Med.*, **275**:580-584 (1966).
269. Marcelle, R., R. Bottin, J. Juchmes, and J. Lecomte, Reactions bronchomotrices de l'homme sain apres blocage des recepteurs β adrenergiques, *Acta Allergol. (Kbh.)*, **23**:11-17 (1968).
270. Tattersfield, A. E., D. G. Leaver, and N. B. Pride, Effects of β-adrenergic blockade and stimulation on normal human airways, *J. Appl. Physiol.*, **35**:613-619 (1973).
271. Townley, R. G., S. McGeady, A. Bewtra, The effect of beta adrenergic blockade on bronchial sensitivity to acetyl-beta-methacholine in normal and allergic rhinitis subjects, *J. Allergy Clin. Immunol.*, **57**:358-366 (1976).
272. Orehek, J., P. Gayrard, Ch. Grimaud, and J. Charpin, Effect of beta adrenergic blockade on bronchial sensitivity to inhaled acetylcholine in normal subjects, *J. Allergy Clin. Immunol.*, **55**:164-169 (1975).
273. McNeill, R. S., and C. G. Ingram, Effect of propranolol on ventilatory function, *Am. J. Cardiol.*, **18**:473-475 (1966).
274. MacDonald, A. G., C. G. Ingram, and R. S. McNeill, The effect of propranolol on airway resistance, *Br. J. Anaesthesiol.*, **39**:919-929 (1967).
275. Grieco, M. H., and R. N. Pierson Jr., Mechanism of bronchoconstriction due to beta adrenergic blockade, *J. Allergy Clin. Immunol.*, **48**:143-152 (1971).
276. Langer, I., The bronchoconstrictor action of propranolol aerosol in asthmatic subjects, *J. Physiol. (London)*, **190**:41P (1967).
277. Colebatch, H. J. H., Adrenergic mechanisms in the effects of histamine in the pulmonary circulation of the cat, *Circ. Res.*, **26**:379-396 (1970).
278. Collier, H. O. J., G. W. L. James, and P. J. Piper, Intensification by adrenalectomy or by β-adrenergic blockade of the bronchoconstrictor action of bradykinin in the guinea-pig, *J. Physiol. (London)*, **180**:13P-14P (1965).
279. Collier, H. O. J., and G. W. L. James, Humoral factors affecting pulmonary inflation during acute anaphylaxis in the guinea pig in vivo, *Br. J. Pharmacol. Chemother.*, **30**:283-301 (1967).

280. Piper, P. J., H. O. J. Collier, and J. R. Vane, Release of catecholamines in the guinea-pig by substances involved in anaphylaxis, *Nature (London)*, **213**:838-840 (1967).
281. Staszewska-Barczak, J., and J. R. Vane, The release of catechol amines from the adrenal medulla by histamine, *Br. J. Pharmacol.*, **25**:728-742 (1965).
282. Feldberg, W., and G. P. Lewis, The action of peptides on the adrenal medulla. Release of adrenaline by bradykinin and angiotensin, *J. Physiol. (London)*, **171**:98-108 (1964).
283. Staszewska-Barczak, J., and J. R. Vane, The release of catecholamines from the adrenal medulla by peptides, *J. Physiol. (London)*, **177**:57P-58P (1965).
284. Collier, H. O. J., G. W. L. James, and P. J. Piper, Intensification by adrenalectomy or by β-adrenergic blockade of the bronchoconstrictor action of bradykinin in the guinea-pig, *J. Physiol. (London)*, **180**:13P (1965).
285. Attinger, E. O., Effects of bronchoconstrictor drugs upon pulmonary circulation, *Arch. Int. Pharmacodyn. Ther.*, **125**:463-485 (1960).

# 6

# Atmospheric Particles
## Behavior and Functional Effects

*DAVID S. COVERT and N. ROBERT FRANK*

University of Washington School of Medicine
Seattle, Washington

This chapter focuses on the properties and functional respiratory effects of airborne particles that are up to 1 or 2 μm in diameter and water soluble. Such particles occur naturally, as a consequence of human activity, and are found throughout the lower troposphere. They may contain a variety of chemical compounds, such as dissolved gases, heavy metals, sulfates, nitrates, and hydrocarbons. When concentrated, as in urban or occupational settings, they pose a significant hazard to health.

Water-soluble particles, whether solid or liquid in the ambient air, undergo physicochemical changes upon entering the warm, humid airways. These changes may affect their pattern of deposition and the response they evoke. Narrowing of the airways is a common response to many noxious particles. The most frequent basis for airway narrowing following brief exposure is likely to be an increase in tracheobronchial smooth muscle tone. With persistent exposure, the airways may become scarred and distorted. Other factors, such as excessive mucoserous secretions, delay in the clearance of secretions, and submucosal edema, may contribute to the narrowing.

Ultimately, the nature of the biologic response to noxious particles, elicited by either brief or prolonged exposure, is a function of the dose. Dosage, particularly as it affects local sites within the respiratory system, is determined by a complex interplay between the particle and host. Some of the commonly recognized determinants of dosage apart from the ambient concentration are:

Physical properties of the particle, including size, shape, and density.

Mode of breathing: The nose is a more efficient scrubber of particles than the mouth, thereby shifting the site of deposition cephalad.

Pattern of ventilation and flow profiles within airways: Slow breathing increases the time for particles to deposit by diffusion and sedimentation. Rapid breathing associated with turbulent flow increases the likelihood for inertial impaction. (A maneuver commonly used to increase the total uptake of therapeutic or bronchoconstrictive aerosols is a rapid, deep inspiration followed by breath holding.)

Size and shape of the airways and parenchyma.

How evenly the dosage is distributed within different regions of the lung should reflect the distribution of mechanical properties and ventilation. Although there is little quantitative information on the subject, it is reasonable to suppose that abnormal lungs with unequally distributed mechanical defects may be subject to regions of intensive exposure, or "hot spots." Hot spots are not adequately reflected in simple measurements of the total uptake of a gas or particle. Conceivably, they contribute to the exaggerated responses of some individuals upon exposure to pollutants, and to the uneven pace at which disease may progress within different regions of the lung.

In healthy individuals the rate of deposition of monodispersed particles in the periphery of the lung during breath holding, a measurement used to assess the size of airspaces, appears to be uniform from one occasion to the next, but varies among individuals [1]. The clearance rate of insoluble particles from the lung also tends to be more consistent within than among individuals [2]. Both findings underscore the role of factors inherent in the lung that determine the level of exposure to particulate matter. Measurements of this type may eventually prove useful in identifying workers in dusty occupations such as coal mining who are at excessive risk.

For comprehensive reviews of the biologic effects of specific air pollutants the reader is referred to several recent monographs [3-6]. Elsewhere in this series are chapters on particle deposition [7] and clearance [8], with emphasis given to insoluble particles, a chapter on ambient pollutants in general [9], and one on the uptake of pollutant gases by the respiratory system [10]. The effects of immunologically active particles are described in Chapter 3 of this volume.

# I. Atmospheric Aerosols

A discussion of the behavior and deposition of atmospheric aerosol particles in the respiratory system requires consideration of their physical and chemical properties. While particle size and density, which determine aerodynamic diameter, primarily govern the deposition efficiency of aerosol particles within the respiratory system, chemical parameters are also important. Chemical composition determines not only the toxicity but also the hygroscopic nature of the particles, thus their potential for growth and for reaction with gaseous compounds before and after inhalation. The relevance of these parameters to the behavior and effect of particles in the respiratory system will be discussed in some detail in the following sections.

The generalizations that will be made about the size distributions and chemical composition of particles apply to anthropogenic aerosols that occur in urban regions or on a subcontinental scale (e.g., the eastern third of the United States or Europe), and even to a large extent on a global scale (the lower troposphere exclusive of polar regions). Thus, the discussion applies to aerosols to which a large fraction of the world's population is exposed. The comments do not necessarily apply to situations in which the aerosol souce is nearby (e.g., in the industrial workplace, on freeways, or during duststorms) or to aerosols used for medical research or clinical treatment, although some of the principles are applicable to them as well.

## A. Aerosol Parameters

Advances in instrumentation have provided detailed information on the size distribution of atmospheric aerosol particles that is of significance to the study of their behavior within the respiratory system. It has been determined that in general the atmospheric size distribution is the sum of two or three separate modes of particles that have different sources, sinks, and physical and chemical properties. To illustrate this, an example of an atmospheric volume-size distribution is presented in Figure 1. In this graph, the volume concentration of the particles [V], expressed as cubic micrometers of particles per cubic centimeter of air, is plotted on a linear scale on the ordinate as a function of the logarithm of particle diameter, $\log D_p$, on the abscissa. Since this is a distribution function, the volume parameter respresents an increment of particle volume per increment of the logarithm of diameter, $d[V]/d \log D_p$. The area under the curve is equal to the total volume concentration, and the area of any size increment is proportional to its fraction of the total volume. In practice the instruments used to measure particle size do not provide continuous data but operate over finite size intervals, $\Delta \log D_p$. Thus, data is of the form $\Delta[V]/\Delta \log D_p$, as shown in

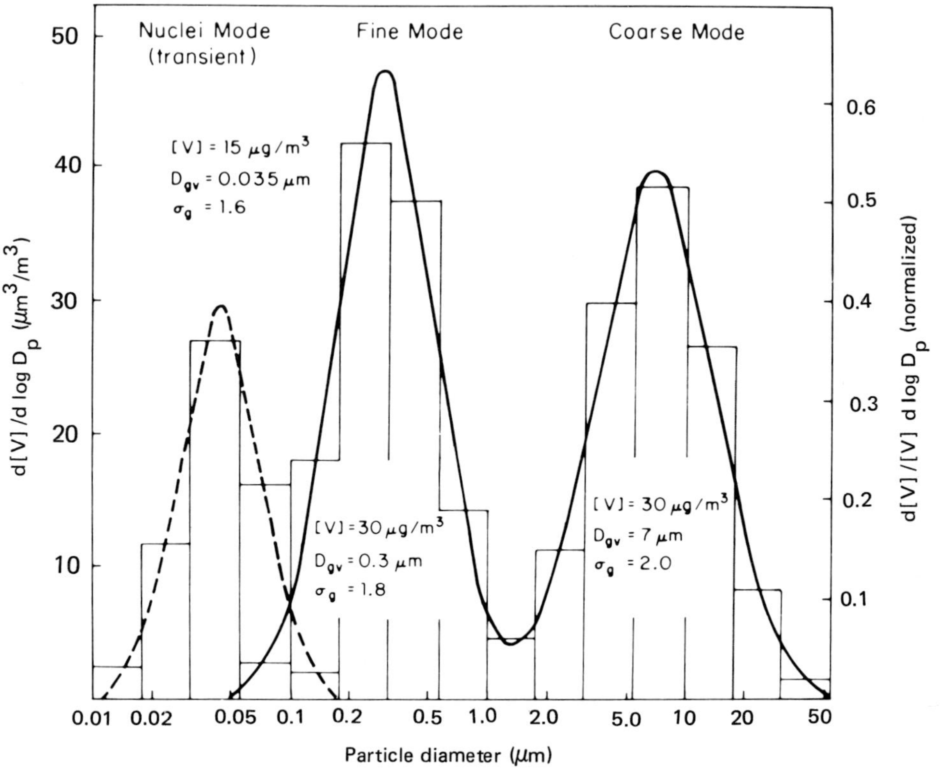


**FIGURE 1** Atmospheric aerosol, volume size distribution. Abscissa: particle diameter $D_p$ ($\mu$m) on a logarithmic scale. Ordinate: (left) incremental particle volume (expressed as concentration) per increment of particle size d[V]/d log $D_p$ ($\mu m^3/cm^3$); (right) normalized volume scale d[V]/[V] d log $D_p$.

the fine print in Figure 1 to which a smooth curve has been fitted. It is often assumed for convenience in the presentation or handling of the data that the modes have a log normal distribution, i.e., that volume (or any other moment) is distributed normally as a function of the log of the diameter. The modes are then described in terms of a geometric mean diameter $D_g$ (in this example, geometric volume mean diameter, $D_{gv}$), and a geometric standard deviation $\sigma_g$. The mass size distribution is the same as the volume-size distribution providing that particle density is independent of particle size. This assumption is valid within each mode but not between modes. For the illustrated distribution, differing particle densities between modes will change the magnitude of the areas of the modes with respect to the volume-size distribution but will not affect the mean or standard deviations. The means and deviations are $D_{gv}$ = 0.035 μm, $\sigma_g$ = 1.6 for the smallest sized or "nuclei" mode; $D_{gv}$ = 0.30 μm, $\sigma_g$ = 1.8 for the central or "fine" mode, and $D_{gv}$ = 7.0 μm and $\sigma_g$ = 2.0 for the largest or "coarse" mode. Often the distribution is normalized in standard statistical fashion so that the area under the curve is equal to unity. This is equivalent to a change of scale on the ordinate. A normalized volume scale is presented on the right-hand ordinate in Figure 1. There are other ways of presenting a size distribution that may be more appropriate depending on the purpose. If a respiratory effect of an aerosol were related to its number or surface area, one would want to study the distribution of these attributes. A more complete description of particle statistics, size distributions, and their relationships can be found in References 11 and 12.

Now that the distribution of atmospheric aerosol particles has been presented, its features and causes can be discussed. The smallest sized nuclei mode is transient, being rapidly transformed by coagulation into the fine mode and dispersed by mixing with air. Consequently, it is found only near its sources, primarily automotive traffic on major highways. The remainder of the discussion will be focused on the fine and coarse modes, which are more prevalent in the atmosphere and more likely to have greater implications for health.

The bimodal form of the volume-size distribution shown in Figure 1 is typical of that found in the atmosphere. However, the total volume concentration of area under the bimodal curve may vary by a factor of 10 or more with time at a particular location or between locations at a particular time. These variations generally occur over relatively long time and space scales, involving days and hundreds of kilometers. The relative magnitude of the two modes may vary by a factor of about 2, depending on the history of the air mass, but the volume-mean sizes of the fine and coarse modes remain between 0.2 to 0.6 μm and 5.0 to 10 μm, respectively. The minimum in the volume-size distribution which separates the two modes, occurs consistently between 1.0 and 2.0 μm.

During periods of high pollution, the elevated particle and reactive gas concentrations can cause an increase in the formation and growth rate of fine particles by coagulation and gas to particle reactions. Under such conditions an increase in the mean size of the fine mode from ~ 0.3 μm to between 0.5 and 0.8 μm has been observed [13].

The chemistry of the particles in these two modes is markedly different and can be related to their sources. The major fraction of particle mass in the fine mode is due to combustive processes associated with human activities, such as fossil fuel power plants, vehicles, industrial processes, domestic heating, hydrocarbon emissions from refineries, and fuel transportation. The emissions consist of gases–sulfur dioxide ($SO_2$), sulfur trioxide ($SO_3$), nitrogen oxides ($NO_X$); hydrocarbons and nuclei mode sized particles; heavy metals such as lead (Pb), vanadium (Vn), and manganese (Mn); and graphitic carbon (soot). In the atmosphere these compounds react in combination with water vapor, ammonia ($NH_3$), and sunlight, all of which occur naturally, as well as with ozone ($O_3$), which occurs naturally but also is a product of photochemical reactions initiated by pollutants. Sulfate and nitrate compounds, and a wide range of hydrocarbons (organic acids, aldehydes, and salts) are formed [14,15].

While it is difficult to generalize about the physical and chemical properties of such a complex mixture as atmospheric aerosols, certain aspects of the fine mode particles have become clear in the last few years. Our present understanding of the structure of these particles is that they consist of a solid water-insoluble core composed of graphitic carbon, hydrocarbons, and heavy metals, which is surrounded by a solid (or liquid) layer of water-soluble organic and inorganic salts and/or acids. At humidities below ~ 70% they are nearly spherical in shape and at higher humidities they become spherical, as will be explained later. Their density is generally considered to be between 1 and 1.5 $g/cm^3$. The water-soluble layer may comprise 50 to 90% of the mass of the particle. Sulfate compounds alone often account for up to 50% of their mass [16-18]. These sulfate compounds may be acid [sulfuric acid ($H_2SO_4$) or ammonium bisulfate ($NH_4HSO_4$)] or nearly neutral ammonium sulfate [$(NH_4)_2SO_4$], depending on the amount of atmospheric ammonia ($NH_3$) which the particles have encountered [19].

The mass of material in the coarse particle mode is more evenly divided between anthropogenic and natural sources than in the fine mode. The primary sources of the coarse mode are soil and sand from the earth's surface, which are raised by the wind either alone or in conjunction with agricultural, mining, or transportation activities. The more strictly anthropogenic components include cement dust, fly ash, and tire fragments. The chemical composition of these particles is generally similar to that of the earth's crust. It includes silicates ($SiO_2$), aluminum (Al), magnesium (Mg), and iron (Fe). Near the coastline, sea salt, which is predominantly sodium chloride (NaCl) in a size range of 3 to 5 $\mu m$, can contribute to the mass of the coarse mode. At times, pollens (> 10 $\mu m$) add significantly to the mass of this size mode.

The physical structure of the particles in the coarse mode is more irregular than that of the fine mode particles. They vary in shape from cubes (NaCl) to needles or plates (asbestos). Their densities range between 2 and 3 $g/cm^3$. Thus, their aerodynamic diameter is ~ 1.5 times their geometric volume mean diameter (as depicted in the size distribution. Fig. 1). They are also less homogeneous chemically.

A summary of the sources, chemical composition, and physical and chemical properties of the fine and coarse modes is presented in Table 1.

**TABLE 1 Chemical Composition and Sources of Atmospheric Aerosol Size Modes**

| Mode | Source | Chemical compounds or classes of compounds | General physical and chemical properties |
|---|---|---|---|
| Accumulation | Combustion of fuels; gas to particle conversion; photochemical oxidation | $SO_4^{2-}$, $NO_3^-$, $NH_3^+$, $H^+$, hydrocarbons, graphitic carbons, heavy metals (Pb, As, Vn) | Water soluble (hygroscopic); low density, 1-1.5; near spherical shape |
| Coarse | Wind-blown dust; grinding processes | Silicates, carbonates, ferric oxides, Al, $Mg^+$, $Ca^{2+}$, pollen, fly ash | Less water soluble (nonhygroscopic); high density, 2-2.5; more irregular shape |

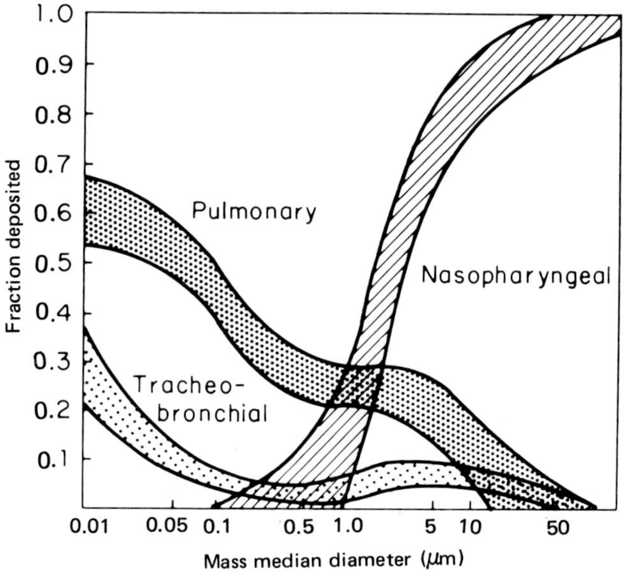


**FIGURE 2** Deposition efficiency curves. Each of the shaded areas (envelopes) indicates the magnitude and variability of deposition for a given mass median (aerodynamic) diameter in each compartment when the distribution parameter $\sigma_g$ varies from 1.2 to 4.5 and the tidal volume is 1450 ml. (From Ref. [26]; © 1966 by Pergamon Press, Ltd., New York.)

### B. Aerosol Deposition

A graph of regional deposition efficiency versus particle size is reproduced from Volume 5 of these series [7] in Figure 2. It is instructive to compare this with the volume-size distribution graph in Figure 1: it can be seen that the fine and coarse modes will deposit in separate regions of the lung. A composite of the functions shown in Figures 1 and 2, which can be thought of as a deposition-size distribution, is illustrated in Figure 3. The coarse mode will deposit primarily in the nasopharyngeal region with a high efficiency of 50 to 100%. The fine mode will deposit primarily in the pulmonary region with a much lower efficiency of 20 to 40%. The transient nuclei mode, when encountered, will deposit primarily in the pulmonary region. Only a small fraction of atmospheric aerosol will ever be deposited in the tracheobronchial region according to these curves. The small fraction of particles deposited in this region may be concentrated in hot spots and thus have a disproportionately large effect. Very little particle mass is ever observed below 0.05 μm in diameter where tracheobronchial deposition theoretically increases to greater than 10%. These statements concerning the deposition of submicrometric particles will be tempered in the following section in which hygroscopic growth is considered. Although seemingly complex. a deposition-size distribution function can provide a simple quantitative estimate of regional dose, which is probably a useful exercise in particle inhalation studies. A regional dose value may be obtained by multiplying the area under the appropriate curve by the total amount of particulate matter inhaled (mass concentration × tidal volume × respiratory frequency).

An interesting point to note is that the primary mechanisms which act to remove particles in the lung (diffusion, gravitational and inertial forces) also act to remove particles from the ambient air. The minimum in deposition efficiency which occurs in the respiratory deposition curves also occurs in the atmosphere and is manifested in the fine mode of the atmospheric particle mass distribution. Indeed, this is often called the "accumulation" mode because particles tend to accumulate at that size for lack of efficient removal mechanisms. Consequently,

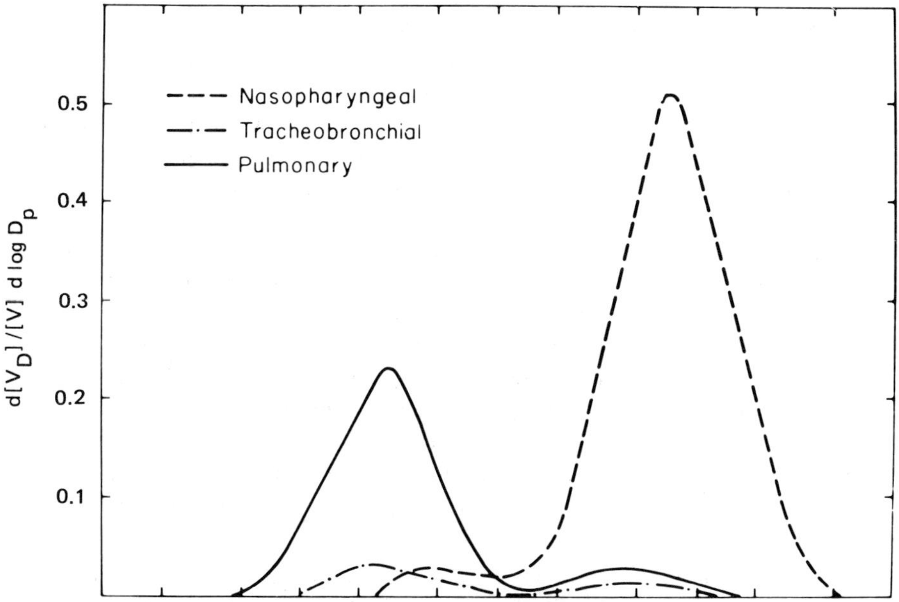


**FIGURE 3** Deposition-size distribution. Abscissa: particle diameter $D_p$ ($\mu$m). Ordinate: increment of aerosol volume deposited per increment of particle size, $dV_D/F \text{ d} \log D_p$ ($\mu g/m^3$), where $V_D$ = particle volume deposited.

although much of the anthropogenic aerosol having potentially toxic effects is concentrated in a size range that has relatively long residence times in the atmosphere, it also collects least efficiently in the respiratory system. Cloud processes in the atmosphere, (i.e., rain, snow, and fog) provide the only effective atmospheric removal mechanisms for the accumulation mode. Similar nucleation processes in the humid respiratory tract may act to increase deposition of hygroscopic accumulation mode aerosol particles.

## II. Aerosol Changes Following Inhalation

### A. Hygroscopic Growth

"Hygroscopic" refers to the ability of certain chemical compounds to adsorb water vapor from the air when exposed to an increase in relative humidity (RH). The uptake of water vapor will proceed until water vapor equilibrium is reached at the phase interface [20]. The reverse process, loss of water vapor to the surroundings, occurs when a hygroscopic compound is exposed to a decrease in RH. Pure hygroscopic compounds are liquids (aqueous solutions such as $H_2SO_4$ or glycerol) and exhibit this behavior continuously over the range of 0 to 100% RH. A different type of hygroscopic behavior, termed deliquescence, applies to compounds, primarily inorganic salts such as NaCl and $(NH_4)_2SO_4$, that exhibit hygroscopic behavior only above a particular RH, which is called the deliquescent point for that compound [20,21]. Below this RH, they exist as the solid crystalline material, that is, there is a discontinuity in their properties at the deliquescent point. Thus, the size of a hygroscopic particle will vary monotonically with ambient RH, while the size of a deliquescent particle will be independent of RH up to the RH that corresponds to its deliquescent point. At that point it will exhibit a step increase in size, and thereafter at higher RH show monotonic behavior. These properties are illustrated for two pure compounds, $H_2SO_4$ and NaCl, in Figure 4. Deliquescent compounds may exhibit hysteresis when exposed to decreasing RH, as illustrated by the dashed line and hatched area in Figure 4. The reverse process, loss of water to form a dry crystal (efflorescence), is unstable and may occur anywhere within the hatched area depending on external parameters.

For pure compounds of $H_2SO_4$, NaCl, or other inorganic salts the magnitude of the increase in particle size between low RH (~ 40%) and the RH found in the respiratory system (95-99.5%) is on the order of a factor of 2 to 5. The ratios illustrated in Figure 4 are valid independently of particle size for paritcles greater than ~ 0.1 $\mu$m in diameter and for RH less than ~ 99.5%. Outside these limits the radius of curvature (i.e., particle size) has an effect on the equilibrium

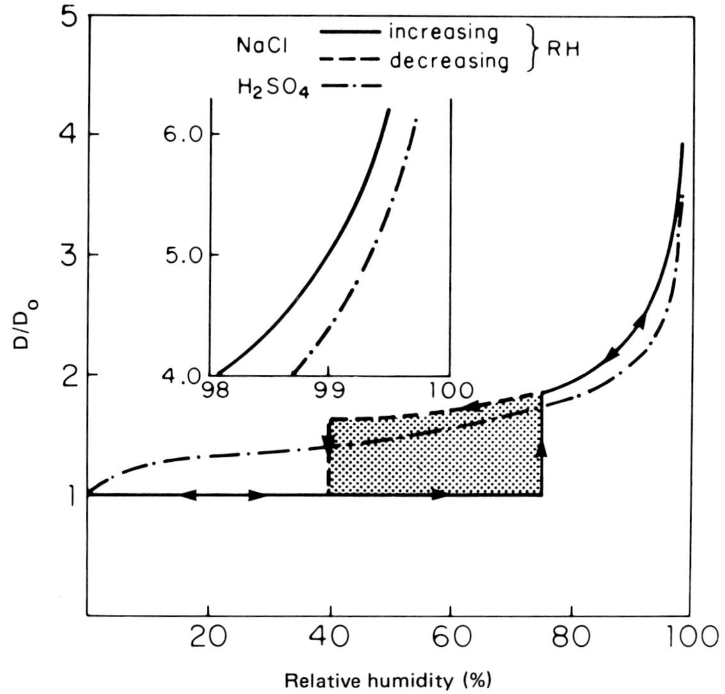


**FIGURE 4** Equilibrium growth factor for hygroscopic particles as a function of relative humidity. Ordinate: ratio of particle diameter at a specified RH (D) to its diameter at 0% RH ($D_0$). Abcissa: percentage of relative humidity (RH). Arrows indicate sense of change in RH, that is, increasing or decreasing. Hatched area is the region of hysteresis for a deliquescent aerosol.

size of hygroscopic aerosols. Particles less than ~ 0.1 μm in diameter will have a smaller equilibrium size and therefore a smaller $D/D_0$ ratio than is shown. Above ~ 99.5% RH but below 100% RH, larger particles will have a larger equilibrium size and larger ratio. For the range of particle sizes and RH under consideration these effects are negligible.

The rate of particle growth is strongly dependent on particle size, however. To a close approximation, the growth rate is inversely proportional to the particle diameter to the second power. The growth rate curves for NaCl particles of two different sizes when suddenly exposed to 99% RH from the dry state are shown in Figure 5. The curves of growth and growth rate shown in Figures 4 and 5 have been determined theoretically and verified by experiment [22-24].

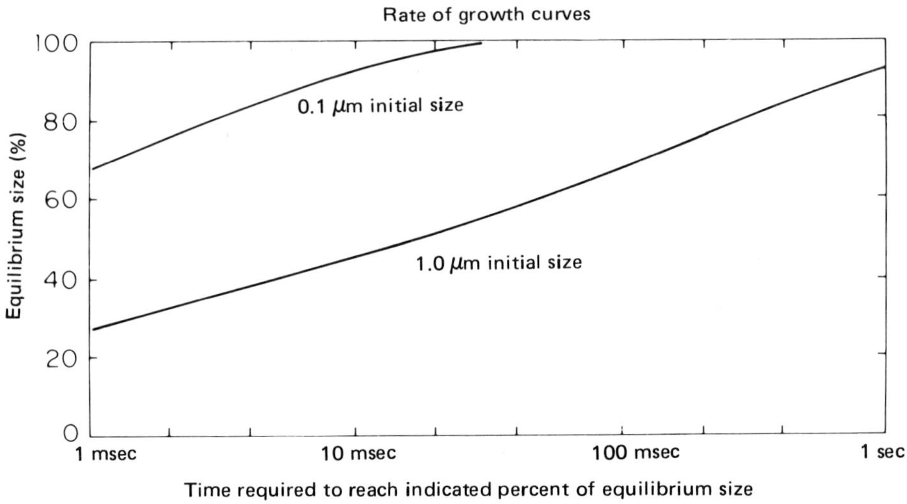


**FIGURE 5** Time dependence of hygroscopic particle growth to 99% RH; percentage of equilibrium size for given initial size.

The fine mode of atmospheric aerosols can be expected to be hygroscopic due to its observed predominant chemical composition, namely, sulfate, nitrate, and organic compounds. Its hygroscopicity has been observed directly in a wide variety of locations [25,26]. However, the magnitude of its increase in equilibrium size with RH is reduced to about half of that observed for pure compounds due to the insoluble compounds which make up part of the mass of fine aerosol particles. In general the particles in the coarse mode are not hygroscopic. Moreover, they are deposited primarily in the upper airways before any significant hygroscopic growth is likely to occur in response to the elevated RH of the upper airways.

There has been much discussion of the possible effect that hygroscopic growth may have on the deposition of inhaled atmospheric aerosol particles in the lung [3,26-28]. However, there are no firm conclusions supported by theory or experiment. Inspection of the deposition curves (Fig. 2) and of the volume-size distribution (Fig. 3) indicates that for fine particles near the modal size of 0.3 μm, growth by a factor of 3 should produce little net change in deposition efficiency. Particles in the smaller half of this mode might be deposited less efficiently were they to grow by a factor of 3. Only those hygroscopic particles in the range of 0.5 to 1.0 μm would be subject to increased deposition efficiency due to hygroscopic growth. Although not well indicated in the deposition curves, pulmonary deposition efficiency in the periphery of the lung increases for particles above 1 $\mu m$ in diameter that have passed through the upper airways [3]. Thus, hygroscopic particles in the size range of 0.5 to 1.0 $\mu m$ that may not grow rapidly enough to be deposited efficiently in the upper airways will grow and be deposited with 30 to 50% efficiency in the pulmonary region due to gravitational settling. This effect may be significant in highly polluted atmospheres [13] where as mentioned earlier the peak of the fine mode shifts to larger sizes (0.5-0.8 $\mu m$). Under such conditions the mass of sulfate compounds, heavy metals, and especially of nitrate compounds has been found at sizes larger than is generally observed for the fine mode.

Perhaps the most significant effect of hygroscopic growth of particles in the respiratory system is the change in chemistry which occurs due to dilution. An acid particle, which may grow in linear dimension by a factor of about 3, grows in volume and is diluted by a factor of about 30. For example, a particle of $NH_4HSO_4$ with a pH $\simeq$ 1 if otherwise unaffected would reach a pH $\simeq$ 2.5. Dilution will increase the activity (reaction rate) of acid particles with certain gases. The increased size will also increase the rate of diffusion of gases to the surface. The point of this will be clear in the next section when reactive gases are discussed.

### B. Chemical Transformation ($NH_3$)

A recent hypothesis proposes that inhaled acid aerosols may be chemically neutralized before they strike the epithelial surfaces [29]. The hypothesis is based on information derived from two scientific fields, atmospheric chemistry and respiratory physiology.

Gaseous $NH_3$ is largely responsible for determining the molecular form of atmospheric sulfate compounds. When trace amounts of this gas on the order of 7 to 20 $\mu g/m^3$ are present in the atmosphere, the molecular composition of atmospheric levels of acid sulfate aerosols is likely to be $NH_4HSO_4$ and/or $(NH_4)_2SO_4$. In the absence of $NH_3$, $H_2SO_4$ predominates. These three sulfate compounds have the following pH values at ordinary ambient RH:

| Compound | pH |
|---|---|
| $H_2SO_4$ | < 0.1 |
| $NH_4HSO_4$ | 1-2 |
| $(NH_4)_2SO_4$ | 5-6 |

It is known that exhaled air contains $NH_3$. An early view held that the pulmonary capillary circulation is the chief source of exhaled $NH_3$. More recent evidence suggests that this $NH_3$ is released chiefly in the upper airways [29].

**TABLE 2 Ammonia ($\mu g/m^3$, 25°C) in Respiratory Gas (Breath Held; Flow Constant)[a]**

| | Mean ± SE | Range |
|---|---|---|
| Nose | 29 ± 4 | 13-46 |
| Mouth | 157 ± 27 | 29-520 |

[a]Sixteen subjects.

If, then, an acid aerosol is inhaled, can it be neutralized by respiratory $NH_3$ while still airborne? Insofar as neutralization occurs, the irritant potential of the particle is likely to be reduced.

Table 2 lists the concentrations of $NH_3$ measured in gas samples drawn at a fixed rate of flow through the nose or mouth of healthy subjects; the subjects held their breath during the procedure. The values are about 5 times higher for the mouth than for the nose. (Microbial deaminases may be chiefly responsible for the rich production of $NH_3$ in the mouth.) The concentration of $NH_3$ at the mouth, and presumably elsewhere in the airways, varies as a function of flow rate (Fig. 6); a rise in inspiratory flow rate, as in exercise, may therefore be expected to dilute the $NH_3$.

In one of the subjects, exhaled air obtained through an endotracheal tube had an $NH_3$ concentration of 32 $\mu g/m^3$, a value similar to that obtained for the nose (Table 2). Based on reported blood ammonium ($NH_4^+$) concentrations, the estimated gas-phase concentration in alveoli may range between 10 and 25 $\mu g/m^3$ [30]. It appears reasonable to conclude that the region of highest concentration within the respiratory system is the oral cavity.

How far the elevated $NH_3$ levels extend beyond the oropharynx during inspiration is yet to be determined. Significant changes in concentration are to be expected in passage owing to the high solubility and diffusivity of the gas. (The concept of a dead space volume for $NH_3$ appears to be untenable.) A technique for the rapid, continuous measurement of $NH_3$ that can be used to sample from several levels of the airways has recently been developed [31]. To test the basic hypothesis, a second sampling and analytical technique is to be added that stops the chemical reaction between $NH_3$ and $H_2SO_4$ aerosol quickly and completely and can then distinguish between $H_2SO_4$ and the ammonium salts, that is, determine the extent of the neutralization.

Four factors should be critical in determining the rate at which $NH_3$ neutralizes an inhaled acid aerosol:

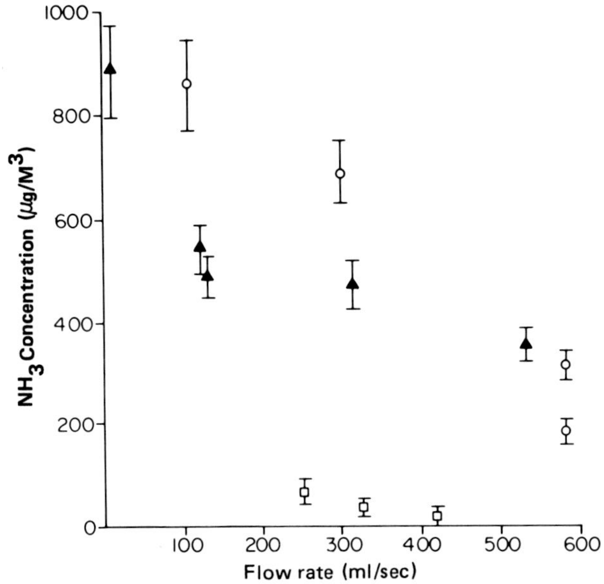


**FIGURE 6** The concentration of ammonia plotted against flow rate in three subjects (□, ○, ▲). Gas was pulled through the nose and out of the mouth at a constant rate. (From Ref. [29]; © 1977 by the American Association for the Advancement of Science.)

1. The rate of diffusion of $NH_3$ to the surface of the particle is dependent on *particle size.*
2. The particle size and its reactivity also depend on *relative humidity* (see section on hygroscopic growth).
3. The higher the *ratio of* $NH_3$ *to acid aerosol,* the faster will be the rate of neutralization.
4. During quiet breathing the transit time of inspired air in the mouth and oropharynx is on the order of 0.1 second. To the extent that high levels of $NH_3$ persist into the tracheobronchial tree and the *residence time* of the aerosol in an $NH_3$-rich environment is prolonged, neutralization should proceed to greater completion.

A theoretical treatment of the role of particle size in regulating the rate of neutralization is shown in Figure 7. Note that after 0.02 sec only the smallest particles have been neutralized, causing a slight reduction in the total mass of

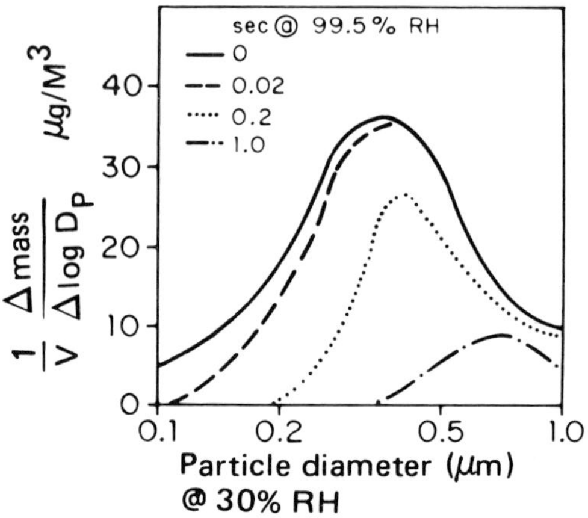


**FIGURE 7** Theoretical mass distribution of sulfuric acid aerosol (accumulation mode) at various intervals during neutralization by ammonia. The relative humidity (RH) is assumed to be 99.5%. The area under each curve represents the estimated mass concentration of sulfuric acid remaining after the indicated period of time, assuming that the rate of reaction is limited by gaseous diffusion. (From Ref. [30].)

$H_2SO_4$. A significant reduction in $H_2SO_4$ mass has occurred by 0.2 sec. Only the largest particles contain a significant fraction of $H_2SO_4$ after 1.0 sec.

Exploratory work on the extent of neutralization that may occur in the airways has been carried out on a single subject who was exposed by mouth to each of two concentrations of $H_2SO_4$. The subject breathed quietly, each respiratory cycle lasting 2 sec. The molar ratio of $NH_4^+/SO_2^{2-}$ was determined in the particles that were exhaled. The findings are shown in Table 3. Whether the neutralization occurred principally during inspiration or expiration or in the 0.5-sec delay needed to make the determination is not known. The concentration of sulfuric acid administered to the subject, that is, 600 and 1200 $\mu g/m^3$, exceed the levels reported in urban air by one or two orders of magnitude.

If respiratory $NH_3$ is shown to be efficient in neutralizing a significant fraction of inhaled acid aerosols, particularly during quiet breathing by mouth, it should be possible to show some correlation between levels of the gas in the mouth and the degree of functional response to these aerosols. As a corollary, the risk of acid sulfate pollution might be increased for individuals with low levels of ammonia. Two populations that might fit this description come to mind, namely, the newborn and the elderly. Both groups, insofar as they are edentate, may lack the microorganisms chiefly responsible for producing ammonia in the

**TABLE 3 Extent of Neutralization of *Expired* Aerosol[a]**

| Expired aerosol concentration ($\mu g/m^3$)[b] | % Neutralized |
|---|---|
| 600 ± 100 | > 50 |
| 1100 ± 200 | 25 ± 5 |
| 1100 ± 200 | 30 ± 5 |

[a]Expired $NH_3$ = 100 $\mu g/m^3$.
[b]Equals ~ 90% of inspired $H_2SO_4$ concentration (0.6 $\mu m$ MMD). Stoichiometrically, 1 $\mu g/m^3$ of ammonia will convert 5.8 $\mu g/m^3$ of sulfuric acid to ammonium bisulfate, or 2.9 $\mu g/m^3$ to ammonium sulfate.
*Source:* From Ref. [30].

mouth. Both groups are considered to be particularly vulnerable to air pollution, perhaps for a variety of reasons.

## III. Interactions with Other Pollutants: $SO_2$ Model

The adverse effects of urban air pollution on health are generally attributed to a mixture of elements. With only infrequent exceptions, individual pollutants are considered to be too low in concentration to exert discrete effects. Instead it is postulated that the pollutants either interact physically or chemically, forming products that are more irritant or toxic than the original ingredients, or that they act additively.

Inhalation toxicology has been testing the former premise for years. The interaction between hygroscopic particles and a soluble gas is a classic example of this type of study [32-35]. Whether the interaction occurs before the mixture is inhaled, following inhalation, or at all, appears to depend on the experimental circumstances. Frequent use has been made of NaCl, a physiologically innocuous aerosol, mixed with $SO_2$. The two agents have been administered to a variety of animals and to human volunteers as well, with somewhat conflicting results. The following discussion is an attempt to resolve some of these conflicts.

As described earlier in the chapter, NaCl is deliquescent (Fig. 8). McJilton et al. [35] reasoned that if the aerosol were mixed with $SO_2$ at an RH below its deliquescent point, there would be virtually no interaction in the ambient air and that the effect of the mixture, if any, would be attributable to the gas alone. However, if the two agents were to be combined at an ambient RH above the deliquescent point of NaCl, the droplet that formed would absorb $SO_2$ to produce an irritant particle.

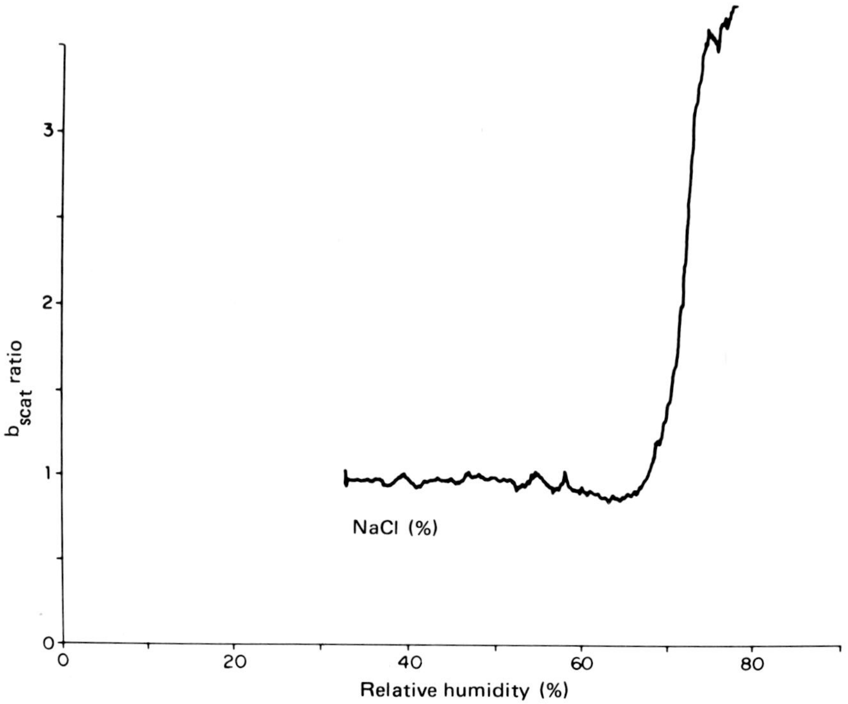


**FIGURE 8** The light-scattering ratio ($b_{scat}$) of NaCl aerosol measured with a nephelometer [85]. The ratio is an index of mass concentration of submicrometric particles. The sharp increase in mass concentration ($b_{scat}$ ratio), starting at a relative humidity of about 68%, occurs as the crystal dissolves in water. (From Ref. [86].)

The experiment was performed on guinea pigs. The concentration of $SO_2$ used, 1 ppm, was too low by itself to alter mechanical function in the animals. Pulmonary flow resistance ($R_L$) was found to increase and compliance ($C_L$) to decrease only when the gas-aerosol mixture was administered at the high RH (Figs. 9a and b). It may be concluded that in this circumstance the gas-aerosol interaction occurred in ambient air.

A second possible basis for synergism, namely, interaction between the particle and gas *following* inhalation, is probably exemplified by Amdur's studies [32,33]. Again, guinea pigs were exposed to NaCl and $SO_2$, separately and in combination. Ambient relative humidity, although not specified, was almost certainly below the deliquescent point of NaCl. The aerosol alone elicited no functional response; $SO_2$, administered in a wide range of concentrations, increased $R_L$, and the effect was magnified by addition of the aerosol. To explain these results, Amdur has postulated that following inhalation the (dry) particles become droplets in the humidified upper airways of the animals and thereupon absorb $SO_2$.

This explanation does pose several problems. $SO_2$ is highly soluble in tissue liquids. Uptake of the gas by the upper airways is therefore rapid and efficient [36,37], and a significant fraction is likely to enter the mucus lining before the aerosol deliquesces. Furthermore, the aerosol, even if administered in high concentrations, has a meager absorptive surface compared with that of the nasal passages against which it must compete for the gas. To illustrate, the mucosal surface between the nares and distal ends of the turbinates is estimated to be about 160 $cm^2$ in adults [38]; if this surface area is assumed to vary directly with body weight among different mammals, the equivalent structure in a 300-g guinea pig should equal about 1 $cm^2$; by comparison the surface area of an aerosol with a mass concentration of 1 $mg/m^3$ and mass median diameter of 1 $\mu m$ is only $3 \times 10^{-5}$ $cm^2$.

Consequently, if synergism is to depend on the reaction between the particle and gas taking place within the airways, large concentrations of the aerosol will be needed to increase its absorptive surface. Amdur's results support this argument. In one report she noted that 10 $mg/m^3$ of NaCl was more effective than 4 $mg/m^3$ [32], and in another report that 3 $mg/m^3$ did not alter the response seen with $SO_2$ alone [39]. It will be recalled that McJilton et al. [35] found no effect when they administered a mixture of 1 $mg/m^3$ of NaCl and $SO_2$ at low ambient relative humidity.

It is not certain which by-products of the interaction may be responsible for the synergism. Solution of sulfur dioxide produces hydrogen, bisulfite ($HSO_3^-$), and sulfite ($SO_3^{2-}$) ions in addition to the physically dissolved gas, all of which are potentially irritating to the mucosal lining:

$$SO_2 + H_2O \leftrightharpoons SO_2 \cdot H_2O$$

$$SO_2 \cdot H_2O \leftrightharpoons H^+ + HSO_3^-$$

$$HSO_3^- \leftrightharpoons H^+ + SO_3^{2-}$$

An intriguing aspect of this type of synergism is that only a small fraction of the total amount of $SO_2$ in the gas phase enters the droplet. One is tempted to conclude that any circumstance causing even a slight change in the solubility of $SO_2$ should therefore also have a significant impact on the degree of synergism. The amount of $SO_2$ that dissolves in an aqueous solution is pH dependent, as shown in Figure 10a. At hydrogen ion concentrations of $10^{-5}$ mol/liter (pH 5), only about $10^{-2}$% of the gas dissolves and the percentage falls below

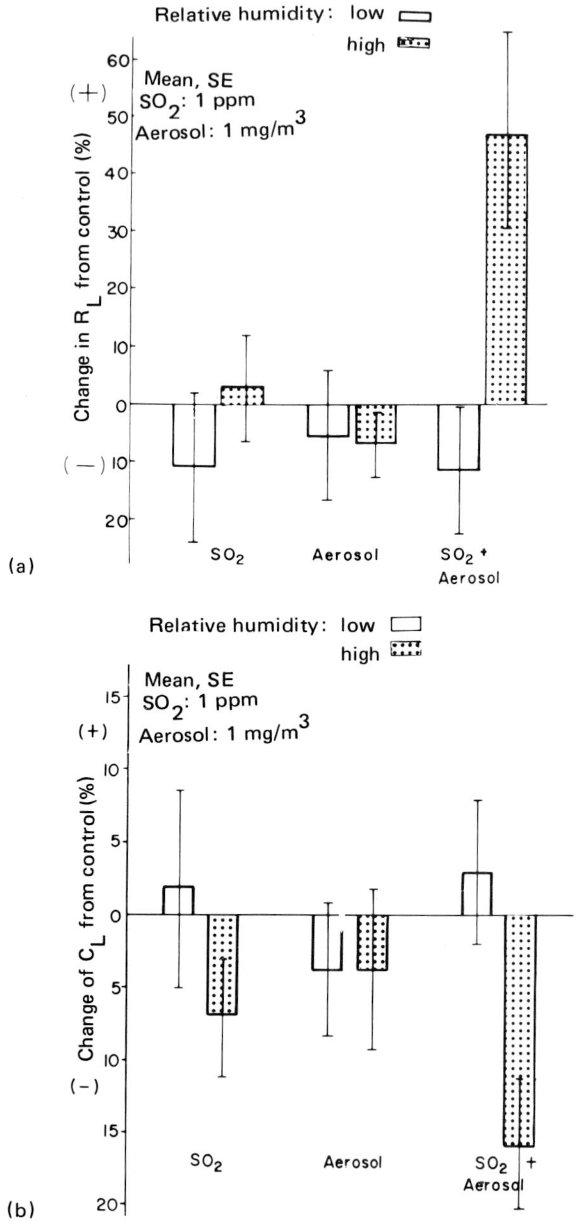
Relative humidity: low
high
Mean, SE
$SO_2$: 1 ppm
Aerosol: 1 mg/m³
Change in $R_L$ from control (%)
(+)
(−)
60
50
40
30
20
10
0
10
20
$SO_2$
Aerosol
$SO_2$ +
Aerosol
(a)
Relative humidity: low
high
Mean, SE
$SO_2$: 1 ppm
Aerosol: 1 mg/m³
Change of $C_L$ from control (%)
(+)
(−)
15
10
5
0
5
10
15
20
$SO_2$
Aerosol
$SO_2$ +
Aerosol
(b)

**FIGURE 9**

$10^{-4}$% at pH $\leqslant 1$ (typical of strong acids). The ratio of bisulfite to sulfite ionic concentrations $[(HSO_3^-)/(SO_3^{2-})]$ is also a function of the pH, as shown in Figure 10b. This ratio increases as the solution becomes more acid, although both ions decrease in absolute concentration.

There is an additional element of complexity to the reaction in that the hydrogen ions produced by the absorption of $SO_2$ (and by carbon dioxide in the ambient air) may be neutralized by respiratory $NH_3$. But if the effect of the $NH_3$ is to raise the pH of the droplet, the solubility of $SO_2$ will then increase (Fig. 10a)!

Amdur and Underhill [33] reported that three factors governed whether and by how much the aerosols they used potentiated the effect of $SO_2$:

1. For potentiation to occur, the aerosol had to be soluble in aqueous solution. Spectrographic carbon, activated carbon, fly ash, and manganese dioxide, all insoluble, were not effective.
2. The degree of potentiation varied roughly with the solubility of $SO_2$ as measured in a bulk solution of the aerosol. In one set of experiments, three inorganic salts were used to generate aerosols, namely, NaCl, potassium chloride (KCl), and ammonium thiocyanate ($NH_4SCN$). The solubility coefficient of $SO_2$, expressed as milliliters of gas at 25°C, 1 atm/ml is lowest for a bulk solution of NaCl, intermediate for KCL, and highest for $NH_4SCN$. The potentiation produced by three aerosols in combination with $SO_2$ was reported to show a similar ranking.
3. Aerosols of metallic salts capable of catalyzing the oxidation of $SO_2$ to $H_2SO_4$ caused the greatest potentiation. Manganese, ferrous, and vanadium aerosols were tested. However, no direct proof was provided that $H_2SO_4$ was formed in the presence of these salts in the experiments.

---

**FIGURE 9**
(a) Average changes ± SE in $R_L$ for each of six exposure modes. The aerosol was polydispersed with a peak particle count at approximately 0.1 μm diameter, and a peak mass at approximately 0.8 μm diameter. Six animals were exposed a total of 12 times per mode. Exposure lasted 1 hr; measurements were made at about 4-min intervals. The increase in $R_L$ for mode 6 ($SO_2$ + NaCl, high RH) exceeds the other changes by the following: compared to mode 2, $P < 0.05$; compared to modes 1, 3, 4, and 5, $P < 0.01$. (b) Average changes ± SE in $C_L$, dynamic pulmonary compliance. Reduction in $C_L$ for mode 6 ($SO_2$ + NaCl, high RH) is significant at $P < 0.01$; average changes in other modes are not significant. (From Ref. [86].)

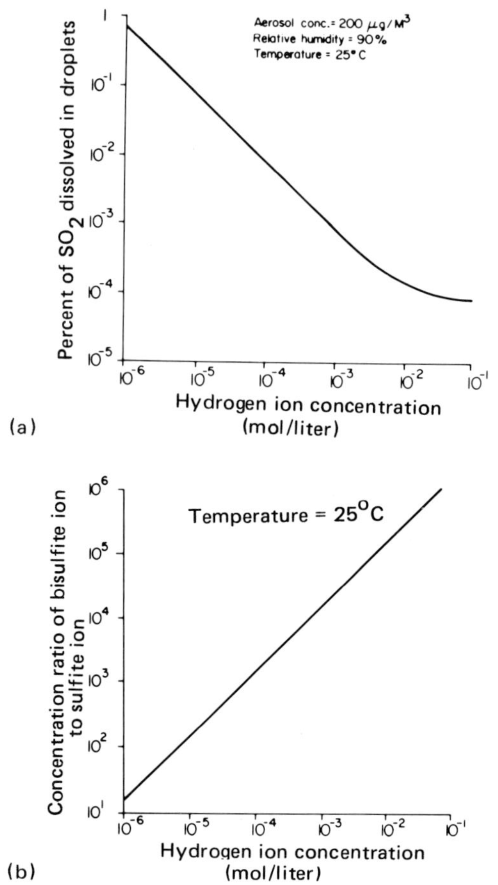


**FIGURE 10** (a) Log-log plot of the molar percentage of $SO_2$ that is physically dissolved versus the hydrogen ion concentration in moles per liter. (A molar concentration of $10^{-4}$ corresponds to a pH of 4.) (b) Log-log plot of the concentration ratio of bisulfite ion to sulfite ion versus the hydrogen ion concentration in moles per liter. For hydrogen ion concentrations greater than $10^{-2}$, the fraction of the dissolved $SO_2$ that dissociates into bisulfite and sulfite decreases significantly. (Courtesy of T. V. Larson.)

Again, the assumption was made in these studies that the interaction between the different aerosols and $SO_2$ occurred in the airways. It is perhaps paradoxical that graphitic carbon (see the first item above) is considered to be an effective catalyst for the oxidation of atmospheric $SO_2$ to $H_2SO_4$ [40], yet it had no potentiating effect. Two other investigative groups have also administered either graphitic [41] or activated [42] carbon in combination with $SO_2$ to animals without finding evidence for synergism. In the latter two studies, the ciliary beat rate in the trachea was measured to test the response.

## IV. Factors That May Modulate Response

This section deals with factors that may control or modify the response of the airways to irritant aerosols. The list is not inclusive. The role that some of these factors may play is speculative, and the intent in presenting them is to encourage further investigation. At the outset it is appropriate to state that bronchoconstriction need not represent the first or most significant response to irritant particles. For example, low doses of sulfuric acid have been shown to depress bronchial clearance in donkeys without altering flow resistance [43].

### A. Reflex Activity

A variety of particles induce reflex bronchoconstriction. They include chemically inert dusts [44-46]; cigarette smoke [45]; citric acid [47]; zinc ammonium sulfate [48], which is an infrequent atmospheric pollutant; and pharmacologic drugs, notably histamine [45,48]. Both afferent and efferent arcs of the reflex appear to run in the pulmonary vagal nerves [48]. Atropine and cooling the vagal nerve prevent or limit the bronchoconstriction.

The nasobronchial reflex has been suggested as an alternative neural pathway for increasing bronchomotor tone, principally to explain the functional effects of sulfur dioxide seen in healthy adults [49]. (Only a small fraction of inhaled $SO_2$ penetrates the nasal passages.) However, in anesthetized animals [50-52], irritation of the nasal mucosa both chemically and mechanically results in bronchial dilatation rather than constriction. The afferent arc of the nasobronchial reflex is formed by the fifth cranial nerve.

Evidence suggests that the sensory component of the bronchoconstrictive reflex is the irritant receptor [46]. This receptor has several other descriptive names, i.e., rapidly adapting, cough, deflation, and expiration receptor. Irritant receptors are most numerous in the larynx and bifurcations of the trachea and bronchi. As noted before, the bifurcations are preferential sites for the deposition of aerosols [53,54]. (There is a close correlation between the deposition efficiency of inhaled particles and the frequency of reported cancer located at bifurcations in the central bronchi [55].) The receptors decrease in number in the peripheral airways. Widdicombe [56] has reviewed evidence that the irritant receptors in central airways are more responsive to mechanical than to chemical stimuli, while the opposite holds for the receptors in small bronchi and bronchioles.

Insoluble dusts are presumed to act as mechanical stimuli. If so, it follows that chemically active aerosols with similar aerodynamic characteristics and (high) mass loadings, may also produce their response through mechanical stimulation. Indeed, changes in the mechanical behavior of the lung from any cause, if associated with distortion, stretching, or distention of the airways, may lead to mechanical stimulation of local irritant receptors. The effect may be cumulative by magnifying any bronchoconstriction that is already present (sometimes referred to as positive feedback) [57]. For this reason it is often difficult to establish primacy between chemical and mechanical stimuli.

There is uncertainty over the size of the field served by a single receptor fiber, an entity that is not easy to delineate. Conceivably the field could vary in size depending on whether the stimulus were mechanical or chemical. Unpublished evidence based on studies of dogs suggests that a field has a diameter of about 1 cm and may overlap its neighbors [58].

The frequency of discharge from isolated irritant receptors has been shown to vary with the type, intensity, and rate of change of the stimulus [57]. Airborne stimuli tested with these preparations include ethyl ether vapor, $NH_3$, histamine, and cigarette smoke; all have been administered in unspecified concentrations [57,59]. Figure 11 shows the increase in the action potentials of a receptor associated with exposure to cigarette smoke (which contains both gases and particulate matter).

### B. Humeral Transmitters

Whether realistic concentrations of soluble particles act directly on tracheobronchial smooth muscle tone, or perhaps cause the release of humeral transmitters, are unresolved questions. (See Chapter 3 for antigen-mediated changes in airway caliber.)

Chares et al. [60] reported that instillation of 1 $\mu$M $(NH_4)_2SO_4$ in isotonic sucrose solution into the tracheas of isolated, perfused, mechanically ventilated rats' lungs was associated with the release of histamine and a decrease in tidal volume. Instilled histamine had the same restrictive effect on ventilation, while isotonic sucrose alone or in combination with 1 $\mu$M sodium sulfate ($Na_2SO_4$) was less effective. They postulated that the ammonium ion acted to depress tidal volume by causing the release of histamine. It should be noted, however, that the dose was considerable. We have estimated that the administration of an equivalent dose of $(NH_4)_2SO_4$ as an aerosol would require about 2 days of continuous exposure, assuming that the aerosol was monodispersed with a diameter of 1 $\mu$m and a density of 2 g/ml, that the ventilatory rate was 100 mg/min, and that all of the inhaled particles were retained. Recent studies in which human volunteers and animals have been exposed acutely to concentrations of $(NH_4)_2SO_4$ aerosol ranging up to several milligrams per cubic meter have failed to demonstrate impairment of pulmonary function [61, 43].

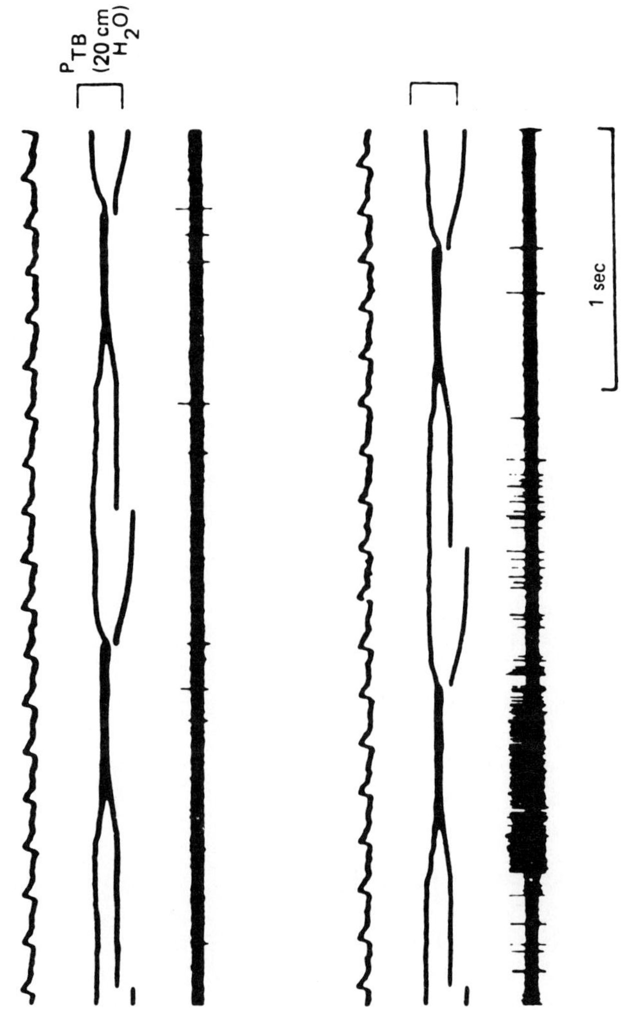


**FIGURE 11** Response of a lung irritant receptor (lowest trace) to inhalation of carbon dust in a rabbit. From above down, blood pressure, tidal volume, transpulmonary pressure, and action potentials in a nerve fiber from the receptor. Upper record, control; lower record, during inhalation of carbon dust, showing increased discharge. (From Ref. [62].)

### C. Mucus

The irritant receptors ramify among the epithelial cells of the airways, apparently within "tight junctions" and may extend virtually to the ciliary layer [62]. (No distinction is made here among the subdivisions of the junctional complex identifiable by electron microscopy.) Consequently, their most superficial terminals are separated from direct contact with airborne contaminants by just the thickness of the mucus layer, plus perhaps the apices of the tight junctions. In rats, the thickness of the mucus is about 8 to 12 $\mu$m (range, 3-15 $\mu$m) in the trachea and diminishes to 2 to 5 $\mu$m (range, 8 $\mu$m to a few tenths of 1 $\mu$m) in the lobar bronchi [63]. There is no information about these dimensions as a function either of airway size or generation for other mammals.

There is controversy at present over whether the mucus layer is continuous and completely covers the underlying epithelium, or is discontinuous so that portions of the epithelial layer come into direct contact with the airstream [64]. If the latter point of view is correct, the likelihood that irritant receptors may be exposed directly to aerosols or gases is of course increased.

It is difficult to judge at what level in the airways mucus, as it is ordinarily defined, ends. The liquid layer in bronchioles is a heterogeneous mixture of reduced "mucoid" consistency that contains secretions from Clara cells and probably also from sources originating in the airspaces [65]. One wonders to what extent the striking vulnerability of the peripheral airways to a variety of contaminants, including cigarette smoke [66,67], ozone [68], and nitrogen dioxide [69,70], is related to the physical and chemical transformations that have overtaken mucus by this level. The alveolar ducts and airspaces just beyond the bronchioles share this vulnerability to pollutants [68-70]. The more distal airspaces are probably buffered from environmental insult by distance (lengthening diffusional pathway) and a sharply expanded surface area.

### D. Host Responsiveness

Orehek et al. [71] have drawn a distinction between the "sensitivity" and "reactivity" of the airways. To do so they established a cumulative dose-response curve to inhaled carbachol with measurements of specific airway conductance ($SG_{aw}$). Bronchial sensitivity was then defined as the estimated dose in milligrams needed to decrease $SG_{aw}$ by 25%. Bronchial reactivity was defined as the slope of the dose-response curve, which was reported to be rectilinear for $SG_{aw}$. They found wide variations in both phenomena among healthy and asthmatic subjects. The two groups were more readily separable in terms of bronchial reactivity than of sensitivity, which was interpreted to mean that different mechanisms were probably involved in the two phenomena. The concept—and the technique—would appear to offer inviting possibilities in assessing the effects of irritant particles among different populations of subjects.

The response of healthy individuals or animals to bronchoconstrictor drugs can be increased either by prior exposure to ozone [72,73] and sulfur dioxide [74], or by upper respiratory viral infections [75]. In some instances the increased responsiveness may persist for weeks [75,72]. It has been suggested that the altered responsiveness is attributable to changes affecting the irritant receptors. Two pieces of supporting evidence are cited. First, the threshold for cough may be lowered in the same individuals [75]; stimulation of irritant receptors is known to induce coughing. Second, inflammation of the epithelial layer of the trachea and bronchi may follow acute exposure to similar concentrations of ozone in animals [76]; such inflammation is likely to involve the receptor directly.

In a similar type of study a group of outpatients with slight to mild asthma were exposed to 0.1 ppm nitrogen dioxide for 1 hr and thereafter exposed to carbachol [77]. There was virtually no effect of the nitrogen dioxide on $SR_{aw}$, but the dose of carbachol needed to raise $SR_{aw}$ by a specified percentage was reduced in over half the subjects. This level of nitrogen dioxide is not uncommonly exceeded in urban air throughout the United States [4]. It may also be exceeded indoors where gas-fueled cooking stoves are used [78].

To date there have been no studies that substituted an irritant atmospheric aerosol for histamine or cholinergic esters to assess altered responsiveness. For example, it would be of interest to determine the response to sulfuric acid following preexposure to ozone, nitrogen, or sulfur dioxide, or in the wake of a viral infection. Such sequences do have their counterparts in daily living. [The concentrations of provocative drugs used in these studies are considerably higher than are the concentrations of sulfate aerosols used in inhalation toxicology. Of course, the sulfates are administered for longer periods of time, so that the total doses in the two circumstances may approach each other. For example, Orehek and associates [71] administered up to 230 $mg/m^3$ carbachol to healthy subjects (total dose about 2 mg), and up to one-tenth that concentration to asthmatic subjects [77]. By contrast, it is unusual for sulfuric acid to be administered to human subjects in concentrations exceeding 1 $mg/m^3$. Acid sulfate levels in and around urban settings have ranged only as high as about 20 $\mu g/m^3$ [17].

Asthma is said to affect about 4% of the population in the United States [79]. How these and other individuals with abnormally reactive airways might respond during controlled exposures to air pollutants is scarcely known. This is due largely to ethical and legal constraints on human experimentation. The need for this information in establishing air quality standards is widely recognized.

### E. Particle pH

A frequently expressed but untested hypothesis to account for the irritant effects of sulfur-containing aerosols is related to pH; that is, the lower the pH of the aerosol the greater will be its irritant potential. The studies of Amdur et al. [80] on guinea pigs provided support for this hypothesis, for $H_2SO_4$ caused the greatest increase in $R_L$ among the sulfates tested at a comparable size and concentration. There were inconsistencies in this theme, however, for $(NH_4)_2SO_4$ (ph $\geqslant 5$) produced a greater rise in $R_L$ than did $NH_4HSO_4$ (pH 1-2). We know of no attempt to measure the changes in the hydrogen ion concentration or electroconductivity of mucus during exposure to acid aerosols or for that matter to $SO_2$, which forms a weakly acid solution upon hydration. The buffering capacity of mucus is not known. Recent developments in microtechniques for the sampling and analysis of mucus should make this information more accessible [81].

Simonsson et al. [47] noted that the bronchoconstrictive reaction to citric acid aerosol in patients with obstructive airway disease occurred within seconds of exposure, but was transient. By contrast, the response to histamine was slower to develop but persisted longer (Fig. 12). The authors suggested that citric acid may have acted by lowering the pH (of mucus) and that the rapid return of flow resistance to control levels may have been attributable to buffering action. The total mass of citric acid delivered to the patients was not specified.

### F. Particle Size

The relation between the size of an inhaled irritant particle and the magnitude of its effect on pulmonary function has been studied in detail by Amdur and associates. They used both zinc ammonium sulfate [$ZnSO_4 \cdot (NH_4)_2SO_4$] and $H_2SO_4$. The results with $ZnSO_4 \cdot (NH_4)_2SO_4$, which ranged in size from 0.3 to 1.4 $\mu$m in diameter by weight, are shown in Figure 13. Guinea pigs were tested.

The increase in $R_L$ per unit mass concentration was greater the smaller the particle. At an equal number of particles per unit volume (different mass concentration), the larger particles were more effective in raising $R_L$.

It is reasonable to assume that a larger irritant particle will evoke more response than a smaller one of identical composition if both land at the same site. Why the larger particles in this study should have been more effective on an equal-number basis, and the smaller particles more effective on an equal-mass basis, is not apparent. The authors pointed out that differences in total uptake and local patterns of deposition might be expected for the various sizes, but that the implications of these differences for changes in $R_L$ were uncertain.

Based on empirical data from human studies [7] and calculations made for an idealized rat lung [82], a lower overall deposition efficiency would be expected

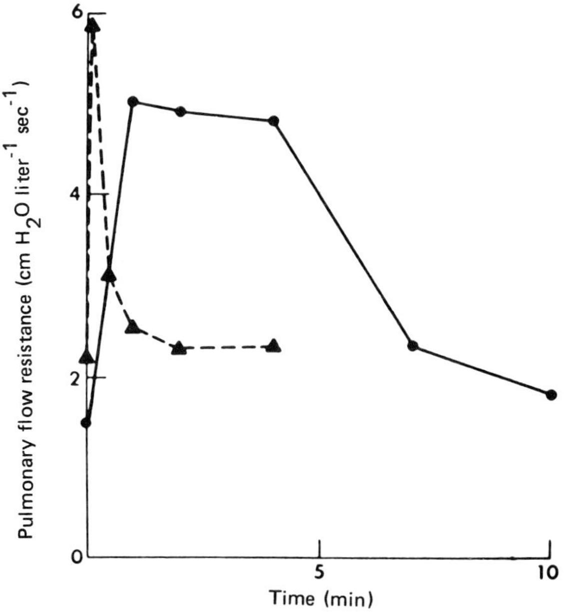


**FIGURE 12** Comparison of time course of changes in total lung resistance ($R_L$) after inhalation of one breath of 20% citric acid aerosol (dashed line) and after inhalation of 10 breaths of 0.01% histamine phosphate aerosol (solid line) in the patient. Added note: The pH of the citric acid solution is estimated to be less than 2. (From Ref. [47].)

for the smallest particle used in the study on guinea pigs, by Amdur and Corn (0.3 $\mu$m), than for the largest one (1.4 $\mu$m), especially following their hygroscopic growth. (Unfortunately, the measurements currently available on particle deposition as a function of size in guinea pigs are meager [82].)

A related parameter that may have bearing on the magnitude of response is the surface area of the irritant particle. For a given mass of particles the total surface area will increase as the diameter is reduced according to the following relation: surface/volume = 6/diameter. (In general, the surface area influences the rate of reaction between liquid particles and surrounding gases. Similarly, if the particles are relatively insoluble, the rate at which they enter solution following deposition in the respiratory system and their reactivity with the surrounding tissues will be proportional to their surface area.)

The changes in $R_L$ induced by $H_2SO_4$ were also influenced by particle size [83]. At equivalent concentrations, particles of 0.3 $\mu$m in mass mean

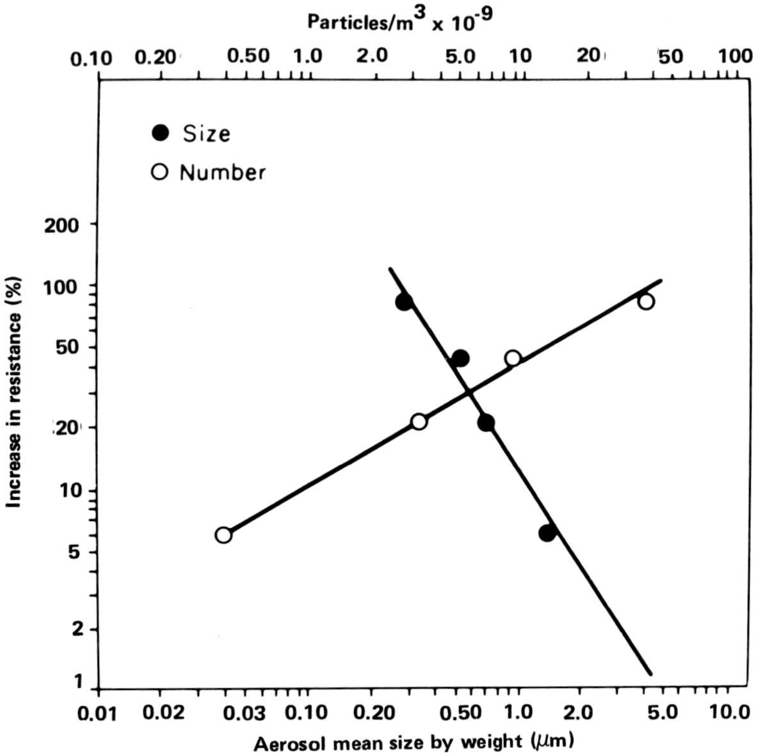


**FIGURE 13** Relationship of the percentage increase in resistance to the diameter of aerosol and to the number of particles at equal mass concentration. (From Ref. [47]. Reprinted with permission; © 1963, Pergamon Press, Ltd., New York.)

diameter (MMD) were more effective in increasing $R_L$ than were particles of 2.6 μm MMD. Again, there is no obvious explanation. Indeed, the larger droplets of $H_2SO_4$ might be expected to be more irritating for reasons that were considered earlier in the chapter: That is, hygroscopic growth and neutralization by $NH_3$, both of which lower the hydrogen ion concentration, would be expected to proceed less rapidly in the larger particles. The larger particles of inhaled $H_2SO_4$ are therefore likely to be more acid than the smaller particles at the instant of deposition. However, an analysis of this sort is complicated by the fact that the deposition efficiencies of the two sizes of particles will vary for different portions of the respiratory tract (see Figs. 2 and 3). The guinea pig, an obligatory nose breather, should filter out a significantly larger fraction of the 2.6-μm particles than of the 0.3-μm particles in the nasopharynx, a factor acting to mitigate the direct effect of the larger particles on the lower airways. On the other hand, of the particles that reach the trachea a greater fraction of the larger ones are expected to deposit within the lower airways, a factor favoring their irritant potential over that of the smaller ones. It would not be surprising if the relative effects of these two sizes were to vary in human subjects depending on whether exposure was by nose or moutn.

## V. Air Quality Standards

The Occupational Safety and Health Administration (OSHA) has established regulations for the working place covering a number of specific airborne particles and dusts. The standard for sulfuric acid is 1 mg/m$^3$ based on a 10-hr workday, 40-hr work week.

The present national ambient air standard for total suspended particulates (TSP) does not specify size distribution or chemical composition. It is set for two averaging times:

| | |
|---|---|
| 75 $\mu$g/m$^3$ | annual geometric mean |
| 260 $\mu$g/m$^3$ | maximum 24-hr mean |

This 24-hr level is not to be exceeded more than once a year at any monitoring station.

There is general agreement that the TSP standard is ambiguous and should be refined. An effort is underway to incorporate into the national air-sampling network (NASN) a sampling method that segregates airborne particles according to size. Out of this effort, which is to be matched with health surveys, should come a standard for the accumulation mode.

Whether the results of toxicological and epidemiological research over the next several years will justify a chemical standard for airborne particles is moot. Currently there are few data on the sulfur-bearing particles except as "total sulfate ions." Explicit information of this type is needed. The technical difficulties of acquiring these data are considerable, so that NASN, which of necessity depends on procedures that are standardized and readily performed, would appear to be an inappropriate instrument for achieving this goal. Instead, research carried out by scientists will be required.

The CHESS Report of 1974 [84] prepared by the Environmental Protection Agency increased concern over the hazards posed by sulfur-containing aerosols. The report has since been severely criticized for deficiencies in its design, execution, and interpretation. Nonetheless, there is still reason for concern. The National Energy Plan of 1977 called for an increasing reliance on coal in the decades immediately ahead, a policy that underscores the need for more information about the biologic effects of these compounds.

## References

1. Lapp, N. L., J. L. Hankinson, H. Amandus, and E. D. Palmes, Variability in the size of airspaces in normal human lungs as estimated by aerosols, *Thorax,* **30**:293-299 (1975).
2. Yeates, D. B., N. Aspin, H. Levison, M. T. Jones, and A. C. Bryan, Mucociliary tracheal transport rates in man, *J. Appl. Physiol.,* **39**:487-495 (1975).
3. National Academy of Sciences, *Airborne Particles.* Subcommittee on Airborne Particles, Committee on Medical and Biologic Effects of Environmental Pollutants, National Academy of Sciences, Washington, D.C. (1977).
4. National Academy of Sciences, *Nitrogen Oxides.* Committee on Medical and Biologic Effects of Environmental Pollutants, National Academy of Sciences, Washington, D.C. (1977).
5. National Academy of Sciences, *Ozone and Other Photochemical Oxidants.* Committee on Medical and Biologic Effects of Environmental Pollutants, National Academy of Sciences, Washington, D.C. (1977).
6. National Academy of Sciences, *Sulfur Oxides.* Committee on Sulfur Oxides, National Academy of Sciences, Washington, D.C. (1978).
7. Hounam, R. F., and A. Morgan, Particle deposition. In *Respiratory Defense Mechanisms,* Vol. 5, Part 1. Edited by J. D. Brain, D. F. Proctor, and L. M. Reid. New York-Basel, Marcel Dekker, 1977, pp. 125-156.
8. Morrow, P. E., Clearance kinetics of inhaled particles. In *Respiratory Defense Mechanisms,* Vol. 5, Part 2. Edited by J. D. Brain, D. F. Proctor, and L. M. Reid. New York-Basel, Marcel Dekker, 1977, pp. 491-543.
9. Andersen, I., The ambient air. In *Respiratory Defense Mechanisms,* Vol. 5, Part 1. Edited by J. D. Brain, D. F. Proctor, and L. M. Reid. New York-Basel, Marcel Dekker, 1977, pp. 25-62.
10. Morgan, M. S., and R. Frank, Uptake of pollutant gases by the respiratory system. In *Respiratory Defense Mechanisms,* Vol. 5, Part 1. Edited by J. D. Brain, D. F. Proctor, and L. M. Reid. New York-Basel, Marcel Dekker, 1977, pp. 157-189.
11. Butcher, S. S., and R. J. Charlson, *An Introduction to Air Chemistry.* New York, Academic, 1972.
12. Herdan, G., *Small Particle Statistics,* 2nd ed. London, Butterworths, 1960.
13. Hidy, G. (ed.), *Characterization of Aerosols in California.* Final Report, Air Resources Board, State of California, 1974.
14. Cronn, D., Analysis of atmospheric aerosols by high resolution mass spectrometry. Ph.D. Dissertation, University of Washington, Seattle, Washington, 1975.
15. Finlayson, B. J., and J. N. Pitts, Jr., Photochemistry of the polluted troposphere, *Science,* **192**:111-119 (1976).

16. Brosset, C., Water-soluble sulphur compounds in aerosols, *Atmos. Environ.*, **12**:25-38 (1978).
17. Charlson, R. J., A. H. Vanderpol, D. S. Covert, A. P. Waggoner, and N. C. Ahlquist, $H_2SO_4/(NH_4)SO_4$ background aerosol: Optical detection in St. Louis region, *Atmos. Environ.*, **8**:1257-1268 (1974).
18. Weiss, R. E., A. P. Waggoner, R. J. Charlson, and N. C. Ahlquist, Sulfate aerosol: Its geographical extent in the midwestern and southern United States, *Science,* **195**:979-981 (1977).
19. Vanderpol, A. H., F. D. Carsey, D. S. Covert, R. J. Charlson, and A. P. Waggoner, Aerosol chemical parameters and air mass character in the St. Louis region, *Science,* **190**:570 (1975).
20. Glasstone, G., *Textbook of Physical Chemistry.* New York, Van Nostrand, 1959, p. 1320.
21. Orr, C., F. K. Hurd, and W. J. Corbett, Aerosol size and relative humidity, *J. Colloid Interface Sci.,* **13**:472-482 (1958).
22. Kerth, C. H., and A. B. Arons, The growth of sea salt particles by condensation of atmospheric water vapor, *J. Meteorol.,* **11**:173-184 (1953).
23. Tang, I. N., Phase transformation and growth of aerosol particles composed of mixed salts, *J. Aerosol Sci.,* **7**:361-371 (1976).
24. Winkler, P., and C. Junge, The growth of atmospheric aerosol particles as a function of the relative humidity. I. Methods and measurements of different locations, *J. Rech. Atmos.,* **6**:617-638 (1972).
25. Charlson, R. J., D. S. Covert, T. V. Larson, and A. P. Waggoner, Chemical properties of tropospheric sulfur aerosols, *Atmos. Environ.,* **12**:39-53 (1978).
26. Task Group on Lung Dynamics for Committee II of the International Commission on Radiological Protection, Deposition and retention models, *Health Phys.,* **12**:173-208 (1966).
27. Morrow, P. E., Aerosol characterization and deposition, *Am. Rev. Respir. Dis.,* **110**(6) Part 2:88-99 (1974).
28. Natusch, D. F. S., and J. R. Wallace, Urban aerosol toxicity: The influence of particle size, *Science,* **186**:695 (1974).
29. Larson, T. V., D. S. Covert, R. Frank, and R. J. Charlson, Ammonia in the human airways: Neutralization of inspired acid sulfate aerosols, *Science,* **197**:161-163 (1977).
30. Larson, T. V., D. S. Covert, and R. Frank, Respiratory $NH_3$: A possible defense against inhaled acid sulfate compounds. In *Environmental Stress: Individual Human Adaptation.* Edited by J. L. Folinsbee, J. A. Wagner, J. F. Borgia, B. L. Drinkwater, J. A. Gliner, and J. F. Beadi. New York, Academic, 1978, pp. 91-99.
31. Larson, T. V., D. S. Covert, and R. Frank, A method for continuous measurement of ammonia in respiratory airways, *J. Appl. Physiol.,* **46**:603-607 (1979).
32. Amdur, M. O., The effect of aerosols on the response to irritant gases. In *Inhaled Particles and Vapours.* Edited by C. M. Davies. Oxford, Pergamon, 1961, pp. 281-292.

33. Amdur, M. O., and D. Underhill, The effect of various aerosols on the response of guinea pigs to sulfur dioxide, *Arch. Environ. Health,* **16**:460–468 (1968).
34. La Belle, C. W., J. E. Long, and E. E. Christofano, Synergistic effects of aerosols, *Arch. Ind. Health,* **11**:297-304 (1955).
35. McJilton, C., R. Frank, and R. Charlson, Role of relative humidity in the synergistic effect of a sulfur dioxide-aerosol mixture on the lung, *Science,* **182**:503-504 (1973).
36. Frank, N. R., R. E. Yoder, J. D. Brain, and E. Yokoyama, $SO_2$ ($^{35}S$ labelled) absorption by the nose and mouth under conditions of varying concentration and flow, *Arch. Environ. Health,* **18**:315-322 (1969).
37. Speizer, F. E., and N. R. Frank, The uptake and release of $SO_2$ by the human nose, *Arch. Environ. Health,* **12**:725-728 (1966).
38. Proctor, D. F., Physiology of the upper airways. In *Handbook of Physiology,* Section 3, *Respiration,* Vol. I. Edited by W. D. Fenn and H. Rahn. Baltimore, Waverly Press, 1965, pp. 309-345.
39. Amdur, M. O., The long road from Donora. 1974 Cummings Memorial Lecture, *Am. Ind. Hyg. Assoc. J.,* **35**:589-597 (1974).
40. Novakov, T., S. G. Chang, and A. B. Harker, Sulfates as pollution particulates: Catalytic formation on carbon (soot) particles, *Science,* **186**:259-261 (1974).
41. Fraser, D. A., M. C. Battigelli, and H. M. Cole, Ciliary activity and pulmonary retention of inhaled dust in rats exposed to sulfur dioxide, *J. Air Pollut. Control Assoc.,* **18**:821-823 (1968).
42. Dalhamn, T., and L. Strandberg, Synergism between $SO_2$ and carbon particles. Studies on adsorption and on ciliary movements in the rabbit trachea in vivo, *Int. J. Air Water Pollut.,* **7**:517-529 (1963).
43. Schlesinger, R. B., M. Lippmann, and R. E. Albert, Effects of short-term exposures to sulfuric acid and ammonium sulfate aerosols upon bronchial airway function in the donkey, *Am. Ind. Hyg. Assoc. J.,* **39**:275-286 (1978).
44. DuBois, A. B., and L. Dautrebande, Acute effects of breathing inert dust particles and carbachol aerosol on the mechanical characteristics of the lungs in man. Changes in response after inhaling sympathomimetic aerosols, *J. Clin. Invest.,* **37**:1746-1755 (1958).
45. Sellick, H., and J. G. Widdicombe, Stimulation of lung irritant receptors by cigarette smoke, carbon dust, and histamine aerosol, *J. Appl. Physiol.,* **31**:15-19 (1971).
46. Widdicombe, J. G., D. C. Kent, and J. A. Nadel, Mechanism of bronchoconstriction during inhalation of dust, *J. Appl. Physiol.,* **17**:613-616 (1962).
47. Simonsson, B. G., F. M. Jacobs, and J. A. Nadel, Role of autonomic nervous system and the cough reflex in the increased responsiveness of airways in patients with obstructive airway disease, *J. Clin. Invest.,* **46**:1812-1818 (1967).
48. Nadel, J. A., M. Corn, S. Zwi, J. Flexch, and P. Graf, Location and mechanism of airway constriction after inhalation of histamine aerosol and inor-

ganic sulfate aerosol. In *Inhaled Particles and Vapours.* Edited by C. N. Davies. Oxford, Pergamon, 1967, pp. 55-67.

49. Andersen, I., G. R. Lundquist, P. L. Jenson, and D. F. Proctor, Human exposure to controlled levels of sulfur dioxide, *Arch. Environ. Health,* **28**: 31-39 (1974).
50. Allison, D. J., T. P. Clay, J. M. B. Hughes, H. A. Jones, and A. Shevis, Effects of nasal stimulation on total respiratory resistance in the rabbit (abstract), *J. Physiol. (London),* **239**:23P-24P (1974).
51. Nadel, J. A., and J. G. Widdicombe, Reflex effects of upper airway irritation on total lung resistance and blood pressure, *J. Appl. Physiol.,* **17**:861-865 (1962).
52. Tomori, Z., and J. G. Widdicombe, Muscular bronchomotor and cardiovascular reflexes elicited by mechanical stimulation of the respiratory tract, *J. Physiol. (London),* **200**:25-49(1969).
53. Bell, K. A., and S. K. Friedlander, Aerosol deposition in models of a human lung bifurcation, *Staub-Reinhalt. Luft,* **33**:178-182 (1973).
54. Schlesinger, R. B., and M. Lippmann, Particle deposition in casts of the human upper tracheobronchial tree, *Am. Ind. Hyg. Assoc. J.,* **33**:237-251 (1972).
55. Schlesinger, R. B., and M. Lippmann, Selective particle deposition and bronchogenic carcinoma, *Environ. Res.,* **15**:424-431 (1978).
56. Widdicombe, J. G., Regulation of tracheobronchial smooth muscle, *Physiol. Rev.,* **43**:1-37 (1963).
57. Mills, J. E., H. Sellick, and J. G. Widdicombe, Activity of lung irritant receptors in pulmonary micro-embolism, anaphylaxis and drug-induced bronchoconstrictions, *J. Physiol. (London),* **203**:337-357 (1969).
58. Widdicombe, J. G., Cited as a personal communication from G. Sant'Ambrogio in Studies on afferent airway innervation, *Am. Rev. Respir. Dis.,* **115**(6) Part 2:99-105 (1977).
59. Widdicombe, J. G., and G. M. Sterling, The autonomic nervous system and breathing, *Arch. Intern. Med.,* **126**:311-329 (1970).
60. Charles, J. M., W. G. Anderson, and D. B. Menzel, Sulfate absorption from the airways of the isolated perfused rat lung, *Toxicol. Appl. Pharmacol.,* **41**:91-99 (1977).
61. Sackner, M. A., D. Ford, R. Fernandez, E. D. Michaelson, R. M. Schreck, and A. Wanner, Effect of sulfate aerosols on cardiopulmonary function of normal humans, *Am. Rev. Respir. Dis.,* **115**(4) Part 2:240 (1977) (abstract)
62. Widdicombe, J. G., Reflex control of airways smooth muscle, *Postgrad. Med. J.,* **51** (Suppl. 7):36-43 (1975).
63. Luchtel, D. L., The mucous layer of the trachea and major bronchi in the rat, *Scanning Electron Microscopy,* **2**:1089-1095 (1978).
64. Van As, A., Pulmonary airway clearance mechanisms: A reappraisal, *Am. Rev. Respir. Dis.,* **115**:721-726 (1977).
65. Faridy, E. E., Effect of ventilation of movement of surfactant in airways, *Respir. Physiol.,* **27**:323-334 (1976).

66. Dosman, J., F. Bode, J. Urbanetti, R. Martin, and P. T. Macklem, The use of a helium-oxygen mixture during maximum expiratory flow to demonstrate obstruction in small airways in smokers, *J. Clin. Invest.*, **55**:1090-1099 (1975).
67. McCarthy, D. S., R. Spencer, R. Guene, and J. Milic-Emili, Measurement of "closing volume" as a simple and sensitive test for early detection of small airway disease, *Am. J. Med.*, **52**:747-753 (1972).
68. Freeman, G., R. J. Stephens, D. L. Coffin, and J. F. Stara, Changes in dogs' lungs after long-term exposure to ozone. Light and electron microscopy, *Arch. Environ. Health,* **26**:209-216 (1973).
69. Evans, M. J., R. J. Stephens, L. J. Cabral, and G. Freeman, Cell renewal in the lungs of rats exposed to low levels of $NO_2$, *Arch. Environ. Health,* **24**: 180-188 (1972).
70. Stephens, R. J., G. Freeman, and M. J. Evans, Early response of lungs to low levels of nitrogen dioxide. Light and electron microscopy, *Arch. Environ. Health,* **24**:160-179 (1972).
71. Orehek, J., P. Gayrard, A. P. Smith, C. Grimaud, and J. Charpin, Airway response to carbachol in normal and asthmatic subjects. Distinction between bronchial sensitivity and reactivity, *Am. Rev. Respir. Dis.*, **115**:937-943 (1977).
72. Golden, J. A., J. A. Nadel, and H. A. Boushey, Bronchial hyperirritability in healthy subjects after exposure to ozone, *Am. Rev. Respir. Dis.*, **118**(2): 287-294 (1978).
73. Lee, L.-Y., E. R. Bleecker, and J. A. Nadel, Effect of ozone on the bronchomotor response to inhaled histamine aerosol in dogs, *J. Appl. Physiol.*, **43**:626-631 (1977).
74. Islam, M. S., E. Vastag, and W. T. Ulmer, Sulfur-dioxide induced bronchial reactivity against acetylcholine, *Int. Arch. Arbeitsmed.*, **29**:221-232 (1972).
75. Empey, D. W., L. A. Laitinen, L. Jacobs, W. M. Gold, and J. A. Nadel, Mechanisms of bronchial hyperreactivity in normal subjects after upper respiratory tract infection, *Am. Rev. Respir. Dis.*, **113**:131-139 (1976).
76. Boatman, E. S., S. Sato, and R. Frank, Acute effects of ozone on cat lungs, *Am. Rev. Respir. Dis.*, **110**:157-169 (1974).
77. Orehek, J., J. P. Masari, P. Gayrard, C. Grimaud, and J. Charpin, Effect of short-term, low-level nitrogen dioxide exposure on bronchial sensitivity of asthmatic patients, *J. Clin. Invest.*, **57**:301-307 (1976).
78. Wade, W. A., III, W. A. Cote, and J. E. Yocom, A study of indoor air quality, *J. Air Pollut. Control Assoc.*, **25**:933-939 (1975).
79. Davis, J. J., NIAID initiatives in allergy research, *J. Allergy Clin. Immunol.*, **49**:323-328 (1972).
80. Amdur, M. E., J. Bayles, V. Ugro, M. Dubriel, and D. W. Underhill, Respiratory response of guinea pigs to sulfuric acid and sulfate salts. Paper presented at the Sumposium on Sulfur Pollution and Research Approaches, May 27-28, 1975. Sponsored by U.S. Environmental Protection Agency and Duke University Medical Center, 1975.

81. Nadel, J. A., Autonomic control of airway smooth muscle and airway secretions, *Am. Rev. Respir. Dis.*, **115**(6) Part 2:117-126 (1977).
82. Granito, S. M., Calculated retention of aerosol particles in the rat lung. M.S. Dissertation, Division of Biological Sciences, Pritzker School of Medicine, University of Chicago, Chicago, Illinois, 1971.
83. Amdur, M. O., Animal studies. In *National Academy of Sciences Proceedings of the Conference on Health Effects of Air Pollutants,* Washington, D.C., October 3-5, 1973. U.S. Government Printing Office, Washington, D.C., 1973, pp. 175-205.
84. CHESS (Community Health and Environmental Surveillance System), *Health Consequences of Sulfur Oxides:* A Report from CHESS, 1970-1971. U.S. Environmental Protection Agency, Office of Research and Development, National Research Center, Research Triangle Park, N.C. 27711, 1974.
85. Charlson, R. J., N. C. Ahlquist, A. Selvidge, and P. B. MacCready, Monitoring of atmospheric aerosol parameters with the integrating nephelometer, *J. Air Pollut. Control Assoc.*, **19**:937-942 (1969).
86. McJilton, C. E., R. Frank, and R. J. Charlson, Influence of relative humidity on functional effects of an inhaled $SO_2$-aerosol mixture, *Am. Rev. Respir. Dis.*, **113**:163-169 (1976).
87. Amdur, M. O., and M. Corn, The irritant potency of zinc ammonium sulfate of different particle sizes, *Am. Ind. Hyg. Assoc. J.*, **24**:326-333 (1963).

# 7

# Clinical Application and Interpretation of Airway Physiology

*E. R. McFADDEN, JR., and ROLAND H. INGRAM, JR.*

Peter Bent Brigham Hospital
and Harvard Medical School
Boston, Massachusetts

The preceding chapters have presented specific details of various aspects of the structure and function of the lung. From this information it is clear that even under normal circumstances the lung is a complicated organ system and to understand its operation requires some knowledge of the interrelations of such diverse areas as morphology, cellular biology, biochemistry, aerobiology, immunology, neuropharmacology, and physiology. In disease states the situation is even more complex in that alterations can occur in any of these indices of respiratory function, and the possible combination of abnormalities due to specific illnesses or lesions of specific sites is almost staggering. However, in practical everyday terms, the basis for functional assessments is not derived from a systematic evaluation of each aspect of the system, but solely from investigating the characteristics of the lung's physiology and neuropharmacology, and, by and large, structure is inferred from the results of this information. Despite the limitations inherent in this approach, appropriate testing and analysis can result in considerable knowledge for

---

Supported in part by Research Career Development Award from the National Heart, Lung, and Blood Institute (McFadden).

both clinical and research purposes about a given individual's problem. The purposes of this chapter are to review the various physiologic assessments of the airways and parenchyma and to analyze the relative contributions of each to the understanding of any functional abnormalities. In addition, the pertinent pharmacologic and physiologic data relevant to understanding the determinants of normal airway caliber, and the sites and mechanisms of airway obstruction, will be explored.

## I. Measurements of Pulmonary Mechanics

From a teleologic standpoint, lungs evolved to allow the human and other species to effect gas exchange for cellular metabolism in a terrestrial environment. Therefore, it would seem reasonable to suppose that the only germane test of lung function would be measurements of the arterial gas tensions. However, since the reserve of the lung is so large, its mechanical function can be seriously compromised by a disease process while its gas-exchanging abilities remain minimally affected. Since this holds true for other parameters as well, there consequently is no single test that can measure, or reflect, all aspects of respiration. For this reason, a multiplicity of methods have evolved, each with unique advantages and disadvantages.

The techniques that are currently in use to measure pulmonary mechanics can be conveniently divided into those that employ submaximal or maximal respiratory efforts on the part of the subject. Examples of the former are measurements of pulmonary resistance, airway resistance, respiratory system resistance, and dynamic compliance. These are all measured during spontaneous tidal respirations and provide a direct assessment of the impedance to breathing. The maximum effort techniques are the oldest and consist of either an analysis of expired volume as a function of time (spirometry) or instantaneous airflow as a function of the volume expelled (maximum expiratory flow volume curves, MEFV). However, these indices of lung function only indirectly assess the state of patency of the airways. As will subsequently be discussed, all the above measures are heavily dependent upon lung volume.

The direct measures make use of the pressure-volume and flow interrelations of the lung. In general terms, to cause any mechanical system to move or change velocity while moving, it is necessary to apply sufficient force to overcome its elastic, frictional, and inertial properties. In the lung inertia is negligible and can be ignored [1] at all but high frequencies [2]. Hence, to move air, the pressure created is dissipated in overcoming only elasticity and resistance.

The elastic properties of the lung are assessed by examining recoil pressures as a function of lung volume under no-flow conditions. This relationship is curvilinear over the volume range and demonstrates that the lungs become stiffer as they approach total lung capacity (TLC). The parameter used to assess elasticity is called compliance and is defined as the change in pressure associated with the change of a given volume of air. In clinical practice this can be measured in two ways. One is by computing the slope of the deflational limb of the pressure-volume curve in the tidal volume range to give static compliance. The second is to relate volume to pressure at points of no flow during spontaneous respiration. The latter has been given the notation "dynamic compliance."

Pulmonary resistance consists of airway and tissue components. The former is an estimate of the friction produced between the air and the conducting airway while the latter represents pressure losses due to the viscosity of the lung parenchyma. Both dynamic compliance and pulmonary resistance can be obtained by estimating pleural pressure with an esophageal balloon while airflow and tidal volume are simultaneously recorded. Airway resistance ($R_{aw}$) can be measured separately with a whole-body plethysmograph by determining the pressure within the alveolus and relating that to airflow.

The indirect measures, spirometry and MEFV curves, are technically simple to perform. Consequently they have enjoyed widespread clinical application. Despite this experience their interpretation can be difficult, for the results are influenced not only by the caliber of the airways, but also by the elastic recoil of the lungs, the volume of air in communication with the airways, the muscle power generated by the subject, and the subject's cooperation.

The physiologic events being measured during a forced exhalation are as follows. The driving force for the movement of air out of the lungs is alveolar pressure, which represents the algebraic sum of the pressure within the pleural space and the elastic reocil. During a maximum forced expiration, pleural pressure becomes positive in sign and increases progressively, as does alveolar pressure. As this happens, the movement of gas from the lungs is accelerated until a point is reached where the pressure surrounding the airways exceeds the pressure within them and they become compressed. In normal subjects this is believed to happen in the bronchi close to the carina [3]. When this narrowing occurs the flow of air reaches a maximum at a given lung volume and then follows a plateau. This has been given the notation of flow limitation. Since flow will not increase further regardless of how much additional effort the subject expends, it is said to be effort independent [4]. This phenomenon is first seen when the lungs have emptied about 15% of their volume, and continues to occur until all the air has been expelled.

Normal individuals cannot generate the critical transbronchial pressure necessary for airway compression high in the vital capacity because of the limitations imposed by respiratory muscle mechanics, properties of the airway walls or lumina, or some combination thereof. Thus, the early part of expiration is said to be effort dependent because flow will increase in proportion to the subject's efforts.

The factors that dominate the early part of a forced expiration (effort-dependent section) are the rapidity of contraction of the expiratory muscles, the elastic recoil at full inflation, and the state of patency of the large central airways [5,6]. The effort-independent portion reflects the resistance within the so-called upstream segment or flow-limiting segment (see below) and the recoil pressure of the lung [6].

## II. Determinants of Maximum Expiratory Flow

From the above it can be appreciated that maximal expiratory flow at any lung volume over the effort-independent range is the result of the dynamic interplay between airway resistance, airway compliance, and the static recoil pressure of the lung. Currently there are three theories regarding the determinants of maximal expiratory flow. These are the "equal pressure point" theory of Mead et al. [6], the "Starling resistor" model of Pride et al. [7] and the "wave speed" theory of Dawson and Elliott [8].

The equal pressure point theory is based upon the fact that during forced expiration, when pleural pressures become quite positive, there are points in the airway where lateral pressure is equal to pleural pressure (i.e., equal pressure points, or EPP). When this occurs the pressure difference from alveoli to EPP is the static recoil pressure of the lung. Airways mouthward from EPP have a greater pressure outside than inside and are thus subjected to a compressive force which causes narrowing to an extent determined by the transbronchial pressure gradient and the compliance of these airways. When the resistance of this compressed segment increases in direct proportion to pleural pressure, further increases in flow at that lung volume are prevented, and EPP become fixed at a location alveolarward from this segment. In this theory the airways can be thought of as being composed of two segments in series: an upstream segment running from the alveoli to the EPP and a downstream segment from EPP to the mouth. At flow limitation the magnitude of the expiratory flow is set by the static recoil pressure and the resistance of the upstream segment. Thus the EPP analysis requires only consideration of events upstream or alveolarward from EPP.

The Starling resistor concept differs from the EPP theory in that it requires consideration of events in the compressed segment downstream from EPP. A Starling resistor most often is composed of a tube that collapses when there is no distending pressure (i.e., zero transmural pressure). If the airways behaved in such a fashion, then collapse would occur at the equal pressure point when it was in the trachea at the thoracic outlet. In such a situation there would be no conflict between the Starling resistor and EPP theories, and by analogy flow would be limited when pleural pressure equaled zero. Since this does not occur, the

Starling resistor model was modified to include a critical transmural pressure at which airways would narrow sufficiently to limit flow. Thus the driving pressure across airways alveolarward from such segments would be the pleural pressure minus the critical transmural pressure. By definition, then, such segments would include all airways upstream from EPP and that portion of the downstream airways between EPP and the point of narrowing. In the final analysis both concepts provide the insight that lung elastic recoil is either the major or the sole driving pressure for maximal flow.

The wave speed theory represents an attempt to explain flow limitation in airways from principles derived from fluid mechanics. It proposes that when the local flow velocity through a tube reaches the local speed of wave propagation within the wall of that tube, flow limitation will occur. Its attraction is that since wave speed propagation is a function of area and the elastic properties of the tube, any process that reduces the cross-sectional area of the airways will reduce propagation and cause flow limitation earlier than normal. In many respects this approach is a more precise quantitation of the Starling resistor model. As of this writing, the principles of this theory have not yet been tested in human lungs.

Given the information presented to date, it would seem that when confronted with the need to obtain an assessment of pulmonary function, a thorough approach would be to evaluate the volume, flow, and pressure characteristics of the lung as well as the integrity of its gas-exchanging abilities to obtain the most complete overview possible. In order to achieve this goal, a battery of tests must be performed, such as static lung volumes, forced exhalation and/or measures of airway resistance or one of its analogs, and arterial blood gases. Although this can be readily accomplished in most clinical settings, interpretation of the results tends to be a function of the patterns of abnormalities found rather than a precise analysis of what each test measures and how they interrelate. For example, diseases associated with airway obstruction will be statistically associated with characteristic changes in lung volumes and spirometric indices. Residual volume (RV), functional residual capacity (FRC), and occasionally TLC will be elevated and the lungs will empty slowly during forced maneuvers so that forced expiratory volumes and flow rates will all be depressed [9]. Consequently, when all or some of these alterations are observed, the patient is said to have an "obstructive ventilatory defect" and severity is judged by the observed degree of deviation from predicted norms. A further limitation is that with this battery it is not possible to determine if the abnormalities encountered are due primarily to involvement of airways or of parenchyma. Therefore, the tests are often repeated after the administration of a bronchodilator and some assessment of "reversibility" is made. The converse approach is also frequently taken. A patient may be given a bronchoconstrictor substance and, if the response exceeds some arbitrary, predetermined limit, he or she is said to show increased airway reactivity and is frequently given the diagnosis of asthma.

Although, at first glance, it may appear difficult to explain why pattern reading is more often used than precise analysis, disease processes involve the lungs and airways nonhomogeneously and often only patterns emerge from these lumped measurements. The more nearly homogeneous the lungs are, the more precise the interpretations of the measurements can be. In analyzing the normal situation, this approach is simplified, since conceptually the above tests can be thought of as dealing with the lung parenchyma and airways in terms of flows as a consequence of a single driving pressure, and lung volume as an index of the geometry of the system. Although not all interpretations will depend upon there being one degree of freedom (i.e., each part moves in the same proportion to its fellows as a direct and repeatable function of a single applied pressure), as a first approximation it is useful to think of there being an airway resistance, a static recoil pressure, and a maximal expiratory flow at any given lung volume. This lumped view of the airways and lung, despite its being an oversimplification, can provide valuable information at both practical and basic levels, and can serve as a framework for examining airway and parenchymal interactions. Further, it allows detection of primary changes in airway caliber independent of concomitant lung volume changes.

Perhaps the most easily understood example of airway parenchymal interactions is the dependency of airway resistance on lung volume [10,11]. Normally, because the airways are imbedded and tethered in the parenchyma and are not rigid structures, they of necessity participate in the volume change of the lungs. During inspiration they lengthen and widen and during expiration they undergo the converse changes. The effects of increasing radial dimensions on resistance far outweighs the axial changes, since in the latter situation resistance is directly proportional to length and in the former situation resistance is inversely proportional to the fourth or fifth power of the radius, depending upon flow regimes [12]. Thus at higher lung volumes resistance is low and increases hyperbolically at lower lung volumes (Fig. 1a). When resistance is expressed as its reciprocal, conductance, the relation between volume and airway dimensions becomes direct and approximately linear (Fig. 1b). [10]. Thus lung size compensation expressed as conductance divided by the volume at which the measurement was made (termed specific conductance, $SG_{aw}$) allows comparisons between individuals and between states in the same subject. For example, in Figure 1b a single conductance value is shown to give two widely different $SG_{aw}$ values, a phenomenon often seen in obstructive airway disease with either acute or chronic hyperinflation. Such an abnormal relation between volume and conductance could mean either that the airways have become stiffer as they become smaller, or that there has been a loss of airway support by the parenchyma. When these changes are observed, the basic issue is whether the patient has primarily an intrinsic airway problem without secondary parenchymal involvement, combined airway-

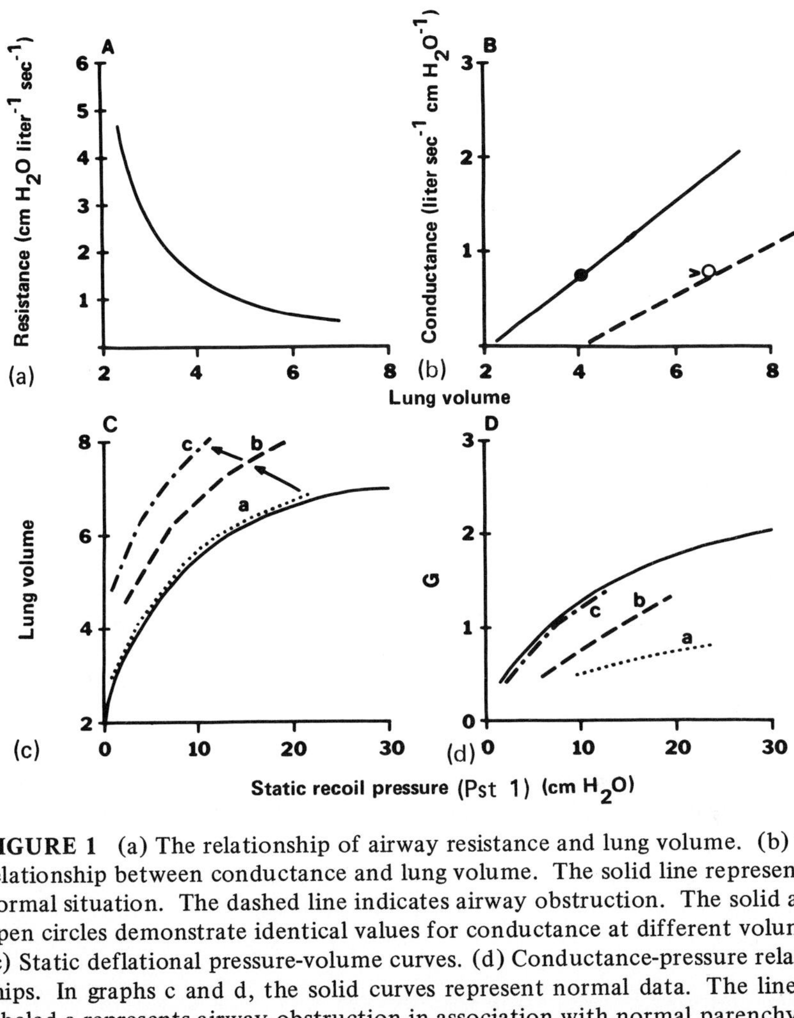


**FIGURE 1** (a) The relationship of airway resistance and lung volume. (b) The relationship between conductance and lung volume. The solid line represents the normal situation. The dashed line indicates airway obstruction. The solid and open circles demonstrate identical values for conductance at different volumes. (c) Static deflational pressure-volume curves. (d) Conductance-pressure relationships. In graphs c and d, the solid curves represent normal data. The line labeled a represents airway obstruction in association with normal parenchymal properties; b indicates combined parenchymal and airway abnormalities; c represents obstruction secondary to loss of recoil only.

parenchymal difficulties, or dimensional changes of airways solely as the result of a parenchymal abnormality.

This differentiation can be approached by relating lung volume to transpulmonary pressure and then relating the latter to conductance [13]. The validity of this manipulation assumes two things. The first is that the volume dependency of airway size is related to static elastic recoil pressures as applied homogeneously throughout the lungs. Evidence to support this idea can be derived from experiments in which the chest was strapped, causing lung volumes to decrease but recoil to increase when this occurred. Maximum flow as a function of recoil pressure remained unchanged [14], indicating that pressure and not volume is the critical variable. The second is that the overall pressure volume curve reflects predominantly parenchymal attributes. This too seems reasonable since it can be readily appreciated that any relative change in airway volume can only be a small percentage of the volume change of the parenchyma. It then follows that significant intrinsic airway changes would have little effect upon the static pressure-volume curve (an exception would be alveolar duct and respiratory bronchiole constriction that would distort the alveoli and directly affect the overall pressure-volume relation [15]). In contrast, the parenchyma cannot be altered without profoundly affecting the airways. The magnitude of the secondary airway dimensional changes observed would then depend upon their compliances.

These considerations are illustrated in Figures 1c and d. Figure 1c plots a normal deflational pressure-volume curve, and in combination with Figure 1b a conductance-pressure plot can be derived (Fig. 1d). If the change in specific conductance shown in Figure 1b were due solely to airway disease (i.e., the lungs' pressure-volume curve remained normal), the resultant conductance-pressure plot would be shifted down and to the right, as illustrated by curve a in Figure 1d. Such alterations are typically observed in chronic bronchitis and asthma [16,17]. A combined airway-parenchymal problem (i.e., intrinsic airway obstruction plus loss of recoil) would be expected to inscribe the curve labeled b in Figure 1d. These types of changes are observed in some cases of acute asthma [16-19], and combined chronic bronchitis and emphysema [20]. If the decrease in specific conductance resulted only from a loss of recoil, curve c would be expected. Note that this curve superimposes on the normal data, although over a more limited pressure range. This alteration would be expected in pure emphysema [17,20,21].

## III. Airway-Parenchyma Interaction

Thus far we have dealt with the lungs as a homogeneous system with one degree of freedom and with recoil pressures inscribed by deflations from TLC. When inspiratory characteristics and time-dependent behavior are considered, the situation becomes more complex, since there is hysteresis in the pressure-volume behavior of the lungs and airways [22,23]. As shown in Figure 2a, a greater distending pressure is required when a volume is reached during inflation from low lung volumes than when the same volume is reached by deflating the lungs from TLC. This means that the volume history of the lungs must be considered because it influences the elastic recoil pressure. For the lungs, hysteresis is due to

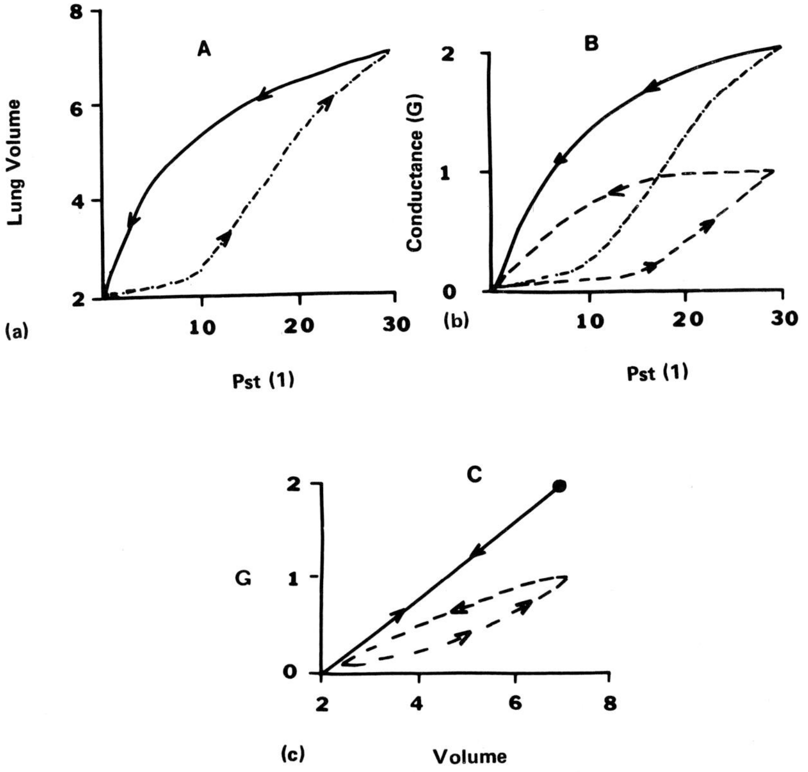


**FIGURE 2** (a) Static inflational and deflational pressure-volume curves of the lung. (b) Expected conductance-pressure relationships of the airways if lung and airway hysteresis were identical (solid and broken curve), or if airways constricted (dashed curve). (c) Expected conductance-volume plot when parenchymal and airway hysteresis were identical (solid line) and when airways constricted (dashed line).

the viscoelastic properties of the gas-liquid interface, connective tissue elements, and possibly to the recruitment of previously closed parallel units [22]. At this point in our discussion we will defer the latter possibility since it violates the constructs of homogeneous behavior.

As discussed earlier, because airways are acted upon by tissue forces as represented by these elastic recoil pressures, they are clearly subjected to different forces at the same lung volume depending on volume history. The resulting effects upon airway dimensions depend upon their hysteresis relative to that of the parenchyma. If the airways were perfectly elastic structures without hysteresis of their own, their dimensions would be uniquely determined by distending pressures. Under these circumstances airways would be larger during inflation and smaller during deflation at the same lung volume. However, this is not the case, and the airways do have hysteresis determined largely by the amount of smooth muscle tone present [24]. This allows for the possibility of the airways varying their size at a point in time relatively independently of parenchymal volume excursions. If airway hysteresis were identical to that of the parenchyma, the shape of the recoil pressure conductance plot (Fig. 2b) would be identical to that of the lung pressure volume curve, and the conductance-lung volume relation would be unaffected by volume history. On the other hand, if airways had greater hysteresis than the parenchyma (such as would occur with bronchoconstriction), then conductance pressure plots would have a greater relative area than lung volume-pressure plots (Fig. 2b) and volume history would influence the relation between conductance and volume in such a manner that isovolume conductance would be greater during deflation than during inflation. If airways had less hysteresis than the parenchyma (such as bronchodilatation), isovolume conductance would be greater when that volume was reached from RV than from TLC (Fig. 2c).

Since hysteresis reflects viscoelastic properties, and since elastic energy dissipates as flow of the viscous elements, time-dependent behavior becomes quite important as well. Consider the situation in which the lungs are inflated to some volume, and flow is stopped; there is a decrease in elastic recoil pressure toward the deflational limb representing the phenomenon of stress relaxation. Conversely, if flow is stopped during deflation, there is an increase in recoil pressure with time (i.e., stress recovery). What does this behavior do to airways and hence to tests of airway function?

Available information suggests that the effects of volume history and time-dependent behavior can be significant. It is known that a single deep inspiration can temporarily decrease induced airway obstruction in normal individuals [25] and by contrast can actually bring about airway obstruction in asthmatics [26]. More recent work has shown that maximal expiratory maneuvers can increase the bronchoconstrictor effects of carbachol [27]. In an effort to avoid these problems, various authors have suggested the use of maximum forced exhalations begun from volumes well below TLC: the so-called partial expiratory flow volume curves [28]. However, this too can present difficulties, depending upon how the studies are performed. Green and Mead have shown that following a maximal inhalation to TLC, breath holding at a lower volume prior to initiation of a forced exhalation can produce a situation in which flow will fall despite an increase in recoil secondary to stress recovery, thus indicating a restoration of, or increase in, airway tone with time [29]. Further, Wellman et al. have shown that when two forced expirations are performed in rapid sequence from lung volumes near FRC, flow on the second maneuver is greater than on the first

[30]. This phenomenon will disappear if a delay of 10 sec or more is interspersed between trials. These findings suggest that time-dependent effects of parenchymal characteristics can overcome or outweigh the effects of dimensional decreases in airways. The practical relevance of these latter observations is that volume history and the timing sequences of studies must be rigidly standardized if intrasubject and intersubject variability is to be kept to acceptable levels and overinterpretation and underinterpretation of the results minimized.

## IV. Regional Nonuniformities of Resistance and Compliance

Thus far we have considered overall pressure-flow-volume relations that require homogeneous behavior in order to be analyzed precisely. Nonetheless, application of these principles to disease states allows some assessment of the predominant sites and mechanisms of airway dysfunction. The following section will deal with nonuniform involvement of the lung as concerns tests of airway function.

Under normal circumstances all the alveoli of the lung are believed to fill and empty in unison even at very high respiratory frequencies [31]. The factors that determine this response are the resistance of the air passages and the compliance of the attendant alveoli. This is called a time constant ($T = R \times C$), and whether all the units of the lung will behave synchronously depends upon the uniformity of distribution of these values. When there are regional changes in either resistance or compliance, this will cause an inequality of time constants, and allow the affected units to behave asynchronously from their fellows.

The available evidence from both pathologic and physiologic investigations indicates that disease states involve the parenchyma and airways in a nonhomogeneous fashion. This can result in inequalities of time constants of parallel lung units or in serially distributed alterations in airway caliber as might happen when there is disease in small versus large airways [31,32]. In the case of parallel inequalities, during respiration the incoming air will take the path of least resistance and be preferentially distributed to the better ventilating units (i.e., those with the lowest time constants). During expiration they will also empty first. Consequently a phase shift will develop, with part of the lung respiring normally and part respiring slowly. In this situation, the rate of change is extremely important. Rapid volume excursions magnify the effect of regions with increases in resistance and slow rates of change emphasize those with compliance abnormalities. This is illustrated in Figure 3. The unit labeled B has a high compliance and resistance. A rapid inflation results in little volume change in this unit due to its high resistance, whereas a prolonged inflation results in full volume change according

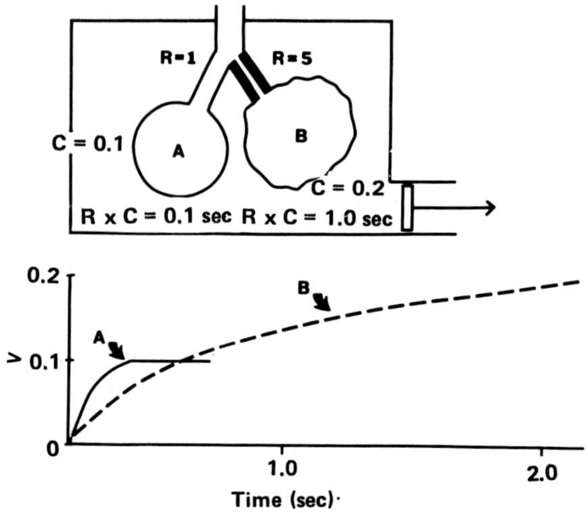


**FIGURE 3** Schematic representation of time constant discrepancies in parallel lung units and the effects of time dependent behavior. R = resistance; C = compliance. Unit B has a time constant 10 times that of unit A. If a square wave of negative pressure is created in the box by pulling the plunger, unit B fills more slowly because of its increased resistance. If the pressure is maintained over time, unit B fills more than A because of its increased compliance. Thus, rapid maneuvers magnify resistive abnormalities, and slow or maintained maneuvers amplify compliance abnormalities.

to the magnitude of the compliance abnormality. The effect that this has on pulmonary function is abnormal nitrogen and/or radioactive xenon washouts [33-35], sequential alveolar emptying during forced expiration [36], frequency dependence of dynamic compliance and resistance [33,34,36-38], and derangements in gas exchange and arterial blood gases [39,40]. In established lung disease these abnormalities are easily demonstrated, but do not serve to distinguish between airway and parenchymal processes. When frequency dependence of compliance, resistance, and distribution of inspired gas are isolated findings, they have been proposed as tests of nonuniform small airway obstruction if overall elastic recoil, maximal flow rate, and resistance are normal [37]. The basic reasoning is that since cross-sectional area of the peripheral airways is so large, significant obstruction could be present without greatly affecting resistance measurements made at the mouth [41]. If elastic properties are within the normal range and frequency-dependent behavior is demonstrated, one could conclude that there are regional inequalities in the time constants of parallel airways secondary to differences in resistances between them [37]. Although the techniques are conceptually well established for the assessment of small airway obstruction, very little morphological evidence exists to support this interpretation.

Collateral airflow channels, if large enough, can eliminate frequency-dependent behavior by providing alternate pathways for filling units with high time constants. Although there is little collateral flow in normal human lungs [42], in chronic obstructive lung disease these channels are sufficiently large [42] that an alternative theory for frequency-dependent behavior has been proposed by Mead [32]. He considered the possibility that the compliance of the larger, more central airways, which is normally less than that of the parenchyma, might act in parallel with the latter (mechanically these two would be in a series configuration, but since there is a common distending pressure operating on both, their electrical analog is parallel). If small airway obstruction is severe, as it can be in chronic obstructive lung disease [43], it could impede alveolar filling so that frequency dependence of compliance could result from airway compliance predominating over parenchymal compliance at higher frequencies. In fact, the Mead analysis would predict frequency dependence of compliance on this basis if small airway obstruction were uniform.

As mentioned above, the total cross-sectional area of each generation of airways beyond the segmental bronchi increases enormously as branching occurs [44]. In canine and human lungs theoretical predictions and experimental measurements have demonstrated that most of the pulmonary resistance is in airways larger than 2 mm in internal diameter [12,41,45]. In point of fact, calculation of the resistive pressure losses as a function of airway size from the morphometric data of Horsfield and Cumming [45] indicates that airways smaller than 2 mm account for less than 12% of viscous pressure losses at inspiratory airflow rates of 0.5 liter/sec. However, since airway resistance depends not only on airway geometry but also on flow rate and gas density and viscosity [46-50], and since these factors may exert different influences on small and large airways [50], by altering the physical properties of inspired gases and the inspiratory flow rates the relative pressure losses of the various generations can be predicted. This could then serve as a basis for utilizing overall pressure-flow relations during submaximal flows as a means of localizing the predominant sites of airway responses.

Figure 4 shows calculated percent pressure drop per generation of airway size for air at flows of 0.5 liter/sec, a mixture of 80% sulfur hexafluoride ($SF_6$) and 20% oxygen (this gas mixture is more than 4 times as dense and 12% less viscous than air when respired) at flows of 1.0 liter/sec, and 80% helium-20% oxygen ($HeO_2$, a mixture one-third as dense as air and 12% more viscous) at 0.25 liter/sec. The expected distribution of pressure losses can be derived by examining tracheal Reynolds' numbers at each flow regime. Reynolds' numbers are defined as:

$$\mathrm{Re} = \frac{DV\rho}{\mu}$$

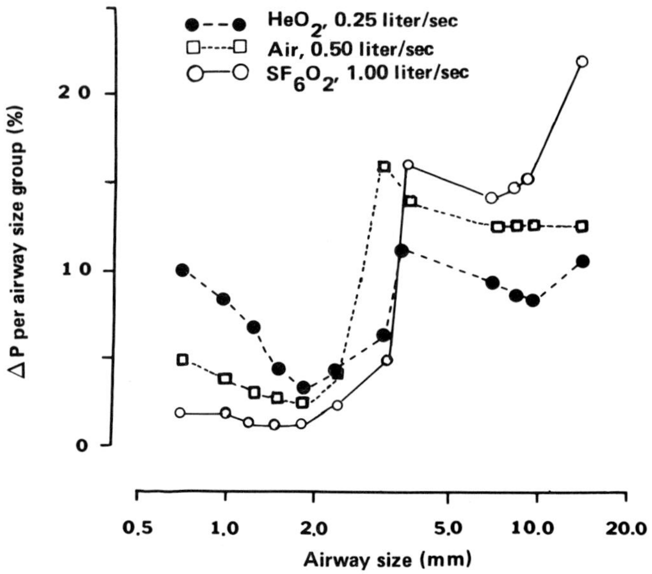


**FIGURE 4** The proportional pressure drop per airway luminal size group on the ordinate is plotted against airway lumen size on the abscissa. $HeO_2$ at 0.25 liter/sec (closed circles) causes a greater proportional pressure drop across small airways and less across larger airways. $SF_6$ at 1.0 liter/sec (open circles) produces just the opposite effect and air at 0.5 liter/sec (open squares) is intermediate. (These calculations are based upon human lung data of Horsfield and Cummings [45] and are redrawn from the data of Drazen et al. [12].)

where D = diameter of the tube
V = velocity
$\rho$ = density
$\mu$ = viscosity

With fixed morphology, the tracheal flow regime serves as an index of the serial distribution of pressure losses down the tracheobronchial tree and the central airways resistance becomes a greater proportion of total resistance when Re are large.

In Figure 4 it can be seen that increased flow rates with $SF_6O_2$ (the more dense, less viscous gas) proportionately increases the pressure drop across large airways, and lower flow rates with a less dense and more viscous gas ($HeO_2$) proportionately increases the pressure drop across small airways. Thus, if constriction were to occur predominantly in large airways, there would be a disproportionate increase in $SF_6O_2$ resistance. Conversely, should obstruction develop predominantly in small airways, the $HeO_2$ resistance would rise. These predictions have been verified in tracheotomized dogs [51,52], but have not been approached in human subjects. The reasons for the lack of systematic human studies are many, and include the large and variable subglottic and glottic contribution to airflow resistance and the fact that bronchoconstrictor challenges with substances like histamine, which can cause edema formation, may affect these structures directly. Because of these upper airway components, most human investigations using gases of differing physical properties have employed maximal expiratory flow maneuvers. The advantages of these techniques are that only the pressure-flow relations of intrathoracic airways are being examined.

It has been known that maximum flow during a forced expiration ($\dot{V}_{max}$) varies inversely with gas density in normal subjects [53]. Of the various gases employed in the past, the one most often used because of its availability and lack of unpleasant side effects is a mixture of 80% He and 20% $O_2$. On the average, at 50% of the vital capacity, the ratio of $\dot{V}_{max}$ $HeO_2$ to $\dot{V}_{max}$ air is 1.50. This high degree of density dependence can be explained by consideration of the location of the flow-limiting segment and the flow regimes within it.

Over most of the forced vital capacity in normal subjects, equal pressure points are located in lobar or segmental bronchi; hence the upstream segment normally is comprised of all the small and many large central airways. These central airways, despite their large individual diameters, have a small total cross-sectional area because there are so few of them. In such airways Reynolds' numbers are large and most of the pressure loss is dissipated in overcoming turbulence and convective accelerative pressure losses, both of which are highly dependent upon gas density. Thus, a higher $\dot{V}_{max}$ with a less dense gas mixture indicates a greater relative contribution of large airways to flow limitation [54].

In contrast to normal subjects, some patients with obstructed airways have been found to have low $\dot{V}_{max}$ $HeO_2$:air ratios, and it has been suggested that this low degree of density dependence represents a relatively greater contribution of small airways to flow limitation [55]. The rationale here is that with increases in the resistance of small airways, equal pressure points are located near the alveoli so that upstream resistance approaches the resistance of the small airways. Under these circumstances, cross-sectional area, although compromised, remains large, and Reynolds' numbers small; consequently, flow will be more nearly laminar and hence less density dependent. Therefore, with the assumption that EPP and static recoil remain the same with both air and $HeO_2$, it is possible to assess the relative contribution of large versus small airways to flow limitation by making isovolume comparisons of $\dot{V}_{max}$ in the midvital capacity range.

As with other tests, decreases in elastic recoil can account for both small airway obstruction and peripheral movement of EPP, especially at low lung volumes. However, if the loss of recoil is only moderate, the density dependence ratios in the mid-VC range are not affected [56]. Therefore, density dependence of $\dot{V}_{max}$ can be used not only as an indicator of the serial distribution of resistance, but also as a test of airway versus parenchymal changes.

## V. Airway Responsivity

The preceding discussion has dealt with ways of interpreting mechanical defects that are found at a given point in time. The following section will deal with ways in which pharmacologic agents and constrictor stimuli can be used to alter lung function to study serial distribution of resistance and the mechanisms accounting for airway responses in both health and disease.

If there are acute changes in pressure flow relations without alterations in parenchymal elastic properties in response to neuropharmacologic agents such as β-adrenergic or parasympathetic agonists or antagonists, and if these changes revert quickly to the control state, it is highly likely that smooth muscle is being altered. Although other processes such as mucosal edema, inflammation, intraluminal secretion secondary to overproduction and/or failure of clearance are frequently present in obstructive pulmonary syndromes, the most effective therapeutic regimens are based on the dilatation of bronchial smooth muscle. Although many kinds of dilator and constrictor substances have enjoyed wide clinical usage in the diagnosis and/or treatment of airway diseases, very little is actually known about their sites of action and the factors that contribute to, or modify, the responses observed. Perhaps it is best to begin with a consideration of bronchial smooth muscle in normals.

There is tonic activity in airway smooth muscle of normal subjects as shown by the distinct bronchodilatation that occurs with the administration of either adrenergic or anticholinergic agents [57-60]. The data in humans are insufficient to state with certainty that normal tone is the result of a balance between parasympathetic and sympathetic influences. However, data in dogs suggest that such a balance exists. In one study [61], stimulation of the parasympathetic system exerted a constriction at all levels of the tracheobronchial tree, but its effect on peripheral airways was magnified by β-adrenergic blockade and inhibited by an intact sympathetic nervous system. This suggests that the major distribution of adrenergic receptors may be in the smaller airways, and raises the possibility of a difference in the predominant distribution of these two opposing influences on airway tone. If this is so, then the bronchodilator effects of atropine and isoproterenol might not only be different in terms of cellular mechanisms but might also act at different sites within the tracheobronchial tree. A recent study suggests that this is the case [60].

In this investigation, atropine and isoproterenol were found to produce identical degrees of bronchodilatation as measured by standard techniques in normal individuals. However, when density dependence was examined, atropine caused a decrease in $HeO_2$:air ratios and isoproterenol caused them to increase. Neither agent changed elastic recoil or lung volumes. The interpretation given these observations was that the effect of atropine was predominantly in the large airways of the upstream segment while that of isoproterenol was in the small peripheral airways. The reasoning employed in reaching this conclusion was based upon the response of $\dot{V}_{max}$ to the gases of different densities described earlier. Since the large density-dependent and small density-independent airways of the upstream segment are in series, and since the driving pressure was constant before and after each agent, if the site of flow limitation was the same after both drugs, increased density dependence could only occur with predominant dilatation of small upstream airways so that more of the pressure was being dissipated in turbulence and convective acceleration in the large airways. Restated in simplistic terms, predominant dilatation of small airways reapportions the overall pressure losses to make the larger airways act as though their relative contribution to flow limitation had increased. Conversely, with atropine, as the larger upstream airways dilated more of the driving pressure was lost overcoming laminar flow and less was spent on density-dependent flow regimes than formerly, i.e., now the relative contribution of small airways to flow limitation had increased.

These findings are of more than physiologic interest since some data indicate that they may have therapeutic application. For example, it has been shown that patients who respond briskly to isoproterenol also increase their density dependence, indicating dilatation of peripheral airways in association with a more mouthward movement of equal pressure points [54]. Further, recent evidence demonstrates that atropine and its congeners are only successful in blocking the bronchospasm that follows exercise in those asthmatics whose obstruction is predominantly in large airways [62].

Perhaps the greatest clinical uses to which changes in airway tone have been put are the assessments of reversibility of obstruction and the degree of responsiveness to the administration of a pharmacologically active bronchoconstrictive agent. In fact it has even been proposed that hyperresponsiveness to such substances be included as a criterion for making the diagnosis of bronchial asthma [63]. It is implicit in such a recommendation that there is a state of hyperresponsiveness of the tracheobronchial tree in asthma. The data upon which this conclusion has been based were originally derived from comparisons of the mean decrements in lung function that occurred when normal subjects and patients with asthma and chronic obstructive lung disease were given standard amounts of histamine or acetylcholine [64-66]. With time, other agents have been studied and dose response curves have been described [26,67-70]. The general conclusion is that there is a spectrum of hyperreactivity, with asthmatics being the most reactive and normals the least; other obstructive syndromes occupy intermediate positions.

Unfortunately, most studies have not critically evaluated the factors that could be contributing to the exaggerated responses observed, and some fundamental questions remain unanswered [70]. In brief, they can be summarized as follows. Since many provocational challenges employ aerosols, despite stated inspiratory concentrations, the retained dose is largely unknown, and that which is retained may have a different site of deposition in different populations. Prechallenge lung function could influence the magnitude of the response. Finally, no uniform methods of assessing the degree of obstruction have been established. Of these, the most significant, and most difficult to standardize, is comparable prechallenge lung function between groups. The importance of this factor has generally been ignored. Yet there are data that point out that the relation between the response to a stimulus and the prestimulus state may be such that responses of different magnitude cannot be simply equated with different sensitivities [71-73]. Part of the reason for this is that the resistance of a tube varies as a function of the radius to the fourth or fifth power. Thus, even though two tubes have similar resistances initially, identical decreases in their radii may result in vastly different absolute changes in resistance. When these factors are taken into consideration, the differences in response between asthmatics and normals become less marked with aerosol challenges [71] and even disappear with intravenous administration of the agents [72,73]. These findings reemphasize the need for learning more about the site of deposition of aerosols and the degree of retention within the airways in disease states as compared to normal individuals.

Despite the handicaps outlined above, real information can be gained from certain types of challenges when the subject is used as his or her own control. A good example is the accentuation of airway responsiveness during mild viral respiratory illness in normal subjects [74,75]. In such subjects there is hyperresponsiveness to histamine which returns to normal with the abatement of the illness. Since this effect can be blocked with prior administration of atropine, and can be reversed with sympathomimetics, it has been postulated that it represents a lowering of the firing threshold of subepithelial receptors which results in reflex contraction of smooth muscle [75]. It is possible that this same phenomenon occurs in patients with airway disease when they have similar illnesses [74]. Although this factor may magnify their problem, it does not necessarily imply a cause and effect relation, for it is not yet known if the underlying disease process causes hyperreactivity or hyperreactivity causes the disease. The problem of airway responsiveness will be discussed in another chapter.

## VI. Clinical Physiology

To this point we have presented the principles which can be used to examine airway and parenchymal function in various circumstances but have not made any systematic attempt to apply them to specific disease entities. The following section will catalog the defects seen in obstructive disease and will examine their interrelations. The best model to employ for this purpose is acute bronchial asthma, for several reasons. First, although asthma is primarily a disease of airways, it causes derangements in virtually all aspects of lung function [16,18,19, 33,39,62,76]. Second, if one begins with a severe episode and makes serial observations during therapy, as the patient improves he or she will invariably pass through multiple phases varying from widespread obstruction through small airway dysfunction to complete normalcy [16,33,77].

The data in Figure 5 were obtained from one asthmatic who is representative of a group previously reported [16] and is offered as a case in point. Studies 1 through 4 represent various stages during the evolution of the disease process in response to treatment. When this individual was acutely ill (study 1), both TLC and RV were elevated, the latter markedly so. Examination of the MEFV curves demonstrated severe difficulty in emptying the lungs during forced expiration. Specific conductance was low and conductance at all lung volumes was depressed despite hyperinflation. In association with these changes there was a loss of elastic recoil. In addition, as shown in Figure 6, there was frequency-dependent behavior. Examination of the conductance-pressure plot in Figure 5 shows it to be down and to the right, demonstrating that even though there is a loss of recoil, the major component responsible for the reduction in maximum expiratory flow was airway obstruction and not loss of parenchymal support. Subsequent analysis will demonstrate that many of the other abnormalities result from this cause as well. At this point in the illness, these data do not give any clue as to the site and nature of the obstruction. It could be due to smooth muscle contraction, mucosal edema, and/or inspissation of secretions, and it could be located anywhere within the tracheobronchial tree.

The alterations listed above are rather typical for acute episodes of asthma and have been observed repeatedly, but the mechanisms underlying each are unknown for the most part. The reduction in maximum expiratory flow probably results from a number of interrelated events: intrinsic airway narrowing, loss of some units because of complete airway closure, changes in bronchial compliance, and loss of recoil.

| STUDY | SGaw | $FEV_1$ | MMF | RV |
|---|---|---|---|---|
| 1 | 0.04 | 23 | 7 | 414 |
| 2 | 0.11 | 67 | 26 | 225 |
| 3 | 0.21 | 86 | 53 | 188 |
| 4 | 0.32 | 106 | 98 | 99 |

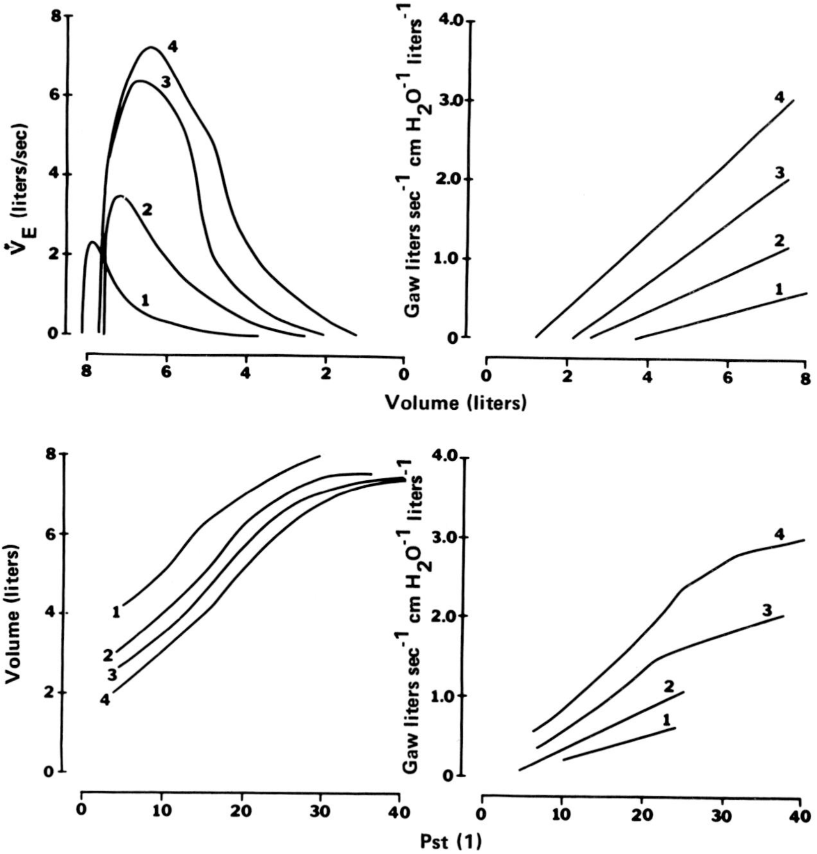


**FIGURE 5** Pulmonary mechanics at various stages of resolution of an acute episode of asthma. The insert at the top of the figure contains routine measures of lung function. The top two panels from left to right display maximum expiratory flow volume curves and conductance-volume relationships, respectively. The bottom contains static deflational pressure-volume curves and conductance-pressure data. The numbers 1 through 4 represent data obtained during acute illness and recovery. $SG_{aw}$ = specific conductance in liters per second per centimeters $H_2O$ per liter; $FEV_1$ = 1-sec forced expiratory volume; MMF = maximum midexpiratory flow; RV = residual volume. These latter three variables are all expressed as a percentage of predicted normal; $\dot{V}_E$ = maximum flow; $G_{aw}$ = conductance; Pst (1) = static recoil pressure.

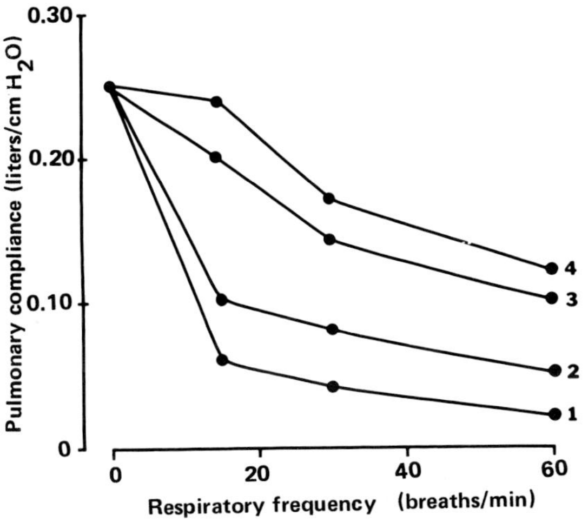


**FIGURE 6** Pulmonary compliance ($C_L$) at various respiratory frequencies (f) during the resolution of an acute episode of asthma. The numbers 1 through 4 correspond to the data in Figure 5.

The acute increase in TLC and the shift in the pressure-volume curve are not due to a destruction of parenchymal tissue in asthma as they are in emphysema, for they can be made to reverse with time and/or with therapy [16,18,76, 78]. It was originally thought that they resulted from stress relaxation secondary to prolonged air trapping [76,78], but this explanation no longer seems tenable, since it has been shown that they can be produced in the laboratory within minutes of a provocational challenge [18,62,79]. Further, there are data that demonstrate that the pressure-volume curve of the lung can be acutely shifted in asthma without concomitant changes in TLC [73,79].

The increase in RV could be due to changes in the elastic properties of the lungs or chest wall, a reduction in muscle power, or an increased tendency of airways to close or to narrow sufficiently to greatly reduce respiratory flow [18,19], suggesting that at least two of these factors contribute. A loss of recoil alone could cause an increase in RV, and the studies of Freedman and colleagues [18] and Colebatch et al. [19] suggest that airway closure or severe retardation of expiration is also operational so that RV is elevated by a dynamic mechanism related to breath-holding time.

Irrespective of the mechanisms of these functional alterations, when treatment is administered there is a progressive improvement in lung function. As this occurs, further insights into the pressure, volume, and flow interrelations can be obtained. It is now generally recognized that the greatest improvements occur early in the treatment period in asthma, and that not all variables improve at the same rate [77]. The latter is clearly shown in Figures 5 and 6. Studies 2 through 4 were made when the patient first became asymptomatic and then 2 and 5 days later, respectively. When the attack had ended clinically (study 2), overall lung function had improved significantly. Specific conductance and 1-sec forced expiratory volumes ($FEV_1$) had almost tripled, and were approaching their normal range. However, flow in the midvital capacity and residual volume were still very abnormal. These data demonstrate that at this stage there is nonuniform involvement of the airways with some behaving normally, or nearly so, and others still involved with the obstructive process. Further, it is unlikely that this residual obstruction represents only smooth muscle contraction.

With continued treatment a stage is reached where $SG_{aw}$, $FEV_1$, conductance-volume and pressure-volume relationships are all within their normal range. Yet RV, MMF, and dynamic compliance remain abnormal (study 3). Detailed studies have shown that, in addition to the above, there is also coexistent maldistribution of inspired air and arterial hypoxemia [33,39,80]. These are fairly characteristic findings in asymptomatic patients with asthma and represent airway obstruction that compromises pulmonary function but is of insufficient magnitude to produce acute symptoms. The next stage is one in which the only abnormality is frequency-dependent behavior (study 4).

The finding of a normal pressure-volume curve in association with studies 3 and 4 indicates that these residual abnormalities are due to persistent airway obstruction and not to changes in elastic properties. The nature of this obstruction is unknown but it probably represents failure to clear inspissated secretions and/or mucosal edema. It is known that the lungs of asthmatics can contain such pathologic findings for prolonged periods [81]. The precise anatomical location is also unknown, but in view of the statistically normal values for $SG_{aw}$ and $FEV_1$, it must be in an area above the alveolar duct and below the central airways. Alveolar duct constriction, although it increases total resistance only slightly and is, therefore, difficult to detect, causes static compliance to decrease and dynamic compliance to remain frequency independent [15]. If these residua were in the central bronchi, it would have been expected to have altered $SG_{aw}$ and $FEV_1$ measurements. Findings similar to these have been reported in asymptomatic smokers and in patients with mild chronic bronchitis and have been interpreted as indicating small airway obstruction [36,37,82].

In light of the previous discussion regarding the effect of baseline lung function on the results of provocational challenges, it seems pertinent to point out that the patterns shown in Figures 5 and 6 can be used to demonstrate this relationship. If a group of asthmatics are repeatedly challenged on different occasions with an identical stimulus, the response is not an all or none event but rather a continuum. In one study [83], when subjects had normal mechanical function prior to challenge the typical response to a given exercise load (a precisely quantifiable nonimmunologic, nonpharmacologic stimulus) was an increase in RV and a fall in airflow in the midvital capacity. However, when the same patients were rechallenged with the same work load at a time when their lung function resembled the third study in Figure 5, they developed a moderately severe attack of asthma. If the preexercise obstruction was of sufficient magnitude to compromise the $FEV_1$, the subsequent response was quite severe and the resultant abnormalities resembled those seen in patients presenting to an emergency room for treatment [77]. The implication of these findings is that they point up the hazards of attempting to determine precise stimulus-response relations without evaluating overall lung function, and may account for the wide variation in response that is often seen in clinical situations.

## VII. Summary

In summary, the mechanical interactions between airways and parenchyma and the strong influence of volume history on these interactions greatly affect the evaluation and interpretation of tests aimed at the physiologic assessment of mechanical lung function. Through the application of various pharmacologic agents, and attention to volume history, much has been learned about the mechanisms of acute airway responses. More recent use of morphometric data and the concepts of fluid mechanics have allowed determination of predominant sites of airway responses that in turn relate to mechanisms. Although the nonhomogeneity of disease processes interferes with precise analysis, appreciation of basic principles in association with the patterns of functional abnormalities with time and treatment permits a reasonable synthesis and understanding of airway diseases.

## References

1. Mead, J., Measurements of the inertia of the lungs at increased ambient pressure, *J. Appl. Physiol.*, **9**:208-212 (1956).
2. Dosman, J., F. Bode, J. Urbanetti, R. Antic, R. Martin, and P. T. Macklem, Role of inertia in the measurement of dynamic compliance, *J. Appl. Physiol.*, **38**:64-69 (1975).
3. Macklem, P. T., and N. J. Wilson, Measurement of intrabronchial pressure in man, *J. Appl. Physiol.*, **20**:653-663 (1965).
4. Fry, D. L., and R. E. Hyatt, Pulmonary mechanics. A unified analysis of the relationships between pressure, volume and gas flow in the lungs of normal and diseased human subjects, *Am. J. Med.*, **29**:672-689 (1960).

5. Hyatt, R. E., D. P. Schilder, and D. L. Fry, Relationship between maximum expiratory flow and degree of lung inflation, *J. Appl. Physiol.,* **13**:331-336 (1958).
6. Mead, J., J. M. Turner, P. T. Macklem, and J. B. Little, Significance of the relationship between lung recoil and maximum expiratory flow, *J. Appl. Physiol.,* **22**:95-108 (1967).
7. Pride, N. B., S. Permutt, and B. Bromberger-Barnea, Determinants of maximum expiratory flow from the lungs, *J. Appl. Physiol.,* **23**:646-662 (1967).
8. Dawson, S. V., and E. A. Elliott, The wave speed limitation of expiratory flow—a unifying concept, *J. Appl. Physiol.,* **43**:498-515 (1977).
9. Bates, D. V., P. T. Macklem, and R. V. Christie, *Respiratory Function in Disease.* Philadelphia, London, Toronto, W. B. Saunders, 1971, pp. 111-218.
10. Briscoe, W. A., and A. B. DuBois, The relationship between airway resistance, airway conductance and lung volumes in subjects of different age and body size, *J. Clin. Invest.,* **37**:1279-1285 (1958).
11. Guyatt, A. R., J. H. Alpers, and A. C. Bromley, Variability of plethysmographic measurements of airway resistance in man, *J. Appl. Physiol.,* **22**: 383-389 (1967).
12. Drazen, J. M., S. H. Loring, and R. H. Ingram, Jr., Distribution of pulmonary resistance: Effects of gas density, viscosity, and flow rate, *J. Appl. Physiol.,* **41**:388-395 (1976).
13. Butler, J., C. G. Caro, R. Alcala, and A. B. DuBois, Physiologic factors affecting airway resistance in normal subjects and in patients with obstructive respiratory disease, *J. Clin. Invest.,* **39**:584-591 (1960).
14. Stubbs, S. E., and R. E. Hyatt, Effects of increased lung recoil pressure on maximal expiratory flow in normal subjects, *J. Appl. Physiol.,* **32**:325-331 (1972).
15. Nadel, J. A., H. J. H. Colebatch, and G. R. Olsen, Location and mechanism of airway constriction after barium sulfate microembolization, *J. Appl. Physiol.,* **19**:387-394 (1964).
16. McFadden, Jr., E. R., and H. A. Lyons, Serial studies of factors influencing airway dynamics during recovery from acute asthma attacks, *J. Appl. Physiol.,* **27**:452-459 (1969).
17. Leaver, D. G., A. E. Tattersfield, and N. B. Pride, Contributions of loss of lung recoil and of enhanced airways collapsibility to the airflow obstruction of chronic bronchitis and emphysema, *J. Clin. Invest.,* **52**:2117-2128 (1973).
18. Freedman, S., A. E. Tattersfield, and N. B. Pride, Changes in lung mechanics during asthma induced by exercise, *J. Appl. Physiol.,* **38**:974-982 (1975).
19. Colebatch, H. J. H., K. E. Finucane, and M. M. Smith, Pulmonary conductance and elastic recoil relationships in asthma and emphysema, *J. Appl. Physiol.,* **34**:143-153 (1973).
20. Duffell, G. M., J. H. Marcus, and R. H. Ingram, Jr., Limitation of expiratory flow in chronic obstructive pulmonary disease. Relationship of clinical

characteristics, pathophysiological type, and mechanisms, *Ann. Intern. Med.*, **72**:365-374 (1970).
21. Black, L. F., R. E. Hyatt, and S. E. Stubbs, Mechanism of expiratory airflow limitation in chronic obstructive pulmonary disease associated with $\alpha_1$-antitrypsin deficiency, *Am. Rev. Respir. Dis.*, **105**:891-899 (1972).
22. Radford, Jr., E. P., Static mechanical properties of mammalian lungs. In *Handbook of Physiology,* Section 3, *Respiration,* Vol. 1. Edited by W. O. Fenn and H. Rahn. Washington, D.C., American Physiological Society, 1964, pp. 429-449.
23. Froeb, H. F., and J. Mead, Relative hysteresis of the dead space and lung in vivo, *J. Appl. Physiol.*, **25**:244-248 (1968).
24. Vincent, N. J., R. Knudson, D. E. Leith, P. T. Macklem, and J. Mead, Factors influencing pulmonary resistance, *J. Appl. Physiol.*, **29**:236-243 (1970).
25. Nadel, J. A., and D. F. Tierney, Effect of a previous deep inspiration on airway resistance in man, *J. Appl. Physiol.*, **16**:717-719 (1961).
26. Simonsson, B. G., F. M. Jacobs, and J. A. Nadel, Role of autonomic nervous system and the cough reflex in the increased responsiveness of airways in patients with obstructive airways disease, *J. Clin. Invest.*, **46**:1812-1818 (1967).
27. Orehek, J., P. Gayrard, C. Grimaud, and J. Charpin, Effect of maximal respiratory maneuvers on bronchial sensitivity of asthmatic patients as compared to normal people, *Br. Med. J.*, **1**:123-125 (1975).
28. Bouhuys, A., V. R. Hunt, B. K. Kim, and Z. Zapletal, Maximum expiratory flow rates in induced bronchoconstriction in man, *J. Clin. Invest.*, **48**:1159-1168 (1969).
29. Green, M., and J. Mead, Time dependence of flow-volume curves, *J. Appl. Physiol.*, **37**:793-797 (1974).
30. Wellman, J. J., R. Brown, R. H. Ingram, Jr., J. Mead, and E. R. McFadden, Jr., Effect of volume history on successive partial expiratory flow-volume maneuvers, *J. Appl. Physiol.*, **41**:153-158 (1976).
31. Otis, A. B., C. B. McKerrow, R. A. Bartlett, J. Mead, M. B. McIlroy, N. J. Selverstone, and E. P. Radford, Jr., Mechanical factors in distribution of pulmonary ventilation, *J. Appl. Physiol.*, **8**:427-443 (1956).
32. Mead, J., Contribution of compliance of airways to frequency-dependent behavior of lungs, *J. Appl. Physiol.*, **26**:670-673 (1969).
33. McFadden, Jr., E. R., and H. A. Lyons, Airway resistance and uneven ventilation in bronchial asthma, *J. Appl. Physiol.*, **25**:365-370 (1968).
34. Ingram, Jr., R. H., and D. P. Schilder, Association of a decrease in dynamic compliance with a change in gas distribution, *J. Appl. Physiol.*, **23**:911-916 (1967).
35. Anthonisen, N. R., H. Bass, A. Oriol, R. E. G. Place, and D. V. Bates, Regional lung function in patients with chronic bronchitis, *Clin. Sci.*, **35**:494-511 (1968).
36. McFadden, Jr., E. R., and D. A. Linden, A reduction in maximum midexpiratory flow rate. A spirographic manifestation of small airway disease, *Am. J. Med.*, **52**:725-737 (1972).

37. Woolcock, A. J., H. J. Vincent, and P. T. Macklem, Frequency dependence of compliance as a test for obstruction in small airways, *J. Clin. Invest.*, **48**: 1097-1106 (1969).
38. Grimby, G. T., T. Takishima, W. Graham, P. T. Macklem, and J. Mead, Frequency dependence of flow resistance in patients with obstructive lung disease, *J. Clin. Invest.*, **47**:1455-1465 (1968).
39. McFadden, Jr., E. R., and H. A. Lyons, Arterial blood gas tensions in asthma, *N. Engl. J. Med.*, **278**:1027-1032 (1968).
40. Levine, G., E. Housley, P. MacLeod, and P. T. Macklem, Gas exchange abnormalities in mild bronchitis and asymptomatic asthma, *N. Engl. J. Med.*, **282**:1277-1282 (1970).
41. Macklem, P. T., and J. Mead, Resistance of central and peripheral airways measured by a retrograde catheter, *J. Appl. Physiol.*, **22**:395-401 (1967).
42. Hogg, J. C., P. T. Macklem, and W. M. Thurlbeck, The resistance of collateral channels in excised human lungs, *J. Clin. Invest.*, **48**:421-431 (1969).
43. Hogg, J. C., P. T. Macklem, and W. M. Thurlbeck, Size and nature of airway obstruction in chronic obstructive lung disease, *N. Engl. J. Med.*, **278**: 1355-1360 (1968).
44. Weibel, E. R., Morphometrics of the lung. In *Handbook of Physiology*, Section 3, *Respiration*, Vol. 1. Edited by W. O. Fenn and H. Rahn. Washington, D.C., American Physiological Society, 1964, pp. 285-307.
45. Horsfield, K., and G. Cumming, Morphology of the bronchial tree in man, *J. Appl. Physiol.*, **24**:373-383 (1968).
46. Jaeger, M. J., and H. Matthys, The pressure flow characteristics of the human airways. In *Airway Dynamics, Physiology and Pharmacology*. Edited by A. Bouhuys. Springfield, Ill., Thomas, 1970, pp. 21-32.
47. Jaffrin, M. Y., and P. Kesic, Airway resistance; a fluid mechanical approach, *J. Appl. Physiol.*, **36**:354-361 (1974).
48. Olsen, D. E., G. A. Dart, and G. F. Filley, Pressure drop and fluid flow regime of air inspired into the human lung, *J. Appl. Physiol.*, **28**:482-494 (1970).
49. Pedley, T. J., R. C. Schroter, and M. F. Sudlow, Energy losses and pressure drop in models in human airways, *Respir. Physiol.*, **9**:371-386 (1970).
50. Wood, L. D. H., L. A. Engel, P. Griffin, P. Despas, and P. T. Macklem, Effect of gas physical properties and flow on lower pulmonary resistance, *J. Appl. Physiol.*, **41**:234-244 (1976).
51. Drazen, J. M., S. H. Loring, and R. H. Ingram, Jr., Localization of airway constriction using gases of varying density and viscosity, *J. Appl. Physiol.*, **41**:396-399 (1976).
52. Barnett, T. B., Effects of helium and oxygen mixtures on pulmonary mechanics during airway constriction, *J. Appl. Physiol.*, **22**:707-713 (1967).
53. Schilder, D. P., A. Roberts, and D. L. Fry, Effect of gas density and viscosity on the maximal expiratory flow-volume relationship, *J. Clin. Invest.*, **42**:1705-1713 (1963).
54. Wellman, J. J., E. R. McFadden, Jr., and R. H. Ingram, Jr., Density-depen-

dence of maximal expiratory flow rates before and after bronchodilators in patients with obstructive airway disease, *Clin. Sci. Mol. Med.*, **51**:133-139 (1976).

55. Despas, P. J., M. Leroux, and P. T. Macklem, Site of airway obstruction in asthma as determined by measuring maximal expiratory flow breathing air and a helium-oxygen mixture, *J. Clin. Invest.*, **51**:3235-3243 (1972).
56. Dosman, J., F. Bode, J. Urbanetti, R. Martin, and P. T. Macklem, The use of a helium-oxygen mixture during maximum expiratory flow to demonstrate obstruction in small airways in smokers, *J. Clin. Invest.*, **55**:1090-1099 (1975).
57. Widdicombe, J. G., D. C. Kent, and J. A. Nadel, Mechanism of bronchoconstriction during inhalation of dust, *J. Appl. Physiol.*, **17**:613-616 (1962).
58. McFadden, Jr., E. R., J. Newton-Howes, and N. B. Pride, Acute effects of inhaled isoproterenol on the mechanical characteristics of the lungs in normal man, *J. Clin. Invest.*, **49**:779-790 (1970).
59. Bouhuys, A., and K. P. van de Woestijne, Mechanical consequences of airway smooth muscle relaxation, *J. Appl. Physiol.*, **30**:670-676 (1971).
60. Ingram, Jr., R. H., J. J. Wellman, E. R. McFadden, Jr., and J. Mead, Relative contributions of large and small airways to flow limitation in normal subjects before and after atropine and isoproterenol, *J. Clin. Invest.*, **59**:696-703 (1977).
61. Woolcock, A. J., P. T. Macklem, J. C. Hogg, and N. J. Wilson, Influence of autonomic nervous system on airway resistance and elastic recoil, *J. Appl. Physiol.*, **26**:814-818 (1969).
62. McFadden, Jr., E. R., R. H. Ingram, Jr., R. L. Haynes, and J. J. Wellman, Predominant site of flow limitation and mechanisms of postexertional asthma, *J. Appl. Physiol. Respir. Environ. Exercise Physiol.*, **42**:746-752 (1977).
63. Scadding, J. G., Definition and clinical categorization. In *Bronchial Asthma. Mechanisms and Therapeutics.* Edited by E. B. Weiss and M. S. Segal. Boston, Little Brown, 1976, pp. 23-30.
64. Curry, J. J., The action of histamine on the respiratory tract in normal and asthmatic subjects, *J. Clin. Invest.*, **25**:785-591 (1946).
65. Itkin, H. I., Bronchial hypersensitivity to mecholyl and histamine in asthma subjects, *J. Allergy*, **40**:245-255 (1967).
66. Herxheimer, H., Bronchial obstruction induced by allergens, histamine and acetyl-beta-methacholine chloride, *Int. Arch. Allergy Appl. Immunol.*, **2**:27-39 (1951).
67. Newball, H. H., and H. R. Keiser, Relative effects of bradykinin and histamine on the respiratory system of man, *J. Appl. Physiol.*, **35**:552-556 (1973).
68. Mathé, A. A., P. Hedquist, A. Holmgren, and N. Svanborg, Bronchial hyperreactivity to prostaglandin $F_{2a}$ and histamine in patients with asthma, *Br. Med. J.*, **1**:193-196 (1973).
69. Fish, J. E., R. R. Rosenthal, W. R. Summer, H. Menkes, P. S. Norman, and

S. Permutt, The effect of atropine on acute antigen-mediated airway constriction in subjects with allergic asthma, *Am. Rev. Respir. Dis.*, **115**:371-379 (1977).

70. Orehek, J., and P. Gayrard, Les tests de provocation bronchique nonspecifiques dans L'asthme, *Bull. Eur. Physiopathol. Respir.*, **12**:565-598 (1976).
71. Orehek, J., P. Gayrard, A. P. Smith, C. Grimaud, and J. Charpin, Airway response to carbachol in normal and asthmatic subjects, *Am. Rev. Respir. Dis.*, **115**:937-943 (1977).
72. Brown, R., R. H. Ingram, Jr., J. J. Wellman, and E. R. McFadden, Jr., Effects of intravenous histamine on pulmonary mechanics in nonasthmatic and asthmatic subjects, *J. Appl. Physiol. Respir. Environ. Exercise Physiol.*, **42**:221-227 (1977).
73. Brown, R., R. H. Ingram, Jr., and E. R. McFadden, Jr., Effects of intravenous prostaglandin $F_{2a}$ on pulmonary mechanics in non-asthmatic and asthmatic subjects, *J. Appl. Physiol. Respir. Environ. Exercise Physiol.*, **44**:150-155 (1978).
74. Parker, C. D., R. E. Bilbo, and C. E. Reed, Methacholine aerosol as a test for bronchial asthma, *Arch. Intern. Med.*, **115**:452-458 (1965).
75. Empey, D. W., L. A. Laitinen, L. Jacobs, W. M. Gold, and J. A. Nadel, Mechanisms of bronchial hyperreactivity in normal subjects after upper respiratory tract infection, *Am. Rev. Respir. Dis.*, **113**:131-139 (1976).
76. Gold, W. M., H. S. Kaufman, and J. A. Nadel, Elastic recoil of the lungs in chronic asthmatic patients before and after therapy, *J. Appl. Physiol.*, **23**:433-438 (1967).
77. McFadden, Jr., E. R., R. Kiser, and W. deGroot, Acute bronchial asthma: Relations between clinical and physiologic manifestations, *N. Engl. J. Med.*, **288**:221-225 (1973).
78. Woolcock, A. J., and J. Read, The static elastic properties of the lungs in asthma, *Am. Rev. Respir. Dis.*, **98**:788-794 (1968).
79. Mansell, A., C. Dubrawsky, H. Levinson, A. C. Bryan, H. Langer, C. Collins-Williams, and R. P. Orange, Lung mechanics in antigen induced asthma, *J. Appl. Physiol.*, **37**:297-301 (1974).
80. Levine, G., E. Housley, P. MacLeod, and P. T. Macklem, Gas exchange abnormalities in mild bronchitis and asymptomatic asthma, *N. Engl. J. Med.*, **282**:1277-1282 (1970).
81. Dunnill, M. S., The pathology of asthma. In *Transactions of World Asthma Conference.* Heart and Chest Association, London, 1965, p. 223.
82. Ingram, Jr., R. H., and C. F. O'Cain, Frequency dependence of compliance in apparently healthy smokers versus non-smokers, *Bull. Physiopathol., Respir. (Nancy)*, **7**:195-212 (1971).
83. Haynes, R. L., R. H. Ingram, Jr., and E. R. McFadden, Jr., An assessment of the pulmonary response to exercise in asthma and an analysis of the factors influencing it, *Am. Rev. Respir. Dis.*, **114**:735-752 (1976).

# AUTHOR INDEX

*Numbers in brackets are reference numbers and indicate that an author's work is referred to although his name is not cited in the text. Italic numbers give the page on which the complete reference is listed.*


## A

Abbott, B. C., 65[89], 76[86], 77 [89], 85, *116*
Abe, C., 9[49], *27*, 66[65,66], 67 [65,66], *115*
Åberg, A. K. G., 86[160], *120*, 197 [69], *210*
Abern, S. B., 195[42], *208*
Ablad, B., 196, *209*
Aboo Zar, M., 126, 172[14], *178*, 221[73], 232[73], *244*
Adams, H. R., 154[137], *186*
Adler, G., 197[69], *210*
Adler, S., 102[126], *118*
Adolphson, R. L., 195, *208*
Adrian, E. D., 233[221], *253*
Adriani, J., 222[118], *247*
Ahlquist, N. C., 264[17,18], 276[85], 285[17], *291, 295*
Ahlquist, R. P., 192, *206*
Aiken, J. W., 199, 200[98,103], *211, 212*
Akasaka, K., 9[49], *27*, 66[65,66], 67[65,66], *115*
Akcasu, A., 193, *207*
Akester, A. R., 14[56], *28*
Alanis, J., 77[90], *116*
Albert, R. E., 281[43], 282[43], *292*
Alcala, R., 233[226], *253*, 303[13], *320*
Aldred, R., 131[51], 171[51], *180*
Aledort, L. M., 105[145], *120*
Allison, D. J., 222[94], 225[94], 226 [94], 239[94], *245*, 281[50], *293*
Alpers, J. H., 230[190], *251*, 302[11], *320*
Altura, B. M., 192[13], *206*
Amandus, H., 260[1], *290*
Amdur, M. O., 230[195], *251*, 275 [32,33], 276[32,33], 277[32,39], 279, 286, 287[83], 288[87], *291, 292, 294, 295*
Amer, S., 124, *177*
Andersen, I., 260[9], 281[49], *290, 293*
Anderson, A. A., 198, *210*
Anderson, I., 229[182], 231[182], *251*
Anderson, J. A., 7[39], *27*
Anderson, J. W., 132, *181*
Anderson, W. G., 282[60], *293*
Anderson, W. H., 222[120], *247*
Andersson, K.-E., 125[7], 158[147], *177, 186*
Andersson, R. G. G., 125[7,8], 126

[Andersson, R. G. G.]
[8,10], 144[116], 145[8,116], 158[8,116,147], 161, 163, 165 [8,116,174,175], 166[8,15,116], 168[8,116], 172[8,116], 173 [8,116], 174[116], 175[116], 176[8,116], *177, 178, 184, 186, 187, 188,* 195[47], *208*
Andres, K. H., 234[230], *253*
Angell, C. S., 197[68], *210*
Anggard, E., 199[97], *211*
Angles d'Auriac, G., 127[19], *178*
Anthonisen, N. R., 308[35], *321*
Anthracite, R. F., 195, *208*
Antic, R., 298[2], *319*
Anton, A. H., 238[262], *255*
Antonissen, L. A., 85[98], 91[98], *117*
Appleman, M. M., 132[60,62], *181*
Arborelius, M. Jr., 222[114], *246*
Ariens, E. J., 221[67], 232[67], *243*
Armstrong, W. McD., 201[121], *213*
Arnold, A., 192[12], 196[12], *206*
Arnold, W. P., 131[51], 171[51], *180*
Arnold, W. V., 131[52], 171[52], *180*
Arnqvist, H. J., 97, *118*
Arons, A. B., 269[22], *291*
Arunlakshana, O., 192, *206*
Asakawa, T., 131[57], *180*
Asano, T., 162[158], *187*
Ashby, C. D., 133[69], 164[167], *181, 188*
Ashmore, J., 142[110], *184*
Aspin, N., 260[2], *290*
Assem, E. S. K., 203[144], *214*
Attinger, E. O., 239[285], *257*
Augstein, J., 202, *213*
Aurbach, G. D., 129[34], *179*
Austen, K. F., 124[1], 142[97,100, 101,102], 143[101], 146[100], 147[1], 148[1], 152[1], 157 [141], 158[141,143], *177, 183, 186,* 202[128,129,132,134,135,
[Austen, K. F.]
136], 203[136], *213, 214,* 231 [208], *252*
Austen, W. G., 142[100], 146[100], *183*
Austin, J. H. M., 217[9], 218[9], 229 [180], *240, 250*
Aviado, D. M., 229[183,184], 230 [183,184,192], 231[205], 236 [253], 238[253], *251, 252, 255*
Avner, B. P., 198[81], *210*
Axline, S. G., 148[124], *185*

## B

Bach, M. K., 157[142], *186*
Bahler, A. S., 66[69], 86[69], *115*
Baigelman, W., 224[153], *249*
Baird, C. E., 130[44], 142[90], 143, 161[44], 165[180], 168[44], 169 [44], 170[44,180], 173[44], 174 [44], *179, 183, 188*
Baird, I. L., 222[104], 223[104], 233[104], *246*
Baker, D. G., 234[241,242], 235[241, 242], *254*
Balchum, O. J., 219[38], 230[194], *242, 251*
Baldwin, C. J., 199[86], *211*
Baltisberger, W., 58, *114*
Bando, T., 16[66], *28*
Banister, J., 230[197], *251*
Bar, H.-P., 158[144], 161[144], 162 [144], 163[144], *186*
Barany, M., 84, 85, *117*
Barnett, D. B., 139[86], 140[86], 141[86], 144, *182*
Barnett, T. B., 311[52], *322*
Baron, G. D., 171[190], *189,* 201 [199], *213*
Barr, L., 66[73], *115*
Barrett-Bee, K. J., 138, 141[84], 146 [84], *182*
Barsinger, G. M., 96[111], 103[111], *117*

Bartlett, D., Jr., 234[229,231], *253, 254*
Bartlett, R. A., 307[31], *321*
Bartlett, S., 220[63], 238[63], *243*
Baruch, D. W., 225[154], *249*
Basbaum, C. B., 221[76], *244*
Bass, H., 308[35], *321*
Bass, P., 16[71], *29*
Basset, F., 3[21], *26*
Bates, D. V., 230[201], *252,* 301 [9], 308[35], *320, 321*
Batten, J. C., 221[82], 230[82], *244*
Battigelli, M. C., 280[41], *292*
Baukal, A., 128[32], 129[32], *179*
Bayles, J., 286[80], *294*
Beall, G. N., 205, *216,* 238[268], *256*
Beall, R. J., 130[36], *179*
Beatty, C. H., 96[111], 103[111], *117*
Beaven, M. A., 195, *208*
Beavo, J. A., 134[75], *182*
Bebb, C., 230[197], *251*
Bechtel, P. J., 134[75], *182*
Becker, J. A., 142[105], *184*
Beland, J., 16[72], *29,* 64, *115,* 201 [113], *212,* 237[257], *255*
Bell, K. A., 281[53], *293*
Benoy, C. J., 199, *211*
Bergen, W., 66[73], *115*
Bergh, N. P., 195[47], *208*
Berkowitz, B. A., 197[62,63,65], *209*
Bernauer, W., 200[106], *212*
Berti, F., 172[193], *189*
Besch, H. R., 128[29], *178*
Beviz, A., 98[122], *118*
Bewta, A., 238[271], *256*
Bhattacharya, B. K., 232[218], *253*
Bianchi, C. P., 164[173], *188*
Bianco, S., 195[44], 196[50], *208*
Bienenstock, J., 23[81,82], *29*
Bihler, I., 97, *118*
Bilbo, R. E., 314[74], *324*
Black, J. W., 192[7], *206*
Black, L. F., 304[21], *321*
Blaksin, A. S., 130[45], 139[45], 171 [45], *180*
Bleecker, E. R., 225[156,157], 231 [213], *249, 252,* 285[73], *294*
Blisard, K. S., 168[188], 171[188], *189*
Blümcke, S., 13, *27,* 219[52], 236 [52], *242*
Blume, A. S., 197[65], *209*
Boatman, E. S., 285[76], *294*
Bocek, R. M., 96[111], 103[111], *117*
Bode, F., 284[66], *294,* 298[2], 312 [56], *319, 323*
Bohr, D. F., 105[149], *120*
Boll, D. E., 46[24], *112*
Borg, K. O., 196[53], *209*
Bose, D., 66[67], 67[67], *115*
Bose, R., 66[67], 67[67], 104[142], 105[142], *115, 119*
Botelho, S. Y., 223[133], *248*
Bottin, R., [269], *256*
Bouchard, T., 2[8], 3[8,18], 4[8], 6 [8], 16[68], 23[8], *25, 26, 28,* 201[112], *212,* 237[255], *255*
Boucher, R. C., 2[7], 6[27], *25, 26,* 156, *186*
Bouhuys, A., 31[1], *111,* 126[17], 172[192], *178, 189,* 196[55], 197[55], 198[76], 200[99,100], *209, 210, 212,* 217[10], 222[10], 229[191], 231[206], 232[206], 237[10], 238[191], 239[191], *240, 251, 252,* 306[28], 312[59], *321, 323*
Bourne, H. R., 128[23], 139[86], 140 [86], 141[86], 144[86], *178, 182,* 203[139], *214*
Boushey, H. A., 222[95,96,122], 226 [95,96], 227[95,96], 229[95], 230[95], 232[96], *245, 247,* 285 [72], *294*
Boussauw, L., 23[84], 24[84], *29*
Bower, A., 227[169], *250*

Bowman, R. H., 104[140], *119*
Bowman, W. C., 192[19], *207*
Boyd, G., 3[18], *26*
Bradley, D. E., 15[62], *28*
Brashler, J. R., 157[142], *186*
Braughler, J. M., 131[58], *180*
Breckenridge, B. M., 130[37], 132[37], *179*
Breeze, R. G., 2[10], *25*
Bremel, R. D., 105, 110, *120*
Brian, J. D., 217[7], 218[7], 237[7], 239[7], *240,* 277[36], *292*
Brink, C., 198[76], *210,* 223[132], 238[132], *247*
Briscoe, W. A., 233[225], *253,* 302[10], *320*
Brittain, R. T., 192[16], *207*
Brocklehurst, W. E., 194, 202[127], *208, 213*
Brodie, B. B., 197[59], *209*
Brodie, T. G., 218[21], 225[21], *241*
Brody, M. J., 143[113], *184*
Brody, T. N., 126[11], *177*
Bromberger-Barnea, B., 300[7], *320*
Bromley, A. C., 302[11], *320*
Bronk, D. W., 218[25], *241*
Brosset, C., 264[16], *291*
Brostrom, C. O., 130[37], 132[37], *179*
Brown, R., 307[30], 314[72,73], 317[73], *321, 324*
Brown, T. G., Jr., 192[12], 196[12], *206*
Brownlee, G., 221[69,70], 232[69, 70], *244*
Bruderman, I., 222[105], *246*
Bryan, A. C., 260[2], *290,* 317[79], *324*
Bryant, L., 219[36], *242*
Bucher, U., 22[80], 23[80], *29*
Buchtal, F., 76[87], *116*
Buckley, R. D., 219[38], *242*
Bueding, E., 163[162], *187*
Bülbring, E., 163[162], 175[201], *187, 190*
Burka, J. F., 202[131], *213*
Burnstock, G., 9[45], 14[45], 16[45], 18[45], 19[45], *27,* 43, 48, 51, 54, 64, 66[70,71,72], *112, 113, 115,* 163[163], *187,* 201, *212,* 217[1], 235[1], 238[1], *239*
Burton, A. C., 76, *116*
Butcher, F. R., 142[106], 143[106], *184*
Butcher, R. W., 124[4], 142[90], 143, 158[148], 159[148], *177, 183, 186*
Butcher, S. S., 263[11], *290*
Butler, J., 233[226], *253,* 303[13], *320*
Butler, T. C., 102, *118*
Butterworth, K. R., 197[73], *210*

## C

Cabezas, G. A., 196[54], *209,* 217[9], 218[9], 221[87], 225[87], 236[87], 237[87], 238[87], *240, 245*
Cabral, L. J., 284[69], *294*
Calkins, D., 133[69], *181*
Calkins, P. J., 193[27], 194[27], 195[37], 197[67], 199[37], 201[27], 204[150,151], *207, 208, 210, 215*
Callas, G., 228[176], *250*
Callerame, M. L., 2[6], *25*
Cameron, A. R., 9[44], 12[44], *27, 62, 115*
Canaday, P. G., 37[8], 75[8], *111*
Caplan, S. R., 48[30], 91[103], *113, 117*
Carlsson, E., 196[53], *209*
Carlsten, A. B., 218[30], *241*
Carlyle, R. F., 219[35], 221[35,88], *242, 245*
Caro, C. G., 233[226], *253,* 303[13], *320*
Caron, M. G., 129[35], *179,* 199[87], *211*
Carr, D. W., 131[55], *180*
Carsey, F. D., 264[19], *291*

Carsten, M. E., 48, 49, 103[130], 110, *113, 119*
Case, R. M., 7[37], *27*
Casnellie, J. E., 164[169], 172 [169], *188*
Cassidy, S. S., 235[244], *254*
Castagna, M., 134[72], *181*
Castelman, W. L., 15[57], *28*
Castillo, J. C., 193, *207,* 221[90], 231[90], *245*
Castro de la Mata, R., 236[253], 238[253], *255*
Catt, K. J., 128[28,32], 129[32], 133[70], 135[70], *178, 179, 181*
Cavanaugh, M. J., 224[148], *248*
Cech, S., 236[251], *255*
Chamberlain, D. A., 224[143], *248*
Chan, W., 2[12], *25*
Chance, B., 94, *117*
Chand, N., 195[39], 202[39], *208*
Chang, S. G., 280[40], *292*
Chan-Yeung, M., 224[149], *248*
Charles, J. M., 282, *293*
Charlson, R. J., 263[11], 264[17,18, 19], 270[25], 271[29], 273[29], 275[35], 276[85,86], 277[35], 279[86], 285[17], *290, 291, 292, 295*
Charpin, J., 197[57], *209,* 238 [272], *256,* 284[71], 285[71, 77], *294,* 306[27], 314[71], *321, 324*
Chesrown, S. E., 139[86], 140[86], 141[86], 144[86], 151[133], *182, 185*
Cheung, W. Y., 132[61,63], *181*
Cho, Y. W., 229[184], 230[184], *251*
Chodosh, S., 224[153], *249*
Choi, J. K., 54, *113*
Chrisman, T. D., 130[43], 172[43], *179*
Christie, R. V., 301[9], 320
Christofano, E. E., 275[34], *292*
Clancy, R. L., 23[82], *29*
Clarke, B. G., 230[190], *251*
Clarke, P. S., 225[158], *249*
Clauser, H., 166[182], *188*
Clay, T. P., 222[94], 225[94], 226 [94], 239[94], *245,* 281[50], *293*
Clement, M. G., 228[175], *250*
Clements, R. S., 97[118], *118*
Clements, R. S., Jr., 97[116], 98[116], *118*
Clinch, N. F., 93, *117*
Clyman, R. I., 130[45], 139[45], 158 [146], 168[146], 171[45], *180, 186*
Coburn, R. F., 15[59], 16[59], *28,* 62, 64, *114,* 201[110], *212,* 237 [258], *255*
Coffey, R. G., 205[162], *215*
Coffin, D. L., 284[68], *294*
Coffino, P., 128[23], *178*
Cohen, M. L., 197[62,63,65], *209*
Cokelaere, M., 2[14], 3[14], *25*
Cole, H. M., 280[41], *292*
Colebatch, H. J. H., 60[51], 61[51], *114,* 217[3,4], 218[4], 221[3,4], 222[97], 223[97], 225[4], 231 [97], 232[97,215], 239[277], *240, 245, 253, 256,* 304[15,19], 315[19], 317[19], 318[15], *320*
Colebatch, J. H. J., 225[158], *249*
Coleman, R. A., 16[67], *28,* 201[111], *212*
Coleridge, H. M., 222[123], 234[238, 239,240,241,242], 235[241,242], *247, 254*
Coleridge, J. C. G., 222[123], 234[238, 239,240,241,242], 235[241,242], *247, 254*
Collela, D. F., 192[17], *207*
Collier, H. O. J., 199[93], *211,* 222 [119], 239[278,279,280,284], *247, 256, 257*
Collins, M. M., [188], *251*
Collins-Williams, C., 317[79], *324*
Colten, H. R., 148[123], *185*
Comroe, J. H., Jr., 223[133], 229 [185], 230[185], 233[227], *248, 251, 253*

Condemi, J. J., 2[6], *25*
Conen, P. E., 2[12], *25*
Conolly, M. E., 198, *210*
Conti, G., 51, 54, *113*
Cook, R. D., 14[53,55], 15[53], *27, 28,* 220[65], *243*
Cooke, P. H., 37[8], 44[21], 75[8], *111, 112*
Cooper, D. M., 224[148], *248*
Cooper, T., 191[1], 193[1], 195[1], *206,* 219[53], 236[53], *243*
Corbett, W. J., 268[21], *291*
Corbin, J. D., 133[68], *181*
Coret, I. A., 197, *210*
Corn, M., 231[210], 232[210], *252,* 281[48], 288[87], *292, 295*
Costa, E., 132[64], 133[71], 134 [73], 142[98], *181, 183*
Costabella, P. M., 57[47], 58[47], 59[47], 60[47], *114*
Cote, W. A., 285[78], *294*
Cotton, D. J., 231[213], *252*
Coupland, R., 3[17], *25*
Covert, D. S., 264[17,19], 270[25], 271[29], 272[30,31], 273[29], 274[30], 285[17], *291*
Cox, J. S. G., 204[154], *215*
Coyle, J. T., 220[56], *243*
Craven, P. A., 131[53], 171[53], *180*
Crawford, K. M., 131[54], 171[54], *180*
Creed, K. E., 126[9], 174[9], *177*
Crompton, G. K., 224[150], *249*
Cronn, D., 264[14], *290*
Cropp, G. J. A., 224[145], *248*
Crouch, C. M., 104, *119*
Cuatrecasas, P., 128[27], *178*
Cubedu, L., 130[39], *179*
Cumming, G., 309[45], 310, *322*
Curry, J. J., 314[64], *323*
Cutz, E., 2[11,12], *25,* 152[134], *186*
Czerniawska-Mysik, G., 200[108], *212*

**D**

Dahlstrom, A., 15[61], 16[61], *28,* 235[248], *255*
Dain, D. S., 222[122], *247*
Dale, H. H., 192, 204, *206, 215,* 223 [127], 231[127], *247*
Dalhamn, T., 3[19], *26,* 280[42], *292*
Daly, I. deB., 63, *115*
Daly, M. De Burghi, 218[22], 219[39], 220[22], 221[22], 237[22], *241,* 242
Daniel, E. E., 66[74], *115*
Daniel, V. L., 66[74], *115*
Dart, G. A., 309[48], *322*
Dautrebande, L., 221[81], 225[163], 226[163], 229[181], 230[163], *244, 249, 250,* 281[44], *292*
Davies, D. S., 198[75], *210*
Davis, B., 224[139], *248*
Davis, H. L., 233[223], *253*
Davis, J. J., 285[79], *294*
Davis, J. W., 130[40], *179*
Davis, L. B., 199[95], *211*
Dawes, G. S., 233[227], *253*
Dawson, S. V., 300, *320*
Dayton, S., 103[136], 104, *119*
Dean, C. M., 192[16], *207*
Debbas, G., 48[28], *113*
DeBeer, E. J., 193, *207,* 221[90], 231 [90], *245*
deCandole, C. A., 221[85], *245*
De Duve, C., 48[29], *113*
DeGroat, W. C., 220[59], *243*
DeGroot, W. J., 228[176], *250,* 315 [77], 318[77], 319[77], *324*
DeKock, M. A., 222[97], 223[97], 231[97], 232[97], 238[266], *245, 256*
Dennis, M. W., 196[55], 197[55], *209*
De Notariis, A., 2[7], *25*

DeRubertis, F. R., 131[53], 171 [53], *180*
Derwall, R., 146[119], *185*
Despas, P. J., 309[50], 311[55], *322, 323*
deTroyer, A., 221[83], *244*
Devine, C. E., 44, 49[35], 54[35], 55[35,43], 57[46], 68[35], *112, 113, 114,* 175[199], *190*
Dewey, M. M., 66[73], *115*
Diamond, J., 126[11], 127[20], 168[185,186,187,188], 170 [117], 171[186,188], *177, 178, 184, 189*
Diamond, L., 196[56], 197[56], *209*
DiBella, F., 151[128], *185*
Dickman, M., 224[152], *249*
Dinsdale, F., 23[83], *29*
Dirken, M. N., 218[26], *241*
Dixon, W. E., 218[21], 221[86], 225[21], 236[86], 237, *241, 245*
Dollery, C. T., 198[75], *210*
Don, H. F., 222[115], 229[115], *246*
Donnelly, T. E., Jr., 138[81], *182*
DoPico, G. A., 224[146], *248*
Dosman, J., 284[66], *294,* 298[2], 312[56], *319, 323*
Douglas, J. S., 172[192], *189,* 196 [55], 197[55], 198, 200[99, 100], *209, 210, 212,* 217[10], 222[10], 223[132], 237[10], 238[132], *240, 247*
Douglas, N. J., 218[16], *240*
Douglas, W. W., 221[85], *245*
Dow, R. S., 13, *27,* 61, *114*
Drakontides, A. B., 221[71], 232 [71], *244*
Drazen, J. M., 202, *214,* 231[208], 233[219,220], 238[267], *252, 253, 256,* 302[12], 309[12],
[Drazen, J. M.]
309[12], 310, 311[51], *320, 322*
Dreyer, A. C., 193, *207*
Dreyfus, C. F., 221[75], 232[75], *244*
Driska, S., 105[144], 106, 110, *120*
Drummond, G. I., 159[151], 173[151], *187*
Dubnick, B., 204[155], *215*
DuBois, A. B., 223[133], 229[181], 233[225,226], *248, 250, 253,* 281 [44], *292,* 302[10], 303[13], *320*
Dubrawsky, C., 317[79], *324*
Dubriel, M., 286[80], *294*
Duchon, G., 66[74], *115*
Duckles, S. P., 222[125], *247*
Dufau, M. L., 128[28], 129[32], 133 [70], *178, 179, 181*
Duffell, G. M., 304[20], *320*
Dumont, J. E., 137[79], *182*
Duncan, L., 159[151], 173[151], *187*
Duncan, P. E., 142[91], *183*
Duncan, W. A. M., 192[7], *206*
Dungworth, D. L., 15[57], *28*
Dunham, E. W., 158[145], *186*
Dunnill, M. S., 7[39], *27,* 318[81], *324*
Durant, C. J., 192[7], *206*
Dybicki, J., 230[194], *251*

## E

Eakins, K. E., 238[260], *255*
Earp, H. S., 127[22], 128[22], 131 [47,59], 132[22], 133, 134[75], *178, 180, 182*
Ebashi, S., 44, 110, *112, 120*
Edmunds, L. H., Jr., 219[41], 236 [41,252], *242, 255*
Eimerl, S., 159[153], *187*
Eiseman, B., 219[36], *242*

Eisen, S. A., 152[136], 153[136], 155[136], *186,* 203[138], *214*
Ekman, M., 193, 195[26], *207*
Ekwall, B., 222[114], *246*
El-Bermani, A., 15[62], *28*
Elbrink, J., 97[120], *118*
El-Fellah, M. S., 199[83], *211*
Elftman, A. G., 233[224], *253*
Elfvin, L. G., 44, *112*
Elliott, E. A., 300, *320*
Ellisman, M. H., 6[31], *26*
Elmer, C., 142[106], 143[106], *184*
Embden, G., 103, *119*
Emery, J. L., 23[83], *29*
Empey, D. W., 285[75], *294,* 314[75], *324*
Engel, L. A., 60, *114,* 309[50], *322*
Epstein, S., 202[133], *214*
Ercan, Z. S., 200, *212*
Ericsson, E., 197[64,69], *209, 210*
Ernster, L., 96[112], *118*
Estensen, R., 127[18], *178*
Evans, C. L., 221[85], *245*
Evans, D. H. L., 175[200], *190,* 219[39], *242*
Evans, M. J., 284[69,70], *294*
Eyre, P., 194[35], 195[35,39], 202[39,131], 204[147], *208, 213 215*

F

Fairbanks, G., 105, *120*
Fanburg, B. L., 199[92], *211*
Faridy, E. E., 284[65], *293*
Farmer, J. B., 202[130], *213*
Farquhar, M. G., 44, *112*
Farr, A. L., 105, *120*
Farr, R. S., 196[49], *208*
Fay, F. S., 37, 44[21], 75, *111, 112,* 201[124], *213*
Fegler, G., 230[197], *251*
Feinstein, M. B., 165[179], *188*
Feldberg, W., 239[282], *257*
Fenn, W. O., 224[137], *248*
Ferguson, C. C., 2[7,8], 3[8], 4[8], 6[8], 9[47], 18[73], 19[73], 23[8], 24[87], *25, 27, 29,* 219[54], *243*
Ferguson, L. K., 218[25], *241*
Fernandez, R., 282[61], *293*
Fertel, R., 162[160], *187*
Fidone, S. F., 227[168], *250*
Figlin, R., 162[160], *187*
Fillenz, M., 218[19], 222[103], 227[103], 228[103], 230[103], 232[103], 233[103], 234[103], *241, 246*
Filley, G. F., 309[48], *322*
Finkel, M. P., 192[18], *207*
Finlayson, B. J., 264[15], *290*
Finnegan, J. K., 224[141], *248*
Finucane, K. E., 304[19], 315[19], 317[19], *320*
Fischer, E. H., 133[69], *181*
Fischer, S. P., 221[66], 223[66], 231[213], 232[66], *243, 252*
Fish, J. E., 314[69], *323*
Fishel, C., 205[161], *215*
Fishman, N. H., 223[136], *248*
Fitzpatrick, D. F., 48[28], *113*
Fleisch, J. H., 160[154], *187,* 191[1], 193[27], 194[27], 195[1,37], 197[58,59,60,66,67,74], 198, 199[37], 201[27], 204[150,151], *206, 207, 208, 209, 210, 215,* 219[53], 222[121], 236[53], *243, 247*
Flenley, D. C., 218[16], *240*
Flesch, J., 231[210], 232[210], *252*
Fletcher, C. M., 230[190], *251*
Flexch, J., 281[48], *292*
Flores, G., 103[134], *119*
Focant, B. W. W., 110[157], *120*
Folkow, B., 218[27,29,30], *241*
Fontaine, R., 94[109], *117*
Ford, D., 282[61], *293*
Ford, L. E., 81[92], *116*
Forman, R., 81[92], *116*
Forn, J., 160[154], *187*

Foster, R. W., 218[33], 220[33], 237[33], *241*
Foster, S. J., 199[89], *211*
Fowler, P. J., 192[17], *207*
Fowler, W. S., 233[223], *253*
Frank, J. S., 42, 88[10], *112*
Frank, N. R., 217[7], 218[7], 222 [111], 226[164,165], 230[195], 237[7], 239[7], *240, 246, 249, 251,* 277[36,37], *292*
Frank, R., 230[199], *252,* 260[10], 271[29], 272[30,31], 273[29], 274[30], 275[35], 276[86], 277[35], 279[86], 285[76], *290, 291, 292, 294, 295*
Franklin, T. J., 199[89,90], *211*
Fraser, D. A., 280[41], *292*
Frearson, N., 110, *120*
Freedman, S., 304[18], 315[18], 317[18], *320*
Freeman, G., 284[68,69,70], *294*
Frey, M. J., 151[133], *185*
Frey, W., 131[55], *180*
Friedlander, S. K., 281[53], *293*
Froeb, H. F., 304[23], *321*
Fry. D. L., 299[4], 300[5], 311 [53], *319, 320, 322*
Furchgott, R. F., 192, 196[10,11], *206, 209*
Fuxe, K., 15[61], 16[61], *28,* 235 [248], *255*

## G

Gabbay, K. H., 148[123], *185*
Gabbiani, G., 57[47], 58[47], 59 [47], 60[47], *114*
Gabella, G., 9[46], 18[74], 19[74], *27, 29,* 44, *112,* 219[40], *242*
Gaddum, J. H., 221[72], 232[72], *244*
Gallin, J. I., 221[68], 232[68], *243*
Gamsu, G., 229[180], *250*
Ganellin, C. R., 192[7], *206*
Gansler, H., 51, *113*
Garbers, D. L., 130[43], 131[46], 162[157], 172[43], *179, 180, 187*
Gardiner, A. J., 218[15], *240*
Gardiner, P. J., 199[94], *211*
Gardner, J. D., 129[34], *179*
Garfield, R. E., 44[20], 48[20], 66 [74], *112, 115*
Garst, J. E., 162[157], *187*
Gasser, H. S., 89[102], *117*
Gay, L. N., 219[43], *242*
Gaylor, J. B., 13, *27*
Gayrard, P., 197[57], *209,* 218[15], 238[272], *240, 256,* 284[71], 285 [71,77], *294,* 306[27], 314[70,71], *321, 324*
George, C. F., 198[75], *210*
George, W. J., 142[111], *184*
Gercken, G., 163[162], *187*
Gershon, M. D., 16[69], *28,* 221[71, 74,75], 232[71,74,75], *244*
Gestenblith, G., 197[68], *210*
Gilbert, N. C., 225[162], *249*
Giles, R. E., 192[18], *207*
Gill, G. N., 134[77], *182*
Gillespie, E., 149[126], *185,* 203[140, 141], 205, *214, 216*
Gillespie, J. S., 126[9], 174[9], *177*
Gillis, C. N., 191[2], *206*
Gilman, A. G., 128[31], *179*
Gilmore, N. J., 156[140], *186*
Gilula, N. B., 6[28], *26*
Ginzel, K. H., 234[241,242], 235 [241,242], *254*
Girling, F., 218[28], *241*
Glass, D. B., 127[18], 131[55], 142 [112], 168[112], *178, 180, 184*
Glasstone, G., 268[20], *291*
Gnegy, M. E., 132[64], *181*
Goddeeris, P., 2[16], *25*
Gold, W. M., 139[86], 140[86], 141 [86], 144[86], 151[133], *182, 185,* 222[122], 229[180], 231 [211,213], *247, 250,* 285[75], *294,* 314[75], 315[76], 317[76], *324*

Goldberg, N. D., 127, 131[55], 142, 158[145], 168[112], *178, 180, 184, 186*
Goldberg, L., 230[203], *252*
Golden, J. A., 285[72], *294*
Goldsmith, J. R., 230[198], *252*
Goldstein, B. D., 219[38], *242*
Golla, F. L., 63, *115*, 194, *207*
Gomori, C. J., 105, *120*
Gonzalez, C., 133[69], *181*
Goodman, A. D., 139, *182*
Goodman, D. B. P., 151[128], *185*
Gordon, A. M., 75[82], 99[82], *116*
Goth, A., 154[137], *186*
Gradley, G. W., 228[178], *250*
Graf, P. D., 196[54], *209*, 219[41], 221[66,87], 222[109,116], 223[66], 225[87], 229[180], 231[210,213], 232[66,210], 236[41,87,252], 237[87], 238[87], *242, 243, 245, 246, 250, 252, 255*, 281[48], *292*
Graham, W., 308[38], *322*
Grand, R. J., 142[109], *184*
Granito, S. M., 286[82], 287[82], *295*
Grant, W. F., 201[123], *213*
Green, L. R., 138, 141[84], 146[84], *182*
Green, M., 217[6], 221[6,79], 224[6], 236[6], *240, 244*, 306[29], *321*
Greengard, P., 124[6], 138[81], 142[6], 151[132], 164[169], 172[169], *177, 182, 185, 188*
Grieco, M. H., [275], *256*
Griffin, J. P., 142[91], *183*, 196[50], *208*
Griffin, P. L., 195[44], *208*, 309[50], *322*
Grimaud, Ch., 238[272], *256*, 284[71], 285[71,77], *294*, 306[27], 314[71], *321, 324*
Grimby, G. T., 308[38], *322*
Grodzinska, L., 200, *212*
Gross, G. N., 196[49], *208*
Gross, N. J., 224[147], *248*
Gryglewski, R. J., 200[101,108], *212*
Guene, R., 284[67], *294*
Guidotti, A., 133[71], 134[73], 142[98], *181, 183*
Gulati, O. D., 197[61], *209*
Guth, L., 219[42], 236[42], *242*
Guthrow, C. E., Jr., 151[128], *185*
Guyatt, A. R., 230[190], *251*, 302[11], *320*
Guz, A., 234[233], *254*

## H

Hackenbrock, C. R., 46[26], 95, *112*
Haddox, M. K., 127[18], 142[112], 158[145], 168[112], *178, 184, 186*
Haenni, B., 51[38], 54[38], *113*
Haga, K., 128[31], *179*
Haga, T., 128[31], *179*
Hagihara, B., 94, *117*
Hahn, H. L., 221[66], 222[101,108, 109], 223[66,101,108], 227[101], 228[101], 231[101], 232[66,101], *246, 243*
Hajdu, S., 42, *112*
Hakansson, C. H., 7[42], *27*, 60, *114*
Hallett, W. Y., 230[200], *252*
Halmagyi, F. J., 217[3], 221[3], *240*
Hamberger, B., 219[49], *242*
Hamberger, C.-A., 218[29,30], *241*
Hamet, P., 160[155], 161[155], 162[155], *187*
Hamill, R. L., 201[120], *213*
Hang, L. M., 2[9], *25*
Hankinson, J. L., 260[1], *290*
Hansell, M. M., 3[22], *26*
Hanson, J. P., 105[145], *120*
Harbon, S., 166[182], *188*
Hardmann, J. G., 130[43,44], 131[46], 137[79], 142[108], 143, 159[108], 160, 161[44], 162[108], 165[180], 168[44,108,183], 169

[Hardmann, J. G.]
[44], 170[44,180], 171[108], 172[43,108], 173[44,108], 174 [44], *179, 180, 182, 184, 187, 188, 189*
Hardy, J. D., 234[237], 236[237], *254*
Harker, A. B., 280[40], *292*
Harper, A. A., 7[37], *27*
Harrison, C., 230[203], *252*
Hartle, D. K., 127[20], 168[185, 187], *178, 189*
Hartshorne, D. J., 105[144], 106, 110[144], *120*
Harwood, J. P., 129[33], *179*
Haselgrove, J. C., 55[45], *114*
Hashimoto, S., 103[136], 104, *119*
Haslam, R. J., 142[103], *183*
Hathaway, D. R., 128[29], *178*
Hawkins, J. T., 163[162], *187*
Hayashi, K., 128[32], 129[32], *179*
Haynes, R. L., 313[62], 315[62], 317[62], 319[83], *323, 324*
Hebb, C., 61, 63, *114, 115,* 218 [18], 235[18], *241*
Hedner, P., 125[7], 158[147], *177, 186*
Hedquist, P., 314[68], *323*
Heisler, N., 102[127], *118*
Herdan, G., 263[12], *290*
Herlihy, J. T., 86[161], *121*
Hertweck, M. S., 234[237], 236 [237], *254*
Herxheimer, H., 231[204], 238 [265], *252, 256,* 314[66], *323*
Herzig, D. J., 204[155], *215*
Heuser, J. E., 221[76], *244*
Hickey, R. F., 222[116], 223[136], *246, 248*
Hidaka, H., 162[158], *187*
Hidy, G., 263[13], 271[13], *290*
Hiestand, P. C., 134[74], *181*
Hill, A. V., 82, 83, 84, 87, 88[94], 89[102], 93, *117*
Hill, I. D., 230[190], *251*
Hillman, C. C., 193[22], *207*
Himori, N., 194[31], 195, *207*
Hiratsuka, K., 195, *208*
Hirsch, J., 202[133], *214*
Hirst, G. D. S., 19[76], *29*
Hladovec, J., 97[115], *118*
Ho, H., 164[170], *188*
Ho, R. J., 131[57], *180*
Hogg, J. C., 2[3], 6[25,26,27], *25, 26,* 156[140], *186,* 217[7,8], 218 [7], 236[8], 237[7], 238[8], 239 [7], *240,* 309[42,43], 312[61], *322, 323*
Hokfelt, T., 15[61], 16[61], *28,* 235 [248], *255*
Holdy, K. E., 134[77], *182*
Holgate, S. T., 199[86], *211*
Holland, D. R., 201[121], *213*
Hollander, W., 105[152], 107[152], 110[152], *120*
Hollands, B. C. S., 235[249], *255*
Holmes, R., 221[85], *245*
Holmes, T. G., 168[186], 171[186], *189*
Holmgren, A., 314[68], *323*
Holroyde, M. C., 204[147], *215*
Holst, P. E., 222[124], *247*
Honjin, R., 218[24], 235[246], *241, 255*
Hooker, C. S., 193, 194, 197[66,67], 201, 204[150,151], *207, 209, 210 215*
Hoppin, F. C., Jr., 221[79], *244*
Hopwood, D., 3[17], *25*
Horng, J. S., 201[120], *213*
Horsfield, K., 309[45], 310, *322*
Horton, D. J., 225[160], *249*
Hounam, R. F., 260[7], 266[7], 286 [7], *290*
Housley, E., 308[40], 318[80], *322, 324*
Huang, Y. C., 130[37], 132[37], *179*
Hubbard, B. D., 46, *112*
Hug, C. C., Jr., 16[71], *29*
Hughes, F., 128[25], *178*

Hughes, J. M. B., 222[94], 225[94], 226[94], 239[94], *245,* 281 [50], *293*
Hukuhara, T., 220[57], *243*
Hung, K.-S., 234[237], 236[237], *254*
Hunt, V. R., 306[28], *321*
Hurd, F. K., 268[21], *291*
Hurwitz, L., 48, *113,* 168[184], 175[198], 176[198], *189,* 198 [81], *210*
Huxley, A. F., 75[82,83], 81, 88 [91], 90[83], 99[82], *116*
Hyatt, R. E., 299[4], 300[5], 304 [14,21], *319, 320, 321*
Hyman, A. L., 144[118], *185,* 199 [95], 200, *211, 212*

## I

Ignarro, L. J., 142[111], *184*
Ingram, C. G., 238[273,274], *256*
Ingram, R. H., Jr., 218[14], 233 [219,220], *240, 253,* 302[12], 304[20], 307[30], 308[34], 309[12], 310[12], 311[51,54], 312[60], 313[54,60,62], 314 [72,73], 315[62], 317[62,73], 318[82], 319[83], *320, 321, 322, 323, 324*
Innes, I. R., 66[67], 67[67], *115,* 229[179], *250*
Inoue, S., 6[25,26,27], *26*
Iravani, J., 234[230], *253*
Ishii, S., 44[13], *112*
Ishikawa, E., 130[40], *179*
Ishikawa, S., 103[40], *179*
Ishizaka, K., 2[4,6], *25*
Islam, M. S., 232[217], *253,* 285 [74], *294*
Isselbacher, K. J., 2[9], *25*
Itkin, H. I., 314[65], *323*
Izutsu, K. I., 102[128], *119*

## J

Jack, D., 192[15,16], *206, 207*
Jackson, D. M., 222[117], *247*
Jacobowitz, D., 219[53], 236[53], *243*
Jacobs, F. M., 222[113], 232[113], 233[113], *246,* 281[47], 286[47], 287[47], *292,* 306[26], 314[26], *321*
Jacobs, K. H., 165[177], *188*
Jacobs, L., 285[75], *294,* 314[75], *324*
Jaeger, M. J., 309[46], *322*
Jaffrin, M. Y., 309[47], *322*
James, G. W. L., 239[278,279,284], *256, 257*
Jamieson, D., 221[89], 235[89], *245*
Jeffrey, P., 6[34], 14[34], *26,* 234 [229], *253*
Jenne, J., 198[81], *210*
Jenson, P. L., 281[49], *293*
Jernerus, R., 222[114], *246*
Johansson, B., 86[162], *121*
Johansson, S. G. O., 2[6], *25,* 125[8], 126[8], 144[8], 145[8], 158[8], 165[8], 168[8], 172[8], 173[8], 175[8], 176[8], *177*
Johnson, E. S., 221[69,70,91], 232 [69,70], *244, 245*
Johnsson, G., 196[53], *209*
Johnston, N., 23[81], *29*
Joiner, P. D., 199[95], *211*
Jones, H. A., 222[94], 225[94], 226 [94], 239[94], *245,* 281[50], *293*
Jones, M. T., 260[2], *290*
Jonsson, R., 231[206], 232[206], *252*
Juchmes, J., [269], *256*
Junge, C., 269[24], *291*
Jungmann, R. A., 134[74], *181*

## K

Kadowitz, P. J., 143[113], 144[118],

[Kadowitz, P. J.]
*184, 185,* 199[95], 200[109], *211, 212*
Kahn, J., 66[72], *115*
Kaiser, E., 76[87], *116*
Kakiuchi, S., 159[152], 170[152], *187*
Kaliner, M. A., 124[2], 139[88], 141[2], 142[97,101,102], 143[2,101], 146[88,120], 148[2], 149[2,127], 150[2,127], *177, 182, 183, 185,* 202[136], 203[136], *214*
Kalisker, A., 205[166], *216*
Kaltreider, H. B., 2[5], 23[5], *25*
Kamburoff, P. L., 195[44], 196[50], *208*
Kamikawa, Y., 201[117], *213*
Kanstein, C. B., 134[77], *182*
Kapanci, Y., 57, 58, 59, 60, *114*
Karczewski, N., 61, *114*
Karczewski, W., 217[5], 221[5], 231[5], 232[5], 234[5], *240*
Kasuya, Y., 198[80], *210*
Katsuki, S., 131[52], 171[52,191], *180, 189*
Katz, A. M., 105[145], *120,* 173[195,196], 174[195,196], *189*
Kaufman, H. S., 315[76], 317[76], *324*
Kaufman, J., 223[134], 226, 229[134], *248*
Keely, S. L., 133[68], *181*
Keiser, H. R., 314[67], *323*
Kellaway, C. H., 202, *213*
Keller, C., 205, *215*
Keltz, H., 195[46], *208*
Kempf, E., 94[109], 97[117], *117, 118*
Kendrick-Jones, J., 110[156], *120*
Kennedy, K. P., 224[143], *248*
Kent, D. C., 221[80], 226[80], 229[80], 239[80], *244,* 281[46], *292,* 312[57], *323*
Kent, K. M., 191[1], 193[1], 195[1], *206,* 219[53], 236[53], *243*
Kerr, J. W., 196[51], *209*
Kerth, C. H., 269[22], *291*
Kesic, P., 309[47], *322*
Kessler, G.-F., 229[180], 231[211], *250, 252*
Kim, B. K., 306[28], *321*
Kimberg, D. V., 142[109], *184*
Kimura, H., 130[41,42], 131[49], 138, 139[83], 141[83,99], 142[99], 143[99], 144[99], 145[99], 158[99], 171[48,49], *179, 180, 182, 183*
Kind, L. S., 193[28], *207*
King, A. S., 14[53,55], 15[53], *27, 28,* 220[65], *243*
Kinsman, R. A., 225[159,160], *249*
Kirchberger, M. A., 173[195,196], 174[195,196], *189*
Kirk, J. E., 67[78], 97, *116*
Kirkpatrick, C. H., 9[44], 12[44], *27,* 62, 66[68], 67[68], 68[68], 104, *115, 119,* 205, *215*
Kiser, R., 315[77], 318[77], 319[77], *324*
Kitamura, S., 235[243], *254*
Klock, L. E., 224[152], *249*
Knapp, P. H., 217[2], *240*
Knapp, P. L., 195[43], *208*
Knoohuizen, M., 154[137], *186*
Knowlton, G. C., 233[222], *253*
Knudson, R., 221[84], *244,* 306[24], *321*
Koelle, G. B., 219[37], *242*
Koide, Y., 134[75], *182*
Konno, K., 9[49], *27,* 66[65,66], 67[65,66], *115*
Kono, T., 132[66], *181*
Konzett, H., 222[107], *246*
Koopman, W. J., 142[97], *183*
Koppanyi, T., 197[71], *210*
Kotani, S., 220[57], *243*
Kotetzky, M. T., 225[159], *249*

Kozar, L. F., 223[126], *247*
Krahl, V. E., 61, *114*
Kramer, G. L., 162[157], *187*
Kratschmer, F., 225, *249*
Krebs, E. G., 133[69], 164[166], *181, 187*
Kreye, V. A. W., 171[190], *189*, 201[119], *213*
Krishnamurty, V. S. R., 197[61], *209*
Kroeger, E. A., 48[31,32], 65[32], 66[75], 67[75,76], 82[93], 83 [93], 89[101], 100[31,101], *113, 115, 117*, 164[171,172,173], 166[172], *188*
Kromer, U., 67[76], 85[98,100], 86[100], 91[98], *115, 117*
Krzanowski, J. J., 139[85], 144[117], *182, 184*
Kuchii, M., 16[70], *28*
Kuehl, F. A., 127[18], *178*
Kuhar, M. J., 220[56], *243*
Kukovetz, W. R., 161, 162[159], *187*
Kumagai, M., 66[65,66], 67[65,66], *115*
Kuo, J. F., 124[6], 134[76], 138[81], 141[94], 142[6,94], 145[94], *177, 182, 183*
Kuo, W.-N., 134[76], 141[94], 142 [94], 145[94], *182, 183*
Kuriyama, H., 9[48], *27*, 37[6], 61 [6], 64[6], 73[6], *111*, 163 [162], *187*, 237[256], *255*
Kuriyama, K., 131[50], 171[50], *180*
Kurosawa, A., 134[73], *181*
Kusner, E. J., 204[155], *215*

## L

La Belle, C. W., 275[34], *292*
Lacey, M., 227[170], *250*
Lad, P. J., 131[54], 171[54], *180*
Lagnado, J. R., 151[129], *185*
Lagunoff, D., 154, *186*
Laidlaw, P. P., 223[127], 231[127], *247*
Laitinen, L. A., 285[75], *294*, 314 [75], *324*
Lakatta, E. G., 197, *210*
Lall, A., 236[252], *255*
Lambert, E. H., 233[223], *253*
Lambley, J. E., 199[96], *211*
Landon, E. S., 48[28], *113*
Lands, A. M., 192, 196[12], *206*
Langer, G. A., 42, 88[10], *112*
Langer, H., 317[79], *324*
Langer, I., 238[276], *256*
Lapp, N. L., 260[1], *290*
Laraia, P. J., 142[97], *183*
Larrabee, M. G., 233[222], *253*
Lars, E., 196[53], *209*
Larsell, G., 13, *27*
Larsell, O., 61, *114*, 218[23], 219 [46], *241, 242*
Larson, C. P., Jr., 222[116], *246*
Larson, T. V., 270[25], 271[29], 272 [30,31], 273[29], 274[30], *291*
Larsson, A. L., 199[85], *211*
Laszt, L., 51[38], 54[38], *113*
Laurent, B., 196[48], *208*
Lauweryns, J. M., 2[14,16], 3[14], 23[84], 24[84], *25, 29*
Lavallee, M., 102[129], *119*
Lazarides, E., 46, *112*
Lazarus, S. C., 151[133], *185*
Leak, L. V., 24[85], *29*
Leaver, D. G., [270], *256*, 304[17], *320*
Lecomte, J., [269], *256*
Le Crom, M., 3[21], *26*
Lee, C. Y., 126[12], *177*
Lee, L.-Y., 285[73], *294*
Lee, T. B., 202[130], *213*
Lee, T. P., 124, 138[81], 142[6], *177, 182*
Lees, G. M., 198, *210*
Lefkowitz, R. J., 128[29,30], 129

[Lefkowitz, R. J.]
[35], 130[38], *178, 179,* 199 [87,88], *211*
Lehman, W., 110[156], *120*
Lehninger, A., 96[113], *118*
Leichter, S. B., 132, *181*
Leith, D. E., 221[84], *244,* 306 [24], *321*
Lenfant, C., 31[2], *111*
Leof, D., 235[247], *255*
Leonard, E. J., 42, *112*
Leroux, M., 311[55], *323*
Leterrier, J. F., 151[130], *185*
Levine, G., 308[40], 318[80], *322, 324*
Levine, R. J., 149[126], *185*
Levison, H., 260[2], *290,* 317[79], *324*
Levitzki, A., 165[178], *188*
Levy, B., 192[14], *206*
Levy, G. P., 201[111], *212*
Lewis, A. J., 172[192], *189,* 198 [76], 200[99], *210, 212*
Lewis, G. P., 239[282], *257*
Lewis, R. A., 158[143], *186,* 202 [129,132], *213, 214*
Libet, B., 219[50], *242*
Lichtenstein, L. M., 148[121], *185,* 203[137,139,140,141,143], 205 [164], *214, 216*
Lichterfeld, A., 199, *211*
Lichtneckert, S., 231[206], 232 [206], *252*
Liebig, R., 200[106], *212*
Limbird, L. E., 128[30], *179*
Lin, C. S., 198, *210*
Lin, M. C., 129[33], *179*
Lindell, S.-E., 231[206], 232[206], *252*
Linden, D. A., 308[36], 318[36], *321*
Lippmann, M., 281[43,54,55], 282 [43], *292, 293*
Lishajko, F., 238[263], *256*
Little, J. B., 300[6], *320*
Lloyd, T. C., 222[110], 229[110], *246*
Lockett, M. F., 238[259,260], *255*
Lodi, C., 219[38], *242*
Loewenstein, J. M., 6[29], *26,* 103, *119*
Loewenstein, W. R., 135[78], *182*
Logsdon, P. J., 205, *215*
Loh, W., 89[101], 100[101], *117*
Lollgen, H., 199, *211*
Londos, C., 129[33], *179*
Long, J. E., 275[34], *292*
Loofbourrow, G. N., 222[104], 223 [104], 233[104], *246*
Loosli, C. G., 234[237], *254*
Loring, S. H., 233[219,220], *253,* 302[12], 309[12], 310[12], 311 [51], *320, 322*
Loten, E. G., 132[65], *181*
Lovejoy, F. W., Jr., 221[81], *244*
Lowry, O. H., 105, *120*
Lowy, J., 55, *114*
Luchtel, D. L., 284[63], *293*
Luck, J. C., 222[123], 234[239], *247, 254*
Luduena, F. P., 192[12], 196[12], *206,* 236[254], *255*
Lulich, K. M., 193, 195, *207*
Lundgren, C., 231[206], 232[206], *252*
Lundgren, G., 231[206], 232[206], *252*
Lundholm, L., 91, 98[104,122], *117, 118,* 125[8], 126[8], 144[8], 145 [8], 158[8], 165[8], 168[8], 172 [8], 173[8], 175[8], 176[8], *177,* 197[64], *209*
Lundin, G., 222[114], *246*
Lundqvist, G. R., 229[182], 231[182], *251,* 281[49], *293*
Luparello, T. J., 225[156,157,159], *249*
Luschka, H., 33, *111*
Lüth, J. B., 171[190], *189*
Lyons, C. A., 151[129], *185*

Lyons, H. A., 225[156,157], *249*, 304[16], 308[33,39], 315[16, 33,39], 317[16], 318[33,39], *320, 321, 322*

## M

Mabif, D. V., 142[104], 160[104], *184*
McAuliffe, J. P., 192[12], 196[12], *206*
McCarthy, D. S., 284[67], *294*
MacCready, P. B., 276[85], *295*
McCredie, R. M., 221[81], *244*
McCulloch, M. W., 238[264], 239 [264], *256*
McDermott, M., [188], *251*
MacDonald, A. G., 238[274], *256*
McDougal, M. D., 232[216], 235 [216], *253*
McFadden, E. R., Jr., 218[14], 225[156,157], *240, 249*, 304 [16], 307[30], 308[33,36,39], 311[54], 312[58,60], 313[54, 60,62], 314[72,73], 315[16,33, 39,62,77], 317[16,62,73], 318 [33,36,39,77], 319[77,83], *320, 321, 322, 323, 324*
McGready, S., 238[271], *256*
McIlroy, M. B., 307[31], *321*
McJilton, C. E., 275[35], 276[86], 277, 279[86], *292, 295*
McKenna, J. M., 156[139], *186*
McKerrow, C. B., 307[31], *321*
McKirdy, H. C., 19[76], *29*
Macklem, P. T., 2[3], *25*, 60, *114*, 217[7,8], 218[7,13,15], 221 [84], 236[8], 237[7], 238[8], 239[7], *240, 244*, 284[66], *294*, 298[2], 299[3], 300[6], 301[9], 306[24], 308[37k38,40,41], 309 [41,42,43,50], 311[55], 312[56, 61], 318[37,80], *319, 320, 321, 322, 323, 324*
McLelland, J., 6[33], 14[33], *26*
McLelland, M., 14[54], *27*
MacLeod, P., 308[40], 318[80], *322, 324*
McManus, G. M., 55[43], *114*
McNary, W. F., 15[62], *28*
McNeill, R. S., 238[273,274], *256*
McNutt, S. N., 6[30], *26*
Maengwyn-Davies, G. D., 195[38], 197[71,72], *208, 210*
Makino, S., 205, *215*
Malaisse, W., 142[110], *184*
Malaisse-Lagae, F., 142[110], *184*
Malawista, S. E., 149[126], *185*
Malhotra, S. K., 66[74], *115*
Malik, K. U., 143[114], *184*
Maling, H. M., 197[59], *209*
Malmfors, T., 196[53], *209*
Malta, E., 203[145], *214*
Manchester, K. L., 103[139], 104 [139], *119*
Mandel, P., 97[117], *118*
Manganiello, V. C., 130[45], 139[45], 141[95,96], 142[95,96], 143[95, 96], 144[96], 145[95,96], 158 [146], 168[146], 171[45], *180, 183, 186*
Mann, S. P., 14[56], 15[63], *28*, 63, *115*, 218[20], 219[20], 235[20], 236[20], *241*
Mansell, A., 317[79], *324*
Marcelle, R., 196[48], *208*, [269], *256*
Marcus, J. H., 304[20], *320*
Margaria, R., 218[25], *241*
Margolis, S., 203[143], *214*
Marquis, N. R., 142[105], *184*
Marshall, J. M., 164[171,172,173], 166[172], *188*
Martin, L. E., 230[203], *252*
Martin, R., 284[66], *294*, 298[2], 312[56], *319, 323*
Masari, J. P., 285[77], *294*
Mason, M. L., 218[23], *241*
Massarella, G. R., 7[39], *27*

Mathé, A. A., 141[115], 143[115], 146[115], *184*, 314[68], *323*
Matsumoto, Y., 76[86], *116*
Matsumura, Y., 230[196], *251*
Matthys, H., 309[46], *322*
Maxwell, L. C., 105[149], *120*
Mayahara, T., 195[45], *208*
Mead, J., 218[13,14], 221[84], 222[111], 224[138], *240, 244, 246, 248,* 298[1], 300[6], 304[23], 306[24,29], 307[30,31,32], 308[38,41], 309[41], 312[60], 313[60], *319, 320, 321, 322, 323*
Mebel, P. E., 60[51], 61[51], *114,* 217[4], 218[4], 221[4], 225[4], *240*
Megerman, J., 83[154], 110[154], *120*
Mehta, J. A., 82[93], 83[93], *116*
Meinrenken, W., 76[85], *116*
Meiss, R. A., 86[159], *120*
Melmon, K. L., 139[86], 140[86], 141[86], 144[86], *182,* 203[139], *214*
Melville, G. N., 226[166], 232[217], *250, 253*
Mendel, P., 94[109], *117*
Meneely, G. B., 230[194], *251*
Menkes, H., 218[15], *240,* 314[69], *323*
Menzel, D. B., 282[60], *293*
Mercke, U., 7[42], *27*
Methew, B. P., 197[61], *209*
Meyer, T. A., 104, 110, *119,* 164[168], *188*
Meyerhof, O., 103, *119*
Meyrick, B., 6[36], 7[36], *27,* 234[236], *254*
Michaelson, E. D., 282[61], *293*
Michio, U., 101[124], *118*
Mickey, J., 130[38], *179,* 199[88], *211*
Middleton, E., Jr., 205[162,166], *215, 216*
Miki, N., 131[50], 171[50], *180*
Milic-Emili, J., 284[67], *294*
Miller, H., 225[154], *249*
Miller, T. D., 224[152], *249*
Millikin, D., 129[35], *179*
Mills, E., 227[167], *250*
Mills, J. E., 192, *207,* 227[173], 228[173], 229[173], 230[173], 231[173,209,212], 232[209], *250, 252,* 282[57], *293*
Minatoya, H., 198, *210,* 236[254], *255*
Minor, L., 199[95], *211*
Miserocchi, G., 234[228], *253*
Mitchell, C. A., 229[191], 238[191], 239[191], *251*
Mitchell, H. W., 193[30], 195[30], *207*
Mitchell, R. W., 85[98], 91[98], *117*
Mittal, C. K., 131[48,49,52,58], 171[48,49,52], *180*
Miyahara, J. T., 16[70], *28*
Mohme-Lundholm, E., 91[104], 97, 98[104,122], *117, 118,* 125[8], 126[8,10], 144[8], 145[8], 158[8], 161, 163, 165[8], 168[8], 172[8], 173[8], 175[8], 176[8], *177*
Molinari, S., 44, *112*
Molliver, M. E., 220[56], *243*
Molony, V., 227[169], *250*
Mongar, J. L., 204[152,153], *215*
Monkhouse, W. S., 24[86], *29*
Mora, J., 103[134], *119*
Moran, N. C., 192[6], *206*
Moretti, R. L., 3[22], *26*
Morgan, A., 260[7], 266[7], 286[7], *290*
Morgan, M. S., 221[79], *244,* 260[10], *290*
Morita, K., 9[48], *27,* 37[6], 61[6], 64[6], 73[6], *111,* 237[256], *255*
Moroz, L. A., 6[27], *26,* 156[140], *186*
Morris, A. H., 224[152], *249*
Morris, W. P., 199[90], *211*

Morrison, A. D., 97[118], 98[116], *118*
Morrison, M. A., 234[241,242], 235 [241,242], *254*
Morrow, P. E., 260[8], 270[27], *290, 291*
Mortola, J. P., 228[175,176], 234 [228,232], *250, 253, 254*
Mount, L. E., 218[22], 220[22], 221[22], 237[22], *241*
Mrhova, O., 97[115], *118*
Mue, S., 9[49], *27,* 66[65,66], 67 [65,66], *115*
Muir, D. C. F., 224[143], *248*
Muir, T. C., 126[9], 174[9], *177*
Mukherjee, C., 199[87], *211*
Mulcahy, P. D., *119*
Murad, F., 130[41,42], 131[48,49, 51,52], 138[80,83], 139[83], 141[83,99], 142[99], 143[99], 144[99], 145[99], 158[99], 171 [48,49,51,52,191], *179, 180, 182, 183, 189*
Murphy, E., 223[126], *247*
Murphy, R. A., 83, 86[161], 110, *120*
Murray, J. J., 201[124], *213*
Mutt, V., 2[15], *25*

## N

Nadel, J. A., 32[4], 59, 60[51], 61 [51], *111, 114,* 126[16], *178,* 196[54], *209,* 217[4,7,9,11], 218[4,7,9,17], 219[41,45], 221 [4,45,66,78,80,87], 222[11,45, 78,93,97,98,101,108,109,112, 113,116,124,125], 223[11,45, 66,93,97,98,101,108,135,136], 224[45,78,93,98,139], 225[4, 87,93], 226[80,93], 227[45, 93,101], 228[101], 229[80,93, 185], 230[11,185,198], 231[97, 101,210,213], 232[66,97,101,
[Nadel, J. A.]
113,210,215], 233[98,112,113], 234[98,112], 236[41,87,252], 237[7,87], 238[87], 239[7,80], *240, 241, 242, 243, 244, 245, 246, 247, 248, 251, 252, 253, 255,* 281 [46,47,48,51], 285[72,73,75], 286 [47,81], 287[47], *292, 293, 294, 295,* 304[15], 306[25,26], 312 [57], 314[26,75], 315[76], 317 [76], 318[15], *320, 321, 323, 324*
Nagaishi, C., 7, 13[41], *27*
Nagano, M., 131[50], 171[50], *180*
Nagasawa, J., 44[14], *112*
Nahas, G. G., 142[104], 160[104], 166[181], *183, 188*
Natusch, D. F. S., 270[28], *291*
Needham, D. M., 54, 105[150], *113, 120*
Nelson, H. E., 205[166], *216*
Nemerovski, M., 142[106], 143[106], *184*
Newball, H. H., 314[67], *323*
Newsholme, E. A., 103[139], 104 [139], *119*
Newton-Howes, J., 312[58], *323*
Ngai, S. H., 142[104], 160[104], *184*
Nicholas, M., 66[74], *115*
Nickerson, M., 229[179], *250*
Nicol, S. E., 127[18], 142[112], 168 [112], *178, 184*
Nilsson, K. B., 125[8], 126[8], 144[8, 116], 145[8,116], 158[8,116], 165 [8,116], 166[116], 168[8,116], 172[8,116], 173[8,116], 174[116], 175[8,116], 176[8,116], *177, 184*
Nisam, M., 139[86], 140[86], 141 [86], 144[86], *182*
Nonomura, Y., 44, 110[155], *112, 120*
Norberg, K.-A., 219[49], 235[248], *242, 255*
Norbet, K., 15[61], 16[61], *28*
Nordenbrand, K., 96[112], *118*
Norman, J., 222[123], *247*

Norman, P. S., 314[69], *323*
Novakov, T., 280[40], *292*
Nunes, J., 151[130], *185*

## O

O'Brien, K. P., 222[120], *247*
O'Cain, C. F., 318[82], *324*
O'Donnell, S. R., 15[60], 16[60], *28*
Offermeier, J., 193, *207,* 221[67], 232[67], *243*
Ohno, Y., 198[80], *210*
Okamoto, E., 1[1], *24*
Okamura, C., 219[47], *242*
Oki, M., 66[74], *115*
Okpako, D. T., 200, *212*
Olsen, C. R., 60, 61, *114,* 217[4], 218[4], 221[4], 222[97], 223 [97], 225[4], 231[97], 232[97, 215], *240, 245, 253*
Olsen, D. E., 309[48], *322*
Olsen, G. R., 304[15], 318[15], *320*
Ong, S. H., 127[21], 131[47], 135 [21], 156[21], 173[194], 174 [194], *178, 179, 189*
Ono, Y., 9[49], *27,* 66[65,66], 67 [65,66], *115*
Oosaki, T., 44[13], *112*
Orange, R. P., 2[11], *25,* 124[1], 142[97,100,102], 146[100], 147[1], 148[1,122,125], 152 [1,134], *177, 183, 185, 186,* 202[128], *213,* 317[79], *324*
Orehek, J., 197[57], 200, *209, 212,* 238[272], *256,* 284, 285[71,77], *294,* 306[27], 314[70,71], *321, 324*
Oriol, A., 308[35], *321*
Orly, J., 128[24], *178*
Orr, C., 268[21], *291*
Otis, A. B., 224[137], *248,* 307 [31], *321*
Ouellette, J. J., 205[161], *215*
Overweg, N. I. A., 142[104], 160[104], *183*

## P

Pagliara, A. S., 139[89], *182*
Paintal, A. S., 234[234,235], *254*
Palacek, F., 229[183], 230[183], *251*
Palade, G. E., 44, *112*
Palmer, G. C., 142[92,93], 143[92, 93], *183*
Palmer, W. K., 134[72], *181*
Palmes, E. D., 260[1], *290*
Panczenko, B., 200[101], *212*
Pantesco, V., 94[109], *117*
Pare, P. D., 6[27], *26,* 156[140], *186*
Parikh, H. M., 197[61], *209*
Park, C. R., 133[68], *181*
Parker, C. D., 314[74], *324*
Parker, C. W., 152[135,136], 153 [136], 155[136], *186,* 203[138], 205, *214, 215*
Parker, K. L., 152[135,136], 153 [136], 155[136], *186,* 203[138], *214*
Parker, S., 227[169], *250*
Parks, M. A., 130[43], 172[43], *179*
Parmeggiani, A., 104[140], *119*
Parnas, J. K., 103, *119*
Parsons, E. M., 192[7], *206*
Pastan, I., 131[56], *180*
Patel, K. R., 196[51], *209*
Paterson, N. A. M., 157, 158[141], *186*
Paton, W. D. M., 126, 163[165], 172 [14], *178, 187,* 220[58], 221[73], 232[73], *243, 244*
Patt, C. S., 131[54], 171[54], *180*
Patterson, R., 156[139], *186,* 193, *207*
Pattle, R. E., 230[202], *252*
Paul, R. J., 48, 91, *113, 117*
Pavelka, M., 6[24], *26*

Pearse, A. G. E., 2[13], *25*
Pearson, B., 219[38], *242*
Pease, D. C., 44, *112*
Pedley, T. J., 309[49], *322*
Penna, M., 236[253], 238[253], *255*
Pepys, J., 204[156], *215*
Perey, D. Y. E., 23[81,82], *29*
Perkins, J. P., 128[26], 130[39], *178, 179*
Perkins, M. E., 192[6], *206*
Permutt, S., 32[3], 33[3], *111,* 300[7], 314[69], *320, 323*
Perrotto, J. L., 2[9], *25*
Perry, S. V., 110[157], *120*
Persson, C. A., 158[147], *186,* 193, 195[26], *207*
Peskar, B. A., 200[106], *212*
Peterson, J. W., 48[30], 91[103], *113, 117*
Petrella, V. J., 128[25], *178*
Phillipson, E. A., 223[126,135], *247, 248*
Phillipson, O., 151[129], *185*
Phipps, R. J., 224[139], *248*
Picarelli, Z. P., 221[72], 232[72], *244*
Pichard, A. L., 132[63], *181*
Pierson, R. N., Jr., [275], *256*
Piiper, J., 102[127], *118*
Piper, P. J., 200[105], *212,* 239 [278,280,284], *256, 257*
Pitts, J. N., Jr., 264[15], *290*
Place, R. E. G., 308[35], *321*
Pöch, G., 161, 162[159], *187*
Poirier, J., 3[21], *26*
Polson, J. B., 139, 144[117], *182, 184*
Poppius, H., 224[144,151], *248, 249*
Poulsen, F. R., 55[44,45], *114*
Powell, C. E., 192[5], *206*
Pride, N. B., [270], *256,* 300, 304 [17,18], 312[58], 315[18], 317[18], *320, 323*
Prime, F. J., 195, 196[50], *208,* [187], *251*
Proctor, C., 238[264], 239[264], *256*
Proctor, D. F., 229[182], 231[182], *251,* 277[38], 281[49], *292, 293*
Prosser, C. L., 66[70,71,72], *115*
Purcell, D. A., 6[23], *26*
Puri, S. K., 141[115], 143[115], 146 [115], *184*

## R

Radford, E. P., Jr., 304[22], 305[22], 307[31], *321*
Rahn, H., 224[137], *248*
Rall, J. E., 225[162], *249*
Rall, T. W., 124[3], 138[82], *177, 182*
Rand, M. J., 238[264], 239[264], *256*
Randall, R. J., 105, *120*
Randle, P. J., 103[139], 104[139], *119*
Ranga, V., 6[27], *26*
Ransom, F., 221[86], 236[86], 237, *245*
Raper, C., 192[19], 203[145], *207, 214*
Rappaport, L., 151[130], *185*
Rash, J. E., 6[31], *26*
Rasmussen, H., 151[128], *185*
Rathbone, L., 198[79], *210*
Rayner, M. D., 222[125], *247*
Read, J., 317[78], *324*
Reaven, E. P., 148[124], *185*
Reed, B. R., 139[86], 140[86], 141 [86], 144[86], 151[133], *182, 185*
Reed, C. E., 205[161], *215,* 224[146], *248,* 314[74], *324*
Reed, P. W., 201[124], *213*
Regardh, C. G., 196[53], *209*
Reid, L., 6[34,36], 7[36], 14[34], 22[79,80], 23[79,80], *26, 27,*

[Reid, L.]
234[236], *254*
Reinhoff, W. F., Jr., 219[43], *242*
Relman, A. S., 102[126], *118*
Remmers, J. E., 228[176], *250*
Repke, D. I., 105[145], *120,* 173 [195], 174[195], *189*
Reyes, P. L., 138[81], *182*
Rhodin, J. A. G., 3[19,20], 6[20], 14[20], 22[20], 23[20], *26*
Rice, R. V., 49[35], 54[35], 55[35], 57[46], 68[35], *113, 114*
Richards, I. M., 222[117], *247*
Richardson, J. B., 2[3,7,8], 3[8,18], 4[8], 6[8], 9[47], 16[68,72], 18[73], 19[73], 23[8], 24[87], *25, 26, 27, 28, 29,* 64, *115,* 201 [112,113], *212,* 219[54], 235 [245], 237[255,257], *243, 255*
Richardson, P. S., 222[95,96], 226 [95,96], 227[95,96], 229[95], 230[95], 232[96], *245*
Rickenberg, H. V., 164[168], *188*
Ridgeway, P., 196[55], 197[55], 198[76], *209, 210,* 223[132], 238[132], *247*
Rikimaru, A., 218[32], 220[32], 236[32], 237[32], *241*
Ringquiat, T. R., 231[206], 232 [206], *252*
Roberts, A., 311[53], *322*
Roberts, D. J., 238[261], *255*
Robillard, E., 225[163], 226[163], 230[163], *249*
Robinson, F. W., 132[66], *181*
Robison, G. A., 124, 158[148], 159[148], *177, 186*
Robson, J. G., 222[115], 229[115], *246*
Robson, R. M., 46[24], *112*
Rodan, G., 165[179], *188*
Rodbell, M., 129[33], *179*
Rodenstein, D., 221[83], *244*
Rogel, S., 222[105], *246*
Rogers, D. C., 48, *113*
Ronge, H. R., 6[24], *26*
Rosado, A., 103, *119*
Rose, B., 135[78], *182*
Rosebrough, N. J., 105, *120*
Rosenbaum, J. L., 151[132], *185*
Rosenblueth, A., 77, *116*
Rosenthal, R. R., 314[69], *323*
Ross, G., 15[58], 16[58], *28,* 37[7], 63, *111,* 220[64], 235[64], 236 [64], *243*
Ross, L. L., 221[74], 232[74], *244*
Rossler, R., 222[107], *246*
Roth, J. A., 191[2], *206*
Rouiller, C. H., 51[38], 54[38], *113*
Rovenstein, E. A., 222[118], *247*
Roy, A., 102[126], *118*
Rubio, R., 77[90], *116*
Rudich, L., 142[106], 143[106], *184*
Rudolph, F. B., 131[46], *180*
Rudolph, S. A., 151[132], *185*
Ruegg, J. C., 76[85], 105[149], *116, 120*
Russell, J. A., 220[63], 238[63], *243*
Russell, T. R., 132[60,62], *181*

## S

Sackner, M. A., 282[61], *293*
Said, J. W., 157[141], 158[141], *186*
Said, S. I., 2[15], *25,* 139[87], *182,* 235[243], *254*
Sala, G., 128[32], 129[32], 133, 135 [70], *179, 181*
Salem, H., 217[11], 222[11], 223[11], 230[11], *240*
Salomon, Y., 129[33], *179*
Salorinne, Y., 224[144,151], *248, 249*
Samanek, M., 229[184], 230[184,192], 231[205], *251, 252*
Sampson, S. R., 222[101], 223[101], 227[101], 228[101], 231[101,214], 232[101], [171], *246, 250, 253*
Samuelsson, B., 199[97], *211*
Sandler, J. A., 158[146], 168[146],

[Sandler, J. A.]
*186,* 221[68], 232[68], *243*
Sands, H., 104, 110, *119,* 164[168], *188*
Sanford, C. H., 127[18], 142[112], 168[112], *178, 184*
Sant' Ambrogio, G., 228[175,176], 234[228,229,231,232], *250, 253, 254*
Sarkar, T. K., 195[46], *208*
Sarr, N., 15[60], 16[60], *28*
Sarver, J. N., 132[66], *181*
Saske, A. T., 107[153], *120*
Sato, G., 220[57], *243*
Sato, S., 285[76], *294*
Saum, W. R., 220[59], *243*
Sawh, P. C., 97[120], *118*
Sayers, G., 130[36], *179*
Sayre, D. F., 238[262], *255*
Scadding, J. G., 313[63], *323*
Scarpa, A., 44[20], 48[20], *112*
Scheinbaum, I., 131[57], *180*
Schild, H. O., 175[200], *190,* 192, 203[144], 204[152,153], *206, 214, 215*
Schilder, D. P., 300[5], 308[34], 311[53], *320, 321, 322*
Schlesinger, R. B., 281[43,54,55], 282[43], *292, 293*
Schmidt, G., 103, 110[133], *119*
Schmidt-Gayk, H., 171[190], *189,* 201[119], *213*
Schmutzler, W., 146[119], *185*
Schneider, R., 199[83], *211*
Schollmayer, J. S., 46[24], *112*
Schönhöfer, P. S., 160[154], *187*
Schramm, M., 128[24], 129[33], 159[153], *178, 179, 187*
Schreck, R. M., 282[61], *293*
Schroter, R. C., 309[49], *322*
Schultz, G., 130, 142, 143, 159[108], 161[44], 162[108], 165[177], 168[44,108,183], 169[44], 170[44], 171[108,189], 172[108], 173[44,108], 174[44], *179, 184, 188, 189*
Schultz, K. D., 171[189], *189,* 130, 161[44], 165[177], 168[44], 169[44], 170[44], 171[189], 173 [44], 174[44], *179, 188, 189*
Schultz, W. H., 142, 143, 169[107], *184,* 204, *215*
Schumacher, H., 103[130], *119*
Schweppe, J. S., 134[74], *181*
Schwieler, G. H., 217[10], 222[10], 237[10], *240*
Scratcherd, T., 7[37], *27*
Seelig, S., 130[36], *179*
Selenger, Z., 159[153], *187*
Sellick, H., 222[99,100], 223[100], 224[100], 227[100,173], 228[99, 100,173], 229[100,173], 230[100, 173], 231[100,173,209], 232[99, 100,209], *245, 250, 252,* 281[45], 282[57], *292, 293*
Selverstone, N. J., 307[31], *321*
Selvidge, A., 276[85], *295*
Severinghaus, J. W., 221[77], *244*
Shaw, D. B., 230[201], *252*
Sheard, P., 202[130], *213,* 230[203], *252*
Sherman, D. L., 221[75], 232[75], *244*
Shetzline, A., 192[17], *207*
Shevis, A., 222[94], 225[94], 226[94], 239[94], *245,* 281[50], *293*
Shibata, N., 105[152], 107[152], 110[152], *120*
Shibata, S., 16[70], *28*
Shimamoto, T., 162[158], *187*
Shimo, Y., 16[66], *28,* 201[117], *213*
Shindo, N., 16[66], *28*
Shock, N. W., 197[68], *210*
Shoenberg, C. F., 54, *113*
Shoji, M., 134[76], *182*
Shuman, H., 44[20], 48[20], *112*
Silva, D. G., 15[58], 16[58], *28,* 37[7], 63, *111,* 220[64], 235[64], 236[64], *243*
Sim, V. M., 230[202], *252*

Simani, A. S., 6[26], *26*
Simmons, R. N., 81, 88[91], *116*
Simonsson, B. G., 195, *208,* 222 [113], 232[113], 233[113], [186], *246, 251,* 281[47], 286, 287[47], *292,* 306[26], 314[26], *321*
Sjoqvist, F., 219[49], *242*
Sjostrand, F. S., 44, *112*
Skidmore, I. F., 160[154], *187*
Skoog, C. M., 91[106], *117*
Skoogh, B. E., 195[47], *208*
Slater, I. H., 192[5], *206*
Sloboda, R. P., 151[132], *185*
Small, J. V., 54, *113*
Smiesko, V., 163[161], *187*
Smith, A. P., 199[91,96], 200, *211, 212,* 284[71], 285[71], *294,* 314[71], *324*
Smith, J. W., 205, *215*
Smith, M. M., 225[158], *249,* 304 [19], 315[19], 317[19], *320*
Smith, P., 131[47], *180*
Smith, P. G., 227[167], *250*
Snapper, J. R., 233[219], *253*
Sobieszek, A., 54, 57, 105, 110, *114, 120*
Sobirn, G., 103[134], *119*
Soiffer, D., 151[131], *185*
Sokol, W. N., 205, *216*
Solandt, D. Y., 218[25], *241*
Solomon, S. S., 142[91], *183*
Somlyo, A. P., 42, 44, 48, 49, 54, 55[9,35,43], 57[46], 68[35], *111, 112, 113, 114,* 159[150], 163[161], 168[150], 174[197], 175[197,199], *187, 189, 190,* 195[36], 201[118], *208, 213*
Somlyo, A. V., 42, 44, 48, 49, 54, 55[9,35], 57[46], 68[35], *111, 112, 113, 114,* 159[150], 163 [161], 168[150], 174[197], 175[197,199], *187, 189, 190,* 195[36], 201[118], *208, 213*
Sonesson, B., 7[42], *27*
Sonnenblick, E. H., 75[81], 83, 86[158], *116, 120*
Sorace, R. A., 196[52], *209*
Sorenby, L., 203[146], *214*
Souhrada, J. F., 196[49], *208,* 225 [159,160], *249*
Spannhake, E. W., 114[118], *185,* 200[109], *212*
Sparrow, M. P., 105, *120,* 193[30], 195[30], *207*
Spector, S. L., 225[159,160], *249*
Speizer, F. E., 226[164,165], *249,* 277[37], *292*
Spencer, H., 235[247], *255*
Spencer, K. E. V., 221[85], *245*
Spencer, R., 284[67], *294*
Spiegel, A. M., 129[34], *179*
Spilker, B. A., 198, *210*
Spruill, W. A., 131[59], *180*
Staehelin, L. A., 6[32], *26*
Stara, J. F., 284[68], *294*
Staszewska-Barczak, J., 239[281,283], *257*
Staub, N. C., 60[51], 61[51], *114,* 217[4], 218[4], 221[4], 225[4], *240*
Stechschulte, D. J., 142[101], 143 [101], *183*
Steck, T. L., 105[148], *120*
Steer, M. L., 165[178], *188*
Stein, O., 103[137], *119*
Stein, Y., 103[137], *119*
Steinberg, M. I., 201[121], *213*
Steiner, A. L., 127[21,22], 128[22], 131[47,59], 132[22], 133, 134, 135[21], 139[89], 156[21], 173 [194], 174[194], *178, 180, 182, 189*
Stensaas, L. J., 227[168], *250*
Stenson, W., 152[135], *186*
Stephens, N. L., 9[43], 12[43], *27,* 46[25], 48[31,32], 65[32], 66 [75], 67[75,76,79], 70[80], 73 [25,80], 82[93], 83, 85[79,98, 100], 86[100], 89[101], 90[83], 91[98,106], 94[25], 96[114],

[Stephens, N. L.]
98[25], 100[31,101], 104[25, 142], 105[142], 110[79,114], *112, 113, 115, 116, 117, 118, 119*
Stephens, R. J., 284[68,69,70], *294*
Sterling, G. M., 221[82], 222[124], 230[82,189], *244, 247, 251,* 282 [59], *293*
Stockinger, G., 6[24], *26*
Stollak, J. S., 196[52], *209*
Stone, D. J., 195[46], *208*
Stone, H., 225[163], 226[163], 230[163], *249*
Stoner, J., 141[95,96], 142[95,96], 143[95,96], 144[96], 145[95, 96], *183*
Stormer, M. H., 46[24], *112*
Storms, W. W., 224[146], *248*
Strandberg, L., 280[42], *292*
Stransky, A., 223[130], *247*
Stransky, M., 223[128], *247*
Stubbs, S. E., 304[14,21], *320, 321*
Stupfel, M., 221[77], *244*
Su, Y. F., 130[39], *179*
Suda, W. L., 225[160], *249*
Sudlow, M. F., 218[16], *240,* 309 [49], *322*
Sudoh, M., 218[32], 220[32], 236 [32], 237[32], *241*
Sullivan, C. E., 223[126], *247*
Sullivan, T. J., 152, 153[136], 154, 155, 156, 157, *186,* 203[138], *214*
Summer, W. R., 314[69], *323*
Suria, A., 168[184], *189*
Suszko, I. M., 156[139], *186*
Sutherland, E. W., 124[3,4], 130[40, 44], 158[148], 159[148], 161 [44], 168[44], 169[44], 170 [44], 173[44], 174[44], *177, 179, 186*
Suzuki, H., 9[48], *27,* 37, 61, 64, 73, *111,* 237[256], *255*
Suzuki, T., 44[14], *112,* 230[196], *251*
Svanberg, L., 222[114], *246*
Svanborg, N., 314[68], *323*
Svedmyr, N., 195[47], 199, *208, 211*
Swamy, V. C., 201[122], *213*
Sweatman, W. J. F., 199[93], *211*
Swi, S., 222[97], 223[97], 231[97], 232[97], *245*
Swift, D. L., 229[182], 231[182], *251*
Symes, W. L., 63, *115,* 194, *207*
Syned, J. G. T., 132[65], *181*
Szaduykis-Szadurski, L., 172[193], *189*
Szczeklik, A., 200, *212*
Szent-Gyorgyi, A. G., 110[156], *120*
Szentivanyi, A., 193[29], 205, *207, 215,* 236[250], *255*
Szentivanyi, Z., 144[117], *184*
Szereda-Przestaszewska, M., 223[128, 129,130,131], 226[129], *247*
Szetivanyi, A., 139[85], *182*
Szmigielski, A., 133[71], *181*

## T

Tada, M., 173[195,196], 174[195, 196], *189*
Tada, T., 2[4], *25*
Taira, N., 194[31], 195, *207*
Takagi, K., 126[13], 161, *178*
Takayanagi, I., 126[13], 161[13], *178*
Takishima, T., 308[38], *322*
Tamplin, B., 217[11], 222[11], 223 [11], 230[11], *240*
Tang, I. N., 269[23], *291*
Tate, R., 130[38], *179,* 199[88], *211*
Tattersall, M. L., 202[130], *213*
Tattersfield, A. E., 199[86], *211,* [270], *256,* 304[17,18], 315[18], 317[18], *320*
Tauber, A. I., 142[101], 143[101], *183*
Taylor, A., 142[103], *183*
Taylor, S. R., 75, *116*

Teo, T. S., 164[170], *188*
Terasaki, W. C., 132[62], *181*
Teshimo, Y., 159[152], 170[152], *187*
Theunynck, P., 2[14], 3[14], *25*
Thiringer, G. K., 199[85], *211*
Thomas, E., 138[83], 139[83], 141[83], *182*
Thompson, E. B., 16[69], *28*
Thompson, W. J., 132[60], *181*
Thornton, J. W., 218[34], *242*
Thurlbeck, W. M., 2[2,3], *24, 25,* 309[42,43], *322*
Ticku, M., 201[122], *213*
Tierney, D. F., 222[112], 233[112], 234[112], *246,* 306[25], *321*
Titus, E., 197[74], 198, *210,* 222 [121], *247*
Tomita, T., 15[59], 16[59], *28,* 62, 64, 67[77], *114, 115,* 201[110], *212,* 237[258], *255*
Tomkins, G. M., 128[23], *178*
Tomori, Z., 217[12], 222[12], 225 [12], 226[12], 227[12], 229 [12], 230[12], 239[12], *240,* 281[52], *293*
Tonomura, T., 107[153], *120*
Toomey, R. E., 193[22], *207*
Toremalm, N. G., 7[42], *27,* 60, *114*
Torrance, R. W., 221[85], *245*
Tos, M. K., 6[35], 7[35,38], *26, 27*
Tothill, A., 198, *210*
Townley, R. G., 195[42], *208,* 238 [271], *256*
Toy-oka, T., 110[155], *120*
Tredelenburg, U., 219[48], 221[48], 231[48], 232[48], *242*
Trenchard, D. W., 234[233], *254*
Trethewie, E. R., 202, *213*
Triggle, C. R., 201[122,123], *213*
Triggle, D. J., 201[122,123], *213*
Triner, L., 140[149], 141[149], 142[104], 158[149], 159[149], 160[104,149], 161[149], 162 [149], 166[181], *183, 186, 188*
Troxell, T. C., 204[150], *215*
Trump, R., 225[162], *249*
Ts'ao, C., 156[139], *186*
Tse, T., 66[65,66], 67[65,66], *115*
Tsuchida, Y., 126[13], 161[13], *178*
Turiaf, J., 3[21], *26*
Turker, R. K., 200, *212*
Turner, J. M., 300[6], *320*
Tuth, J. B., 201[119], *213*
Tuttle, R. R., 192, 193, *207*
Twose, P. A., 199[90], *211*
Tyler, W. S., 15[57], *28*
Tyll, J., 198, *210*

## U

Ueda, T., 1[1], *24*
Uenishi, K., 159[152], 170[152], *187*
Ugro, V., 286[80], *294*
Ulmer, W. T., 232[217], *253,* 285[74], *294*
Underhill, D. W., 275[33], 276[33], 279, 286[80], *292, 294*
Urbanetti, J., 284[66], *294,* 298[2], 312[56], *319, 323*
Uzunov, P., 132[64], 162[160], *181, 187*

## V

Vachon, L., 195[43], *208*
Valentine, M. D., 205[164], *216*
Vallieres, J., 44[20], 48[20], *112*
Vamos, N., 98[122], *118*
Van As, A., 284[64], *293*
Van Cauter, E., 137, 138, *182*
Vanderpol, A. H., 264[17,19], 285 [17], *291*
van de Woestijne, K. P., 312[59], *323*
Van Dorben-Broekema, M., 218[26], *241*
van During, M., 234[230], *253*
Van Dyke, H. B., 197, *210*
Vane, J. R., 165[176], *188,* 200[105],

[Vane, J. R.]
*212,* 239[280,281,283], *257*
Vanhoutte, P. M., 220[60,61,62], *243*
Vanov, S., 235[249], *255*
Vanpeperstraete, F., 22[78], 23[78], *29*
Vastag, E., 285[74], *294*
Vaughan, J. H., 2[6], *25*
Vaughan, M., 130[45], 138[82], 139[45], 141[95,96], 142[95, 96], 143[95,96], 144[96], 145 [95,96], 158[146], 168[146], 171[45], *180, 182, 183, 186,* 221[68], 232[68], *243*
Vermiere, P. A., 220[60], *243*
Verosky, M., 140[149], 141[149], 142[104], 158[149], 159[149], 160[104,149], 161[149], 162 [149], 166[181], *183, 186, 188*
Vibert, P. J., 55[44,45], *114*
Vidruk, E. H., 222[101], 223[101], 227[101], 228[101], 231[101, 214], 232[101], *246, 253*
Vigdahl, R. L., 142[105], *184*
Viljanen, A. A., 224[144], *248*
Vincent, H. J., 308[37], 318[37], *322*
Vincent, N. J., 221[84], *244,* 306 [24], *321*
Vinogradova, M. I., 222[106], 233 [106], *246*
Virlon, A., 151[130], *185*
Vizi, E. S., 163[165], *187,* 220[58], *243*
Vogel, J., 96[114], 110[114], *118*
Volicer, L., 141[115], 143[115], 146[115], *184*
Von Euler, U. S., 238[263], *256*
von Hayek, H., 57, 58, 59, 61, *114*
Vriem, C., 235[243], *254*
Vulliemoz, Y., 140[149], 141[149], 142[104], 158, 159, 160[104, 149], 161, 162[149], 166[181], *183, 186, 188*

**W**

Waddell, J. E., 199, 200[98], *211*
Waddell, W. J., 102, *118*
Wade, O. L., 199[83], *211*
Wade, W. A., III, 285[78], *294*
Waggoner, A. P., 264[17,18,19], 270 [25], 285[17], *291*
Wakaboyashi, K., 195[45], *208*
Wakade, T. D., 196[52], *209*
Wallace, J. R., 270[28], *291*
Wallach, D. F. H., 105[148], *120,* 131[56], *180*
Waller, M., 151[129], *185*
Wallis, D. I., 219[51], 221[51], 232 [51], *242*
Walsh, C., 6[33], 14[33], *26*
Walsh, D. A., 133[69], 134[72], 164 [167], *181, 188*
Walton, G. M., 134[77], *182*
Walton, K. G., 138[81], *182*
Waltuch, T., 219[36], *242*
Walz, D. T., 197[71], *210*
Wang, J. H., 164[170], *188*
Wanner, A., 202, *214,* 282[61], *293*
Wardell, J. R., 192[17], *207*
Warren, K. S., 2[9], *25*
Wasserman, M. A., 192[14], *206,* 231 [207], *252*
Wasserman, S. I., 157[141], 158[141], *186,* 202[132], *214*
Watanabe, A. M., 128[29], *178*
Watanabe, M., 198, *210*
Watanabe, S., 224[152], 230[199], *249, 252*
Wedner, H. J., 127[21], 135[21], 156 [21], *178*
Weibel, E. R., 309[44], *322*
Weibrodt, N. W., 16[71], *29*
Weimann, G., 172[193], *189*
Weiner, N., 15[64], *28*
Weinstein, R. S., 6[30], *26*
Weisenthal, L. M., 16[71], *29*
Weisfeldt, M. L., 197[68], *210*
Weiss, B., 142[98], 162[160], *183, 187*

Weiss, E. B., 222[120], *247*
Weiss, R. E., 264[18], *291*
Wellman, J. J., 218[14], *240,* 307 [30], 311[54], 312[60], 313 [54,60,62], 314[72], 315[62], 317[62], *321, 322, 323, 324*
Wells, J. N., 160[155], 161[155], 162[155,157], 165[180], 170 [180], *187, 188*
West, G. B., 232[216], 235[216], *253*
Wheeldon, E. B., 2[10], *25*
Whimster, W. P., 24[86], *29*
White, A. A., 131[54], 171[54], *180*
Whittenberger, J. L., 222[111], 230 [195], *246, 251*
Widdicombe, J. G., 7[40], 16[65], 22[77], *27, 28, 29,* 59, 61[58], *114,* 217[5,6,12], 218[31], 219 [31,44,45], 221[5,6,31,44,45, 78,80], 222[12,31,45,78,92,93, 95,96,98,99,100,102,103], 223 [45,93,98,100,129,130,131,135], 224[6,45,78,93,98,100,140], 225[12,93], 226[12,80,93,95,96, 129], 227[12,31,45,93,95,96, 100,103,172,173,174], 228[99, 100,103,173,177], 229[12,31, 44,80,93,95,100,172,173], 230 [12,31,44,95,100,103,172,173], 231[5,100,173,209,212], 232 [5,96,99,100,103,209], 233[31, 44,98,103,140,172], 234[5,31, 98,103,172], 235[31], 236[6,31], 237[31], 239[12,31,80], *240, 241, 242, 244, 245, 246, 247, 248, 250, 252,* 281[45,46,51,52], 282[57,58,59], 283[62], 284 [62], *292, 293,* 312[57], *323*
Wikberg, J., 125[8], 126[8], 144 [8], 145[8], 158[8], 165[8], 168[8], 172[8], 173[8], 175 [8], 176[8], *177*
Wilke, D. R., 65[89], 77[89], 85, *116*
Wilkinson, J. R., 201[120], *213*
Williams, H. L., 225[155], *249*
Williams, J. C., 2[3], *25,* 192[18], *207*
Williams, L. T., 128[29], *178*
Willman, E., 198[79], *210*
Wilsin, A. G., 221[66], 223[66], 232 [66], *243*
Wilson, K. M., 221[85], *245*
Wilson, N. J., 217[7,8], 218[7], 236 [8], 237[7], 238[8], 239[7], *240,* 299[3], 312[61], *319, 323*
Winegrad, A. I., 97[116,118], 98[116], *118, 119*
Winkler, P., 269[24], *291*
Wise, J. C. M., 222[96], 226[96], 227 [96], 232[96], 234[229,231], *245, 253, 254*
Wojcik, J. D., 142[109], *184*
Woledge, R. C., 84[96], 93, *117*
Wolff, D. J., 130[37], 132[37], *179*
Wolff, J., 129[33], *179*
Wong, D. T., 201[120], *213*
Wong, V., 2[12], *25*
Wood, J. D., 19[75], *29,* 220[55], 231[55], *243*
Wood, L. D. H., 218[15], *240,* 309 [50], *322*
Wood, W. B., 222[104], 223[104], 233[104], *246*
Woodward, B., 219[51], 221[51], 232[51], *242*
Woolcock, A. J., 217[7,8], 218[7], 236[8], 237[7], 238[8], 239[7], *240,* 308[37], 312[61], 317[78], 318[37], *322, 323, 324*
Worcel, M., 127[19], *178*
Worcester, J., 230[195], *251*
Wright, G. W., 222[110], 223[134], 226, 229[110,134], *246, 248*
Wright, P. H., 142[110], *184*
Wrogemann, K., 46[25], 73[25], 94 [25], 98[25], 104[25], *112*
Wu, Y. J., 165[180], 170[180], *188*

## Y

Yalein, S., *119*
Yamado, S., 195[45], *208*
Yamaraki, R., 159[152], 170[152], *187*
Yamauchi, A., 48, 51, 54, *113*
Yeates, D. B., 260[2], *290*
Yernault, J.-C., 221[83], *244*
Yocom, J. E., 285[78], *294*
Yoder, R. E., 277[36], *292*
Yokiwa, Y., 217[11], 222[11], 223[11], 230[11], *240*
Yokoyama, E., 230[193,196,199], *251, 252,* 277[36], *292*
Young, W. A., 230[201], *252*
Youssef, H. H., [187], *251*
Yu, D. Y. C., 231[211], *252*

## Z

Zaid, G., 238[268], *256*
Zamel, N., 223[126], [187], *247, 251*
Zapata, P., 227[168], *250*
Zapletal, A., 306[28], *321*
Zarzecki, S., 202[133], *214*
Zbinden, A. F., 139[86], 140[86], 141[86], 144[86], *182*
Zebe, E., 76[85], *116*
Zemplenyi, T., 97, *118*
Zenser, T. V., 128[25], *178*
Zuskin, E., 229[191], 238[191], 239 [191], *251*
Zwi, S., 231[210], 232[210], *252,* 281[48], *292*

# SUBJECT INDEX


### A

Acetylcholine, 72, 124, 132, 219
  314
Actin filaments, 37, 52, 55, 107
Activator $Ca^{2+}$, 68
Active state, 81, 89
Active tension, 75
Actomyosin, 105
Adenosine triphosphate, 100
Adenylate cyclase, 128
Adenylate deaminase, 103
ADP: $O_2$ ratio, 46, 95
Adrenergic nerves, 14, 15, 16, 18,
  61, 63, 219, 236
Adrenergic receptors, 192, 312
Aerosol
  atmospheric, 264
  deposition, 266
  hygroscopic growth, 268
  particle size distribution, 261
  physical and chemical properties,
   264
Air quality standards, 289
Airway
  epithelium, 2
  morphology, 2, 24
  obstruction, 301, 304
  parenchymal interactions, 302
  reflexes, 225, 227
  resistance, 301, 302, 307
α-Actin, 46
α-Adrenergic receptors, 195
Airway smooth muscle, 191, 220
  β-adrenergic antagonists, 236
  β-adrenergic blocking agents, 239
  hydrogen ion concentration, 222
  sleep and neural control, 222-223
Anaerobic glycolysis, 97
Anatomical dead space, 59
Antigen-induced mediator release,
  202
Asthma (*see* Bronchoconstriction)
Atelectasis, 59
Atmospheric aerosols, 261
Atmospheric particles, 259
Atropine, 66, 139, 313
Axon(s)
  adrenergic, 220
  cholinergic, 220
  ultrastructure, 14, 15, 18
  unmyelinated, 22
  vesicles, 14, 15, 18

### B

Basement membrane, 41
$\beta_1$ and $\beta_2$ receptors, 196
β-acrenoceptor, 62
β-adrenergic receptors, 196, 239
β-receptor desensitization, 197
β-receptors, 64
Blocking agents
  guinea pig ileum, 218
  rabbit trachea, 219
Bradykinin, 144
Bronchi, 2, 19
Bronchial artery
  histamine and, 231
  *See* also Histamine, receptors
Bronchial smooth muscle, 57, 312
Bronchoconstriction
  asthma and, 223
  chemical irritants and, 230
  chemoreceptors and, 224

[Bronchoconstriction]
cigarette smoke and, 229
dead space, 223
drug-induced, 233
efferent fibers and, 224
feedback mechanisms and, 224
propranolol-induced, 238
reflex conditioning and, 221-222, 224
sensitization and, 224
$SO_2$ and, 223
vagus nerves and, 217
Bronchomotor, response to dust, 226, 228, 229
Bronchomotor reflexes, methods
local anesthetics, 222
general anesthetics, 222
respiratory maneuvers, 222

## C

$Ca^{2+}$ pumps, 88
Ca-ATPase, 110
Ca-spikes, 67
Calcium ion sensitivity, 108
Carbohydrate metabolism, 91
Cartilage
bronchial, 22, 23
rings, 33
tracheal, 22, 23
Catecholamines
release of acetylcholine and, 220
Cell-to-cell junctions, 42
Chemical irritants (*see* Bronchoconstriction)
Cholinergic nerves, 14, 15, 60, 61, 219
Chromatin, 52
Cigar-shaped nucleus, 33
Clara cell, 2
Collagen, 23
fibrils, 37
Collateral airflow channels, 309
Compliance, 276, 299, 307, 308, 309, 315, 317, 318
Conductance, 303, 306, 318
Connective tissue, 23
Contractile and regulatory proteins, 104
Contractile apparatus, 52
Contractile element, 80
Control of carbohydrate metabolism, 98
Cristae, 46
Current-voltage relation, 67
Cyclic AMP, 98, 123, 164
Cyclic GMP, 123
Cyclic nucleotides, 135, 203

## D

Dense bodies, 37, 44, 52
Desmin, 46
Distribution of inspired gas, 308
DP/dt, 78
Drug receptors, 192
Dynamic muscle constants, 83

## E

Elastic properties, 298, 308, 312
Elastic recoil, 304, 306
Epithelium
airway, 2
cell types, 2, 3
neuroepithelial bodies, 2
ultrastructure, 6
Equal pressure point, 300, 311, 312

## F

Fatty acid metabolism, 103
$FEV_2$, 318, 319
Field stimulation
atropine and, 218
tetrodotoxin, 218
Force-velocity relationships, 80
Forced vital capacity, 311
Frank-Starling relation, 75
Functional residual capacity, 301, 306

## G

Ganglia, 13, 18, 19, 22, 219
Ganglion cells, 61
Gap junctions, 6, 9, 43
Gas uptake, 277
Glands
  epithelial, 6
  ultrastructure, 7
Glycogen, 99
  breakdown, 98
  granules, 46
Glycose transport, 97
Golgi bodies, 48
Guanylate cyclase, 130

## H

$H_1$ and $H_2$ receptors, 195
Hexamethonium, 232
Histamine, 123, 143, 223, 232, 314
  receptors, 194
Host responsiveness, 284
Humeral transmitters, 282
Hygroscopic growth, 268, 270
Hyperreactivity, 314
Hyperresponsiveness, 313
Hypoxia, 96, 100

## I

Inhibitors and uncouplers, 96
Innervation
  adrenergic, 14, 15, 16, 235, 236
  afferent, 13, 14
  efferent, 13, 14
  vagal, 14, 15, 217
Intermediate filaments, 44, 57
Intermediate junctions, 44
Interstitial smooth muscle cells, 58
Intracellular pH, 101
Intraneuronal vesicles, 63
Isometric tetanic curve, 77
Isoproterenol, 313
Isoproterenol reversal, 197
Isotonic curves, 77

## K

$K^+$ conductance, 67
Kultschitzky's cells, 2

## L

Length-tension relationships, 73
Light and dark cells, 51
Lung elastic recoil, 301
Lung size, 302
Lymphatics, 23
Lymphoid tissue, 23
Lysosomes, 48

## M

Maximum expiratory flow, 299, 315
  determinants of, 300
Measurements of pulmonary mechanics, 298
Membrane rectification, 66
Mg-ATPase activity, 105
Microtubules, 57
Mitochondria, 42, 46, 94
Mucus, 284
Mucus cells, 6
Mucous glands, 1
Musculus transversus trachea, 33
Myogenic response, 42, 67
Myosin, 53, 55

## N

Nerves
  adrenergic, 14, 15, 16, 18, 60, 61, 219, 236
  cholinergic, 14, 15, 60, 61, 219
  nonadrenergic, 16, 62, 64, 236, 237
  purinergic, 16, 64
Neuroepithelial bodies, 2

Neurotransmitters
β-adrenergic, 235
regulation of airway smooth muscle and, 220
Neutralization of $H_2SO_4$, 272, 274
Nexus, 6, 43
Nonadrenergic, 16, 62, 64, 236, 237
Nuclear membrane, 52
Nuclear pores, 52
Nucleoli, 52
Nucleus, 52

**O**

Opaque, vesicles, 18
Oxidative phosphorylation, 46, 94, 95

**P**

$pA_2$ and $K_B$ values, 192
Pacemaker cells, 9
Parallel elastic component, 81
Parasympathetic fibers, 63, 217, 312
Particle pH, 286
Particle size, 286
Pasteur effect, 98
Peg-and-socket (PS) junctions, 43
Pentose shunt, 97
Pharmacologic receptors, 125, 191
Pharmacomechanical coupling, 68
Phasic electrical activity, 66
Phosphocreatine, 100
Phosphofructokinase, 98, 298
Pinocytotic vesicles, 37, 42
Plasma membrane, 37
Pollutants, 275
additive effects, 275
discrete effects, 274
synergism, 275
Polyol pathway, 97
Power curve, 84
Pressure-flow relations, 311, 312
Pressure-volume relations, 304, 305, 316, 318
Prostaglandin receptors, 199
Prostaglandins, 143
Pulmonary mechanics, 316
Pulmonary receptors, 222
Purinergic nerves, 16, 64

**Q**

$Q_{10}$ values, 87
$Q_{10}$ values derived from force-velocity measurements, 89

**R**

Rate of particle growth, 269
Receptors, slowly adapting and irritant, 223
circulation, 234
cough receptors, 227, 229
rapidly adapting receptors, 227
stretch receptors, 223, 227
type-C receptors, 227
type-J receptors, 227
use of aerosols and, 232
Recoil, 315, 317
Recoil pressure, 302, 304, 306
Recurrent laryngeal, 61
Reflex activity, 281
Regulatory proteins, 110
Reimplantation in dogs, 219
Residual volume, 301, 305, 315, 317, 319
Resistance, 299, 307, 308, 309, 310, 314
Respiratory control rate, 95
Respiratory control ratio, 46
Reynolds' number, 309, 311
Rough reticulum, 51

**S**

Sarcolemma, 37
Sarcoplasmic reticulum, 42, 48
Series-elastic component, 81, 85, 89

Serotonin, 221
Small airway obstruction, 309
Smooth muscle
 action potentials, 9
 biochemistry, 90
 bronchial, 57, 312
 electrophysiology, 65
 force-velocity relations, 80, 82
 length-tension relations, 73
 parenchymal, 58
 tracheal, 32
 ultrastructure, 9, 37
Spirally cut trachea, 193
SRS-A receptor, 148, 202
Starling resistor, 300, 301
Static recoil, 311
Stimulus-response relationship, 71
Suprachondral plexus, 63
Sympathetic innervation, 13
Sympathetic nerves, 61

**T**

Tetraethylammonium chloride (TEA), 67
Tight junctions or nexuses, 6, 43
Total lung capacity (TLC), 299, 301, 304, 306, 315, 317
Trachea, 2, 19
Tracheal smooth muscle
 atropine, 218
 field stimulation, 218
 tetrodotoxin, 218
Transbronchial pressure, 299
Transverse tubular structures, 48
Tropomyosin, 107
Troponin, 110, 132

**V**

$V_{max}$, 84, 311, 313
Vagal bradycardia
 nasal irritation and, 225
Vagal efferent pathways (*see* Bronchomotor reflexes)
Vagal nuclei, 13
Vagus nerve, 1, 14, 61, 217
Ventilation perfusion ratios, 60
Vesicles, 14, 15, 18
Viscoelastic properties, 305

**W**

Wave speed theory, 300

**Z**

Z-line material, 46
Zonula adherens, 44